Progress in
Cancer Research and Therapy
Volume 13

COLORECTAL CANCER:
PREVENTION, EPIDEMIOLOGY, AND SCREENING

Progress in
Cancer Research and Therapy

Progress in
Cancer Research and Therapy
Volume 13

Colorectal Cancer: Prevention, Epidemiology, and Screening

Editors

Sidney J. Winawer, M.D.
Chief, Gastroenterology Service
Memorial Sloan-Kettering Cancer Center
Professor of Clinical Medicine
Cornell University
Medical College
New York, New York

David Schottenfeld, M.D.
Chief of Epidemology and
Preventive Medicine
Memorial Sloan-Kettering
Cancer Center
and Professor of Public Health
Cornell University Medical College
New York, New York

Paul Sherlock, M.D.
Chairman, Department of Medicine
Memorial Sloan-Kettering Cancer Center
and Professor of Medicine
Cornell University Medical College
New York, New York

Raven Press ■ New York

Raven Press, 1140 Avenue of the Americas, New York, New York 10036

Made in the United States of America

International Standard Book Number 0–89004–477–3
Library of Congress Catalog Card Number 79–62974

Great care has been taken to maintain the accuracy of the information contained in the volume. However, Raven Press cannot be held responsible for errors or for any consequences arising from the use of the information contained herein.

Materials appearing in this book prepared by individuals as part of their official duties as U.S. Government employees are not covered by the above-mentioned copyright.

Preface

Colorectal cancer has become a major worldwide health problem of concern to primary practicing physicians, epidemiologists, gastroenterologists, surgeons, endoscopists, pathologists, economists, health officials, legislators, laboratory scientists, radiologists, and others. This volume represents a unique effort to bring together contributors of international stature to address comprehensively the critical issue of screening for colorectal cancer. The big question of whether or not to screen for colorectal cancer is being debated actively today. In order to answer this question, each element must be considered individually. These elements are treated in depth in the various sections in this book.

The background for screening is set by an evaluation of current epidemiologic and etiologic considerations. Epidemiologic considerations are especially critical in a particular country in order to justify embarking on a national screening program. The etiologic factors of fiber, fat, bile acids, and fecal flora are discussed by the key proponents. Within high-risk countries there are individual groups that are especially susceptible to colorectal cancer. The genetic high-risk groups, i.e., those with familial polyposis or with nonpolyposis inherited colon cancer, including clinical and theoretical considerations and the status of biological markers, are discussed in detail by the key investigators in this field. Their personal views are interwoven into their discussions.

The extremely broad and complex issues related to screening are presented in a series of chapters including clinical and laboratory considerations, cost, use of the health belief model to examine patient compliance and motivation, and the important area of physician awareness of the concepts and technology currently available. This is followed by an in-depth review of important ongoing screening programs around the world, or those completed within the last few years, written by the organizers and directors of these programs. The consistencies of the data are examined and future needs suggested.

The final section deals with inflammatory bowel disease, mainly ulcerative colitis. In addition to an examination of risk factors, epidemiology, and etiology, there are multiple presentations related to the controversial and potentially useful concept of dysplasia. Most of the important international groups working in this area have been specifically included in order to identify areas of agreement and disagreement on this topic.

This volume provides a challenge to the international community to establish a collaborative effort for the prevention of cancer at this anatomic site. Prevention may be defined as primary—the identification and eradication of causal factors, and secondary—the detection of early cancer and identification and control of premalignant conditions. The importance of focusing on a prevention approach is underscored by newer understanding of environmental factors and genetic susceptibility, conceptual understanding of underlying risk factors, and recent developments of newer technology for screening and diagnosis.

Sidney J. Winawer
David Schottenfeld
Paul Sherlock

Acknowledgments

This volume is based on an International Symposium on Colorectal Cancer held in New York on March 6–7, 1979. The major thrust of the symposium was epidemiology and screening.

Much effort must go into the planning of an international symposium. This could not have been accomplished without the organizational expertise of Mr. S. Wayne Kay of SmithKline Diagnostics and his able staff. The symposium was made possible through support in part by an education grant from Smith-Kline Diagnostics. The administrative assistance of the Program Chairman cannot be acknowledged too strongly. In this capacity, Ms. Florence Lefcourt provided invaluable efforts. We are also grateful for the help provided by Ms. Barbara LePorte.

We wish to acknowledge the important role of the Chairman of our International Scientific Advisory Committee, Dr. Rulon W. Rawson, and the members of his Committee, Drs. Kenneth C. Calman, John Christodoulopoulos, Massimo Crespi, L. Demling, Richard G. Farmer, Alfonso Fraise, Peter Frühmorgen, Angelita Habr-Gama, Victor Gilbertsen, Philip Gold, Seibi Kobayashi, H. Kulke, Basil Morson, Paul Rozen, William Silen, Parviz Sorouri, V. Varro, Jerome D. Waye, and Norman Zamcheck. This committee provided invaluable input into the planning of the program and identification of many superb workers in the field around the world.

The work of the Program Committee is always basic to the development of a successful scientific program. To this end, considerable time and effort were devoted by its members, Drs. Thomas P. Almy, Reinhard Gnauck, Kerry Goulston, David Greegor, LaSalle Leffall, David G. Illingworth, Daniel G. Miller, David Schottenfeld, and Paul Sherlock.

Finally, a "working" symposium achieves its objectives only by active participation of those present. The objectives of this symposium were assured, given the impressive group of people who agreed to come and interact with their colleagues from around the world.

Contents

ix

Clinical and Laboratory Considerations in Screening

Screening of the General Population

Risk of Cancer in Inflammatory Bowel Disease

Contributors

Thor Alm
St. Erik's Hospital
Department of Gastroenterology
S-11282 Stockholm, Sweden

Thomas P. Almy
Dartmouth Medical School
Hanover, New Hampshire 03755

David E. Anderson
M.D. Anderson Hospital
Houston, Texas 77030

Margo Andrews
Preventive Medicine Institute
Strang Clinic
New York, New York 10016

Henry D. Appelman
University of Michigan Medical School
Ann Arbor, Michigan 48104

M. Earl Balis
Memorial Hospital
Memorial Sloan-Kettering Cancer Center
New York, New York 10021

George H. Barrows
Bayfront Medical Center
St. Petersburg, Florida 33701

Theodore M. Bayless
Johns Hopkins Hospital
Baltimore, Maryland 21205

Norman Berlinger
Department of Otolaryngology
National Naval Medical Center
Bethesda, Maryland 20014

J. G. Brecht
Zentralinstitut für die Kassenärztliche
  Versorgung
Cologne, West Germany

R. S. Brody
North Shore Hospital
Manhasset, New York 11030

Denis P. Burkitt
St. Thomas's Hospital Medical School
London, England

Glenys Burton
Memorial Sloan-Kettering Cancer Center
New York, New York 10021

H. J. R. Bussey
St. Mark's Hospital
London EVIV 2 PS England

Kenneth C. Calman
University of Glasgow
Glasgow, Scotland

Edward Cooper
University of Leeds
Department of Oncology
Leeds, England

Betty Shannon Danes
Cornell University Medical College
New York, New York 10021

Jerome J. DeCosse
Memorial Sloan-Kettering Cancer Center
New York, New York 10021

L. Demling
Medizinische Klinik mit
  Poliklinik
Erlangen, West Germany

Owen Dent
Department of Sociology
Australian National University
Cambria, Australia

Eleanor Deschner
Memorial Sloan-Kettering Cancer Center
New York, New York 10021

Ghislain Devroede
CT Hospital Universitaire
Sherbrooke, P.Q., J1H 5N4 Canada

Mark P. Diamond
Johns Hopkins Hospital
Baltimore, Maryland 21205

William O. Dobbins III
Department of Medicine
University of Michigan Medical Center
Ann Arbor, Michigan 48105

Sir Richard Doll
University of Oxford
Oxford, OX 26 PS England

David M. Eddy
Engineering-Economic Systems
Terman Engineering Center /
Stanford University
Stanford, California 94305

Göran R. Ekelund
Malmo Allm. Sjukhus
Kir. Klin.
Malmo, Sweden S21401

Anthony A. Eyers
St Mark's Hospital
London EVIV 2 PS England

Zvi Fireman
Ichilov Hospital
Tel Aviv, Israel

M. Fleisher
Memorial Sloan-Kettering Cancer Center
New York, New York 10021

P. Frank
University of Chicago Hospital
Chicago, Illinois 60637

Peter Frühmorgen
Medizinische Klinik mit Poliklinik
Erlangen, West Germany

Eldon J. Gardner
Department of Biology
Utah State University
Logan, Utah 84322

Tuvia Gilat
Department of Gastroenterology
Tel Aviv University Medical School
Tel Aviv, Israel

Victor Gilbertsen
University of Minnesota Health Center
Minneapolis, Minnesota 55455

Jane E. Gilpin
University of Chicago Hospital
Chicago, Illinois 60637

Reinhard Gnauck
Deutsche Klinik für Diagnostik
Weisbaden, West Germany 6200

D. M. Goldenberg
11837 Gainesborough
Potomac, Maryland 20854

Barry Goldin
Department of Medicine
New England Medical Center Hospital
Boston, Massachusetts 02111

Kerry Goulston
Concord General Hospital
New South Wales, Australia

David H. Greegor
840 Michigan Avenue
Columbus, Ohio 43215

M. Snyder Halper
Preventive Medicine Institute
Strang Clinic
New York, New York 10016

Shlomo M. Hellerstein
Ichilov Hospital
Tel Aviv, Israel

H. Holstein
Zentralinstitut für die Kassenarztliche
Versorgung
D-5000 Koln, Germany 41

T. Iwama
Tokyo Medical and Dental University
School of Medicine
Bunkyo-Ka Tokyo 113, Japan

Diane D. Jarrett
Bayfront Medical Center
St. Petersburg, Florida 33701

Joseph B. Kirsner
The University of Chicago Hospitals and
Clinics
Chicago, Illinois 60637

Levy Kopelovich
Sloan-Kettering Institute
New York, New York 10021

LaSalle D. Leffall, Jr.
Howard University Hospital
Washington, D.C. 20060

Bernard Levin
University of Chicago Hospital
Chicago, Illinois 60637

Charles J. Lightdale
Memorial Sloan-Kettering Cancer Center
New York, New York 10021

Martin Lipkin
Memorial Sloan-Kettering Cancer Center
New York, New York 10021

Henry T. Lynch
Creighton University Medical School
Omaha, Nebraska 68178

Jane F. Lynch
Creighton University Medical School
Omaha, Nebraska 68178

Patrick M. Lynch
Creighton University Medical School
Omaha, Nebraska 68178

Richard B. McConnell
University of Liverpool
Liverpool, England

Richard B. McHugh
University of Minnesota
Minneapolis, Minnesota 55455

Carlyle H. Miller
Memorial Sloan-Kettering Cancer Center
New York, New York 10021

Daniel G. Miller
Preventive Medicine Institute
Strang Clinic
New York, New York 10016

Basil C. Morson
St. Mark's Hospital
London EVIV 2 PS, England

F. Warren Nugent
Lahey Clinic
Boston, Massachusetts 02215

J. Donald Ostrow
Northwestern University Medical School
Chicago, Illinois 60611

Moses Paulson
Johns Hopkins Hospital
Baltimore, Maryland 21205

Jacob Rattan
Ichilov Hospital
Tel Aviv, Israel

Bandaru S. Reddy
American Health Foundation
Valhalla, New York 10595

Robert H. Riddell
University of Chicago Hospital
Chicago, Illinois 60637

Sheila M. Ritchie
St. Mark's Hospital
London EVIV 2 PS , England

David Roth
Memorial Sloan-Kettering Cancer Center
New York, New York 10021

Paul Rozen
Ichilov Hospital
Tel Aviv, Israel

Josephine S. Salser
Memorial Sloan-Kettering Cancer Center
New York, New York 10021

David Schottenfeld
Memorial Sloan-Kettering Cancer Center
New York, New York 10021

Leonard M. Schuman
University of Minnesota Health Science
   Center
Minneapolis, Minnesota 55455

F. W. Schwartz
Zentralinstitut für die Kassenarztliche
   Versorgung
D-5000 Koln, Germany 41

Morton K. Schwartz
Memorial Sloan-Kettering Cancer Center
New York, New York 10021

Daniel G. Sheahan
Trinity College
Dublin 2, Ireland

Paul Sherlock
Memorial Sloan-Kettering Cancer Center
New York, New York 10021

Curtis L. Songster
Bayfront Medical Center
St. Petersburg, Florida 33701

Neil E. Spingarn
American Health Foundation
Valhalla, New York 10595

Reuven Terdiman
Ichilov Hospital
Tel Aviv, Israel

James P. S. Thomson
St. Mark's Hospital
London EVIV 2 PS, England

R. Turner
University of Leeds
Leeds, England

Joji Utsunomiya
Second Department of Surgery
Tokyo Medical and Dental University
   School of Medicine
Bunkyo-ka Tokyo 113, Japan

A. M. O. Veale
Department of Community Health
School of Medicine
University of Auckland
Auckland, New Zealand

Jerome D. Waye
Mt. Sinai School of Medicine of the City
   University of New York
Gastrointestinal Endoscopy Unit
Mt. Sinai Hospital
New York, New York 10028

J. Weisburger
American Health Foundation
Valhalla, New York 10595

Stanley Williams
University of Minnesota Health Center
Minneapolis, Minnesota 55455

Sidney J. Winawer
Memorial Sloan-Kettering Cancer Center
New York, New York 10021

Ernst J. Wynder
American Health Foundation
Valhalla, New York 10595

John H. Yardley
Johns Hopkins Hospital
Baltimore, Maryland 21205

Norman Zamcheck
Boston City Hospital
Boston, Massachusetts 02118

Morris S. Zedeck
Memorial Sloan-Kettering Cancer Center
New York, New York 10021

Foreword

To achieve their important and ambitious goals, the planners of the recent International Symposium on Colorectal Cancer, held in New York City in 1979, brought together a multitude of active investigators otherwise separated by geography or by formal scientific disciplines. That the participants communicated so freely and effectively is in part the consequence of the great social importance of the problem of colonic cancer in the modern world, yet at the same time, an indication of the breadth and openness of their minds. The process of cross-fertilization, begun years ago under conditions far less favorable than the present, can be credited with many of the advances in this field. The resulting hybrid vigor justifies an optimistic forecast of further progress. Many of the participants in the symposium were invited to give of themselves once again by preparing a critical contribution to this volume. Although this book was inspired by the symposium, it was created *de novo* as an independent work.

The information presented in this volume richly illustrates the complexity of the task of colon cancer control and the potential wastefulness of simplistic approaches based on incomplete understanding of the facts. Although fecal testing for occult blood would appear, by certain criteria, an almost ideal measure of population screening, it is apparent that its benefits must be weighed even more carefully than heretofore against the aggregate risks and costs of the whole procedure it entails. This judgment still depends on literally dozens of procedural choices yet to be made. These must be supported by national and international consensus if the best possible method is to be recognized and made widely available.

We can anticipate, for any fully recommended detection procedure, major problems in securing the compliance of those who stand to benefit. In a world where, we are told, the average person does not realistically plan beyond the next payday, how many will sacrifice present convenience for future health? Clearly, a large-scale and continued effort in public education will be required, one sufficient to overcome the persisting cultural obstacles to open an objective consideration of gastrointestinal functions, in general, and bowel function, in particular.

The contributors to this volume have together outlined these formidable agenda for translational research and have suggested a means of achieving the desired results. We can hope that, through continued and ever closer international cooperation in protocols for clinical research, much confusion can be avoided and the lag time for the emergence of a fully satisfactory screening procedure can be reduced.

Although no one questions the desirability of detection of asymptomatic colon cancer in individuals at high risk, the methods to be used, the frequency of their application, and the criteria for recognition of minimal neoplastic change must be subjects of continued investigation. In this field, as well, the prospective advantages of cooperative protocol-based studies are regarded as substantial.

Further benefits can be expected from the observation of large numbers of high-risk patients in multiple centers according to standardized protocols. They can, to their own advantage, become the subjects of clinical trials of measures of primary prevention. The hypotheses regarding environmental risk factors of colon cancer, now being generated by the findings of epidemiologists and laboratory investigators, cannot be directly translated with confidence into measures of cancer control applicable to the population as a whole. Yet the fruits of basic research, applied in a conscientious and scientifically sound fashion, should be first offered to those at greatest risk from this disease. They would thereby be guaranteed optimal practices of disease detection and the earliest access to valid strategies of primary prevention while hastening the day when these measures can be wisely recommended to the general public.

The recent symposium and this volume certainly will not have been the last efforts before effective control of colonic cancer is at hand. The need for more hard-won progress is ever more plain. Yet the likelihood of ultimate success, and to a considerable extent, the diverse means by which it may be achieved, have become clearer than ever before.

Thomas P. Almy

Colorectal Cancer: Prevention, Epidemiology, and Screening, edited by S. Winawer, D. Schottenfeld, and P. Sherlock. Raven Press, New York © 1980.

Introduction: Future Thrusts in Epidemiology of Colorectal Cancer

Kenneth C. Calman

Glasgow, Scotland

The study of colorectal cancer is a fast developing one in the field of cancer epidemiology and preventive oncology. Numerous clues are already available and are well summarized in the following chapters. Yet all answers are not available, and it is appropriate therefore to look for gaps in our knowledge and understanding of the epidemiology of colorectal cancer, and to try to define future studies in this area.

Perhaps the first important point to make is a plea for standardization of the reporting of results in colorectal cancer. This applies not only to the site of the lesion, the pathology, and the staging procedures, but also to the type of demographic data required. It is also essential to separate, from the epidemiological point of view, colon and rectal cancer, even if this means a synthesis of information at some later stage.

From the point of view of descriptive epidemiology, a great deal of information must be obtained. Thus the relationships among the incidence, site, and number of adenomas must be defined in a number of clinical situations. Migrant studies have clearly indicated the changing incidence of colorectal cancer, with risks approaching those of the new host country. As these cancers, however, appear predominantly in the developed countries, there is a tremendous need for careful monitoring of incidence in the developing countries where an increase in the incidence and mortality may be expected. This provides a natural experiment which should be exploited. There is also need for further international studies on the natural history of these cancers. The clinical presentation, pathology, and progression in different countries may offer further information on the pathogenesis of colorectal cancer.

A number of diseases are now recognized to predispose to colorectal cancer. For the epidemiologist they can be useful in several ways. First, they allow the progression from premalignant to malignant lesions to be studied, and thus the epidemiological factors of importance can be defined. Second, if such high-risk groups can be identified, they can be used for appropriate screening studies. Third, such high-risk groups can be used to study preventive measures with the hope of achieving results more rapidly than with an average risk population. This latter aspect is especially relevant in relation to the adenomas and the

1

subsequent development of carcinoma. The whole area of the relationship between adenomas and carcinomas requires careful study at the epidemiological level. In such studies the role of the host must not be neglected, and this indeed may be a fruitful area of study.

A major area for future study will clearly be the definition of the carcinogen(s) in the environment which are associated with the development of colorectal cancer. Many such factors have been identified and thoroughly reviewed in this volume. The fat-fiber hypotheses are not antagonistic, and indeed the interrelationship between the two may be of considerable importance. Other factors, however, have also been suggested, and as the area of metabolic epidemiology develops, so does an understanding of the process of carcinogenesis at a cellular and molecular level.

This naturally raises the question of the role of animal models in epidemiological studies. The experimental models for the development of colonic cancer in rodents have allowed a number of studies to be performed. The dangers of extrapolation from mouse to man are well known. However, animal models may give clues to etiology and allow the development of the appropriate clinical clinical questions. Of perhaps more interest are the spontaneously occurring questions. Of perhaps more interest are the spontaneously occurring adenocarcinomas of the gastrointestinal tract in large animals. No full epidemiological studies have been mounted comparing the incidence of such tumors in man and animals in defined geographical areas. Certain factors, including the diet of both man and animals, indicate that such studies might be rewarding.

There are many loose threads surrounding the epidemiology and pathogenesis of colorectal cancer. Some of the ways in which they may be drawn together are suggested above. A great deal of work remains to be done, but the leads are already there; they now require elucidation.

Colorectal Cancer: Prevention, Epidemiology,
and Screening, edited by S. Winawer, D. Schottenfeld,
and P. Sherlock. Raven Press, New York © 1980.

General Epidemiologic Considerations in Etiology of Colorectal Cancer

Richard Doll

University of Oxford, Oxford, England

Sixteen years ago, an international group met in London, under the auspices of the World Organization of Gastro-Enterology, to discuss the epidemiology of gastrointestinal cancers with special reference to their causation (13). Its report, which had the merit of brevity, began:

> A great deal of evidence is now available to show that the incidence of gastrointestinal cancer varies from place to place and from time to time. Moreover, the incidence among migrant populations is, in general, intermediate between that found in their original homeland, and that in the country to which they have emigrated. It is evident, therefore, that environmental factors play an important part in the development of these cancers and that many of them may be preventable.

And there, so far as cancer of the large bowel was concerned, it nearly ended. "There is very little evidence," the report went on to say, "to implicate any particular factor as a cause of cancer of the large bowel. Study of the use of purgatives has been negative, except for some slight evidence to suggest that liquid paraffin may contribute to the development of a small proportion of cases. . . . Variations in diet which lead to differences in faecal transit through the bowel and to differences in faecal bulk, which might affect the concentration of a carcinogen in contact with the mucosa and the duration of contact, deserve investigation. In many African countries, where there is a very low incidence of large bowel cancer, it is customary to have the bowels open three or four times a day and the faecal bulk is high." Rather surprisingly, the group added that there was evidence to suggest that "transit times, at least in some of these populations, are not notably different from those observed in Europe and North America." One line of investigation that was suggested was to study the incidence of bowel cancer in patients with ulcerative colitis, who, it was recognized, were particularly susceptible to cancer of the colon. Many of these patients took restricted diets, so that there might be an opportunity for relating the occurrence of the disease to variations in diet that were maintained under medical observation. And that was about all.

Now the situation has changed dramatically. New ideas about the possible roles of dietary fat, meat, vegetables, and fiber, and about the metabolic activity of the bacterial flora and the presence of mutagens in the feces, have opened up lines of research that may reasonably be hoped to provide the basis for a program for prevention within the next decade. They are discussed in detail in other chapters, and I shall attempt to give here only the epidemiological background against which they were developed.

DISTINCTION BETWEEN CANCERS OF COLON AND RECTUM

First we have to consider whether there is any need to separate cancers of the colon and rectum, or whether, for etiological inquiry, they can be regarded as constituting a single entity.

That they should be considered together is suggested by their common relationship to polyps and ulcerative colitis, the correlation between their incidence rates in different populations, and the similarity of the structure and functions of the two organs. Moreover, many tumors occur at the rectosigmoid junction and are difficult to classify as arising in one or another site. There are, however, some reasons for maintaining the separation, even though the principal causes of both diseases may be the same. The most important is the difference in sex ratio; others are minor differences in their distribution with age, place, and time.

RELATIONSHIP OF INCIDENCE TO AGE

Relationships with age are shown in Fig. 1. A double logarithmic scale has been used so that a linear relationship indicates that incidence increases in proportion to a power of the age, the actual power being indicated by the slope of the line. Between 50 and 80 years of age the male age-specific incidence rates for each condition are practically equal. At these ages, both sets of data increase approximately in proportion to the sixth power of the age. This type of relationship—but with the power of age varying from the fourth to the seventh—is characteristic of all epithelial cancers that are not obviously affected by hormonal activity and is thought to result from continuing exposure to an environmental carcinogen (3), as with lung cancer in cigarette smokers, skin cancer in men exposed to ultraviolet light, and many tumors produced by animal experiments.

Under 35 years of age, the rates, particularly those for colon cancer, are higher than would be predicted by the relationship at older ages. This can be accounted for by the inclusion in the population of a small proportion of people with grossly increased susceptibility. It would be produced if approximately 1 in 10,000 people suffered from polyposis coli, a figure that agrees reasonably well with estimates of the polyposis gene frequency (16,17).

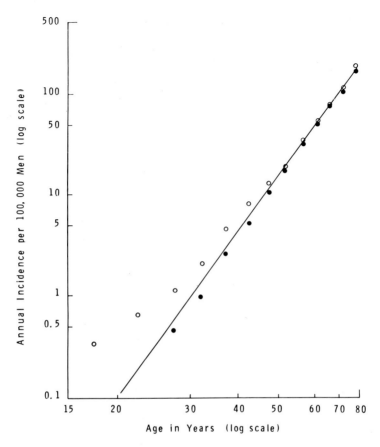

FIG. 1. Relationship between incidence of cancers of the colon and rectum and age: data obtained by pooling figures for men in 5 regions in England and Wales between 15 and 80 years of age (9). Incidence rates and age are both shown in logarithmic scales.

RELATIVE INCIDENCE IN MEN AND WOMEN

Cancers of the large bowel are distinguished by occurring almost equally in both sexes. There are, however, a few differences that may be important etiologically. First, cancer of the rectum occurs slightly more often in men than in women in nearly all countries, whereas cancer of the colon tends to be commoner in women. More interestingly, the sex ratios change with age. In England, for example, cancer of colon is commoner in women up to 60 years of age and is then slightly commoner in men; whereas cancer of the rectum occurs equally in both sexes up to 45 years of age, but becomes nearly twice as common in men after 65 years of age. For some reason it appears that men become progressively more heavily exposed than women as age increases.

GEOGRAPHICAL VARIATION

By far, the most interesting observation is the variation in the incidence of the two diseases in different countries. Male incidence rates collected by the International Union against Cancer (22,23) and the International Agency for Research on Cancer (9) are listed in Table 1. The rates are standardized for age, using the standard world population (23), and are limited to ages 35 to 64 years, because data for areas with undeveloped health services are unreliable at old ages.

TABLE 1. *Geographical variation in incidence from cancers of the colon and rectum: men aged 35–64 years standardized for age (9)*

Population	Incidence per 100,000 men per year	
	Colon	Rectum
Hawaii, Chinese	57.7	36.0
" Japanese	37.1	29.7
" Caucasian	36.8	20.4
New Zealand, white	36.1	23.8
Connecticut	35.8	26.0
Detroit, black	35.3	24.8
Alameda, black	34.9	15.9
Iowa	34.5	19.6
Detroit, white	33.5	23.2
San Francisco, black	33.2	15.6
Newfoundland	32.4	19.1
San Francisco, white	32.3	20.0
New York State	30.2	18.9
British Columbia	29.6	21.5
Alameda, white	29.4	21.7
Manitoba	27.8	22.2
New Mexico, white[a]	27.0	15.9
San Francisco, Chinese	26.8	24.4
Canada, Maritime Provinces	26.0	19.8
Switzerland, Geneva	24.1	15.0
Utah	23.9	13.0
El Paso, white[a]	23.6	12.8
Saskatchewan	22.5	21.4
U.K., Liverpool	22.3	19.8
Alberta	22.0	15.2
Quebec	21.6	17.5
U.K., Birmingham	21.3	20.5
U.K., Ayrshire	20.6	19.8
U.K., Oxford	20.4	17.1
U.K., S.W.	20.1	17.1
Cape, white[b]	20.0	6.0
Sweden	19.2	13.2
U.K., S. metropolitan	19.0	14.3
Denmark	18.9	20.6
U.K., Sheffield	17.7	18.0

TABLE 1. *(Continued)*

Population	Incidence per 100,000 men per year	
	Colon	Rectum
Hawaii, Hawaiian	17.3	18.7
Iceland	17.0	10.4
Norway	16.7	13.3
Germany, Hamburg	16.6	13.6
" Saarland	16.6	21.8
Singapore, Chinese	16.6	16.3
Israel, Jews	15.9	15.1
Jamaica	15.5	7.5
Hawaii, Filippino	15.5	18.1
New Zealand, Maori	14.8	5.8
Hungary, Vas	14.6	
Poland, Warsaw	14.4	10.1
Germany, G.D.R.	14.1	15.9
Singapore, Indian	12.4	11.7
Brazil, Sao Paulo	12.1	12.8
New Mexico, Spanish	11.2	8.6
El Paso, Spanish	11.2	4.1
Poland, Katowice	10.6	11.4
Puerto Rico	9.9	7.5
Poland, Cracow	9.9	8.5
Finland	9.7	9.3
Malta	9.0	9.9
Yugoslavia, Slovenia	8.8	16.7
Japan, Osaka	8.7	9.0
Spain, Zaragoza	7.9	9.4
Japan, Mujagi	7.8	9.5
Cuba	7.7	5.1
Poland, Warsaw rural	7.1	5.3
Singapore, Malay	6.8	9.9
Japan, Okayama	6.4	10.9
Hungary, Szaboles	6.1	7.5
Colombia, Cali	5.8	5.4
Chile[c]	5.8	6.4
India, Bombay	5.7	6.1
Cape, colored[b]	5.5	5.0
Mozambique, L.M.[c]	5.3	(0.0)
Romania, Timis	5.1	16.0
Natal, black[b]	5.1	3.5
Bulawayo	4.5	3.6
Johannesburg, black[c]	4.0	2.4
Israel, non-Jews	3.8	6.0
New Mexico, Indian	3.7	12.1
Brazil, Recife	3.5	4.3
Cape, black[b]	3.5	(0.0)
Nigeria	3.4	3.4
Natal, Indian[b]	2.5	5.1
Uganda, Kampala[c]	(0.0)	3.5

[a] White population refers to white other than Spanish.
[b] See ref. 23.
[c] See ref. 22.

Very low rates are recorded generally in black Africa, south of the Sahara, and among the non-Jewish population of Israel, whereas somewhat higher, but still low rates are found in Asia and Eastern and Southern Europe. Low or very low rates are also common in most parts of South America and Spain. High rates, in contrast, are found in Western Europe and North America, whereas very high rates are found only in Canada, the United States (including its black and Asiatic populations), and in the white population of New Zealand. Mortality data show that high rates are also found in Argentina and Uruguay.

Table 1 also shows that the geographical distribution of rectal cancer is similar to that of cancer of the colon. That the correlation with colon cancer is not exact must be due in part to random variation of small numbers since adequate diagnostic facilities were available for only small populations in many of the areas in which low incidence rates for colon cancer were recorded. It seems, however, that the variability of rectal cancer is somewhat less than that of colonic cancer (coefficient of variation 44% against 58%), and that its incidence in developed countries is disproportionately high in comparison to that of colon cancer only in Denmark and, perhaps, Germany and the United Kingdom.

For the most part these national differences in the incidence of colorectal cancer correlate with the differences in economic status of the countries at the start of World War II.

MIGRANT STUDIES

That the differences are not genetic in origin is shown by migrant groups whose experience of disease changes when they change their way of life in a new country—the most obvious examples being the black Africans in the United States and the Japanese and Chinese who more recently migrated to California and Hawaii. Observations on Japanese migrants, in particular, have shown that their colon cancer risk progressively diverged from that in Japan until it now approximates the high risk among U.S. whites (6,7,19). Other examples include Poles and Norwegians who migrated to America before World War II (5,20) and Poles who migrated to Australia shortly after it (21).

TEMPORAL VARIATION

If some aspect of industrialized society is responsible for high incidence rates, the question arises whether we have to look for a factor that was introduced recently, or one that was introduced with industrialization in the nineteenth century. We have, therefore, to inquire about changes in the incidence of large bowel cancer in time.

Such data are less easy to come by than those illustrating geographical differences because a high standard of case registration has been obtained in only a few places for more than 10 years. We have therefore to rely to a large extent on trends in mortality, which may be influenced not only by changes in diagnostic

TABLE 2. *Trends in mortality from cancers of the colon and rectum in England and Wales 1911–1975: ages 35–64 years, standardized for age*[a]

| Period | Mortality per 100,000 per year from cancer of: | | | |
| | Colon | | Rectum | |
	Men	Women	Men	Women
1911–1915	8.6[b]	9.8[b]	8.7	6.0
1916–1920	8.9[b]	10.3[b]	9.1	5.9
1921–1925	9.7[b]	10.4[b]	9.4	5.8
1926–1930	10.3[b]	10.8[b]	9.2	5.4
1931–1935	9.2	9.4	9.2	5.2
1936–1940	9.8	10.0	8.8	9.1
1941–1945	9.7	10.2	8.4	5.1
1946–1950	8.6	9.4	7.4	4.6
1951–1955	7.1	7.9	6.0	4.0
1956–1960	6.3	7.3	5.2	3.5
1961–1965	6.0	6.9	4.8	3.3
1966–1970	6.4	6.8	4.7	3.2
1971–1975	6.5	6.7	4.6	3.1

[a] Standardized in 5 year age groups on the standard European population (23).
[b] Estimated from data for cancer of the intestines, including duodenum.

standards, but also by changes in the efficacy of treatment. Nevertheless, the general picture is fairly clear. In England and Wales, for example, the mortality rate standardized for age, and once again limited to ages 35 to 64 years because of the unreliability of death certification at old ages before the war, remained fairly constant from 1911 to 1941 for both types of cancer and then fell by between 30 and 40% due, possibly, to improvements in treatment (Table 2). In the last few years, the mortality from colon cancer has shown a tendency to increase in men, but the change is very slight and the overall impression is that the factors that are responsible for these cancers must have been present in the environment to much the same extent since the end of the nineteenth century.

Incidence data for Connecticut and Denmark, which provide the longest series, show little evidence of change over the last 30 years and no reason to modify the conclusion derived from the British mortality data. In contrast, Japanese data show a substantial increase, particularly in the elderly (10), which has accompanied a dramatic increase in the consumption of meat and milk products.

SPECIFIC ETIOLOGICAL FACTORS

Epidemiological data have not, by themselves, carried us much further. Only one study has implicated the use of a drug, and this was a case-control study of 614 patients with gastrointestinal cancer whose past histories were compared with those of twice as many patients with nongastrointestinal diseases (2). No differences were found in purgative use in general—but the proportion of patients with both gastric and intestinal cancer who had used liquid paraffin regularly for more than 5 years was about double that in the control group, and the relative excess was greater still for those few patients who had used it for more than 20 years. Liquid paraffin is made from petroleum by distillation between 360° and 390°. Twenty-five years ago, when the results of the study were reported, it contained fluorescent substances that could have been carcinogenic. Since then the product has been purified further and it no longer contains such substances.

There is evidence also for only one occupational factor. Many large studies, particularly in the United States, have demonstrated an increased mortality from cancer of the large bowel in asbestos workers (for example, ref. 18); but other studies have not (14), and the evidence for a causal relationship is incomplete. Asbestos workers have a much greater risk from cancer of the lung and some are liable to develop mesothelioma of the peritoneum. The reported excess of bowel cancer is based on certified causes of death, and the question arises whether it could be due to diagnostic confusion; for example, in the attribution of the site of the primary cancer when patients present with secondaries in the liver. Newhouse and Wagner (12) found several unreported cases of mesothelioma in the only study in which autopsy data were reviewed extensively, and asbestos ought not to be regarded as a cause of large bowel cancer without more definite evidence than we now have.

Those current hypotheses concerning the etiology of the disease that seem likely to be most fruitful relate, in one way or another, to aspects of diet. These, unfortunately, are all extremely difficult to investigate by epidemiologic methods. Not only do the components of diet change during an individual's life, but the individual may not know what some of the components are. In developed countries the food that is eaten varies from day to day and the individual has great difficulty in recording what he eats in a consistent fashion. Moreover, variations in one item are often closely correlated with variations in another (as, for example, the consumption of animal protein and fat). Other items, in contrast, are consumed so uniformly that it may be extremely difficult to tell whether associations exist in individuals that have been suggested by comparisons between broad social or national groups.

It may not be surprising, therefore, that epidemiologic studies which have concentrated on individual items of diet have given rise to conflicting results. On an international scale, for example, colorectal cancer is closely associated with the consumption of both meat and fat (1), whereas case-control studies, which have investigated personal eating habits, have nearly always been negative (4,8,27,28). One study alone, which was confined to Japanese migrants in Hawaii (6), suggested that those who ate more than the average amount of meat might have about twice the risk of developing colorectal cancer as those who ate less. If the consumption of meat does involve a specific risk, vegetarians ought to be spared even though they lived in a society in which the disease is common.

Evidence that this might be so was obtained when Seventh-Day Adventists, who are mostly vegetarian, were found to have about half as great a risk of colorectal cancer as other residents of California (15), but this observation became less impressive when Lyon et al. (11) pointed out that a similar deficiency occurred in the Mormons of Utah, who are among the biggest beef eaters in the United States. If the consumption of meat does increase the risk, it can hardly be a very specific effect as Kinlen *(personal communication)* has found that the mortality from intestinal and rectal cancer in women belonging to strict religious orders in Britain, grouped as either completely or partially abstaining from meat, was 80 and 93% of that expected from the experience of single women in the country as a whole.

If a vegetarian diet does diminish the risk of colorectal cancer, it might be not because of the absence of meat but because of an excess of vegetables. That this might be so was postulated by Wattenberg (25) when he found that addition of a variety of vegetables to the diet (including Brussels sprouts, cabbage, turnips, cauliflower, and broccoli) induced benzo[*a*]pyrene hydroxylase activity in the small intestine of rats. This action appears to be due to the presence of indoles, and when a selection of these was added to the diet, Wattenberg and Loub (26) found that the incidence of mammary tumors in rats given dimethylbenzanthracene was reduced, as was the incidence of tumors of the forestomach in mice given benzo[*a*]pyrene. That vegetables may have a protective effect against colorectal cancer in man is suggested by Bjelke's (1) finding, in case-control studies in Norway and the United States, that the risk of colon cancer was reduced by about 25% in men who ate large amounts of vegetables and by a similar (but more striking) finding by Graham et al. (4) among patients at Roswell Park.

Further progress is, perhaps, less likely to come from detailed studies concentrating on one aspect of diet than from collaborative studies between epidemiologists and laboratory workers in which individuals are characterized by the way food is metabolized and the end-product in the stools. Many such studies have been stimulated by Burkitt and by Wynder, and the results are reviewed elsewhere in this volume.

REFERENCES

1. Armstrong, B., and Doll, R. (1975): Environmental factors and cancer incidence and mortality in different countries, with special reference to dietary practices. *Int. J. Cancer,* 15:617–631.
1a. Bjelke, E., (1973): *Epidemiologic Studies of Cancer of the Stomach, Colon, and Rectum, with Special Emphasis on the Role of Diet, Vol. III & IV.* University Microfilm, Ann Arbor, Michigan.
2. Boyd, J. T., and Doll, R. (1954): Gastro-intestinal cancer and the use of liquid paraffin. *Br. J. Cancer,* 8:231–237.
3. Cook, P., Doll, R., and Fellingham, S. A. (1969): A mathematical model for the age distribution of cancer in man. *Int. J. Cancer,* 4:93–112.
4. Graham, S., Dayal, H., Swanson, M., Mittelman, A., and Wilkinson, G. (1978): Diet in the epidemiology of cancer of the colon and rectum. *J. Natl. Cancer Inst.,* 61:709–714.
5. Haenszel, W. (1961): Cancer mortality among foreign-born in the United States. *J. Natl. Cancer Inst.,* 26:37–132.

6. Haenszel, W., Berg, J. W., Kurihara, M., and Locke, F. B. (1973): Large bowel cancer in Hawaiian Japanese. *J. Natl. Cancer Inst.,* 51:1965–1779.
7. Haenszel, W., and Kurihara, M. (1968): Studies of Japanese migrants, 1. Mortality from cancer and other diseases among Japanese in the United States. *J. Natl. Cancer Inst.,* 40:43–68.
8. Higginson, J. (1966): Aetiological factors in gastrointestinal cancer in man. *J. Natl. Cancer Inst.,* 37:527–545.
9. I.A.R.C. (1976): *Cancer Incidence in Five Continents,* vol. III, edited by J. Waterhouse, C. Muir, P. Correa, and J. Powell. International Agency for Research on Cancer, Lyon.
10. Lee, J. A. H. (1976): Recent trends of large bowel cancer in Japan compared to United States and England and Wales. *Int. J. Epidemiol.,* 5:187–194.
11. Lyon, J. L., Klauber, M. R., Gardner, J. W., and Smart, C. R. (1976): Cancer incidence in Mormons and non-Mormons in Utah, 1966–1970. *N. Engl. J. Med.,* 294:129–133.
12. Newhouse, M. L., and Wagner, J. C. (1969): Validation of death certificate in asbestos workers. *Br. J. Ind. Med.,* 26:302–307.
13. O.M.G.E. (1964): The epidemiology of gastrointestinal cancer with special reference to causation. *Gut,* 5:196–200.
14. Peto, J., Doll, R., Howard, S. V., Kinlen, L. J., and Lewinsohn, H. C. (1977): A mortality study among workers in an English asbestos factory. *Br. J. Ind. Med.,* 34:169–173.
15. Phillips, R. L. (1975): Role of life style and dietary habits in risk of cancer among Seventh Day Adventists. *Cancer Res.,* 35:3515–3522.
16. Pierce, E. R. (1968): Some genetic aspects of familial multiple polyposis of the colon in a kindred of 1,422 members. *Dis. Colon Rectum,* 11:321–329.
17. Reed, T. E., and Neel, J. B. (1955): A genetic study of multiple polyposis of the colon (with an appendix deriving a method of estimating relative fitness). *Am. J. Hum. Genet.,* 7:236–263.
18. Selikoff, I. J., and Hammond, E. L. (1978): Asbestos-associated disease in United States shipyards. *Cancer,* 28:87–99.
19. Smith, R. L. (1956): Recorded and expected mortality among Japanese of the United States and Hawaii, with special reference to cancer. *J. Natl. Cancer Inst.,* 17:459–473.
20. Staszewski, J., and Haenszel, W. (1968): Cancer mortality among the Polish-born in the United States. *J. Natl. Cancer Inst.,* 35:291–297.
21. Staszewski, J., McCall, M. G., and Stenhouse, N. S. (1971): Cancer mortality in 1962–66 among Polish immigrants to Australia. *Br. J. Cancer,* 25:599–610.
22. U.I.C.C. (1966): *Cancer Incidence in Five Continents,* edited by R. Doll, P. Payne, and J. Waterhouse. Union Internationale contre le Cancer, Geneva.
23. U.I.C.C. (1970): *Cancer Incidence in Five Continents, Vol. II,* edited by R. Doll, C. S. Muir, and J. A. H. Waterhouse. Union Internationale contre le Cancer, Geneva.
24. Veale, A. M. O. (1965): *Intestinal Polyposis.* Cambridge University Press, Cambridge.
25. Wattenberg, L. W. (1971): Studies of polycyclic hydrocarbon hydroxylases of the intestine possibly related to cancer. *Cancer,* 28:99–102.
26. Wattenberg, L. W., and Loub, W. D. (1978): Inhibition of polycyclic aromatic hydrocarbon-induced neoplasia by naturally occurring indoles. *Cancer Res.,* 38:1410–1413.
27. Wynder, E. L., Kajitani, T., Ishikawa, S., Dodo, H., and Takano, A. (1969): Environmental factors of cancer of the colon and rectum, II. Japanese epidemiological data. *Cancer,* 23:1210–1220.
28. Wynder, E. L., and Shigematsu, T. (1967): Environmental factors of cancer of the colon and rectum. *Cancer,* 20:1520–1561.

*Colorectal Cancer: Prevention, Epidemiology,
and Screening,* edited by S. Winawer, D. Schottenfeld,
and P. Sherlock. Raven Press, New York © 1980.

Fiber in the Etiology of Colorectal Cancer

Denis P. Burkitt

Unit of Geographical Pathology, St. Thomas's Hospital Medical School, London, England

Probably every illness depends on a balance between the factors causative of and protective against that particular disease, and both of these are likely to be multiple. Cancer is no exception, and immunological and surveillance mechanisms have received much attention of late. In spite of this, there has been a tendency to focus attention almost exclusively on possible causes of colorectal cancer to the exclusion of possible protective factors. As a result, the hypothesis that fiber-depleted diets may predispose to the development of large bowel cancer has been viewed as an alternative to that which implicates diets rich in fat. These have in fact been considered as competing and even as opposing theories. It is now realized that this was a faulty approach and the theories incriminating high fat or low fiber diets as the causation of colorectal cancer are complementary to rather than in opposition to one another. They are "both and" rather than "either or" hypotheses.

Large bowel cancer is now viewed as one of a number of diseases characteristic of modern western culture against which fiber-rich diets may afford protection (30). Other bowel diseases against which dietary fiber has been postulated to confer protection include appendicitis (3,28), diverticular disease (24), and hemorrhoids (5). Cholelithiasis (13), hiatus hernia (4), and diabetes (1,15) have also been included in the list.

EPIDEMIOLOGICAL EVIDENCE

It must be emphasized that the distribution, both geographic and socioeconomic, of high fat diets is almost inevitably the same as that of low fiber diets. Nearly all communities derive 10 to 15% of their energy requirements from protein and the remaining 85 to 90% from fat and carbohyrates combined. Consequently, these two main sources of energy are reciprocally related to one another. Moreover, carbohydrate-rich diets are almost invariably fiber-rich and vice versa.

Colorectal cancer is more closely related to economic development than is any other form of cancer. Minimal rates occur in communities subsisting largely on fiber-rich starchy carbohydrate foods, and rates are maximal in those with diets rich in fat and refined carbohydrates and depleted in fiber. These dietary

13

changes are also characteristic of subgroups within communities who have lower than average rates of colorectal cancer. This applies to Seventh-Day Adventists who are mainly vegetarians (32) and Mormons (18) who have a high intake of cereal fiber consumed in home-ground wholemeal flour.

All communities in which large bowel cancer has increased following immigration from a low- to a high-risk area have both increased the fat and reduced the fiber in their diets. This applies to Japanese immigrants to Hawaii and California, to the Jews who emigrated from North Africa and the Yemen to Israel, and in a large scale to American slaves, whose descendants became the black Americans of today whose dietary customs and bowel cancer rates now correspond to those of white Americans.

The possible protective role of cereal fiber in particular has been suggested by studies comparing the diets of both Copenhagen Danes (22), and New Yorkers (26) with those of rural Fins. Although the incidence of bowel cancer in the Danes and Americans is four times greater than that in the Fins, their fat intakes are comparable. The Fins, however, consume nearly twice as much fiber, mainly in the form of rye bread, and as a result pass twice the volume of stools. Epidemiological studies indicate that colon cancer risk is inversely related to stool volume and is directly related to intestinal transit time, and these are related to fiber intake.

ANIMAL EXPERIMENTS

Many of the experimental studies undertaken to estimate the effect of dietary fiber and bowel tumor incidence have involved the use of injected 1,2/dimethyl-hydrazine (DMH). A number of recent studies have shown what appears to be a significant protective action of fiber against colon cancer. Chen et. al. (6) showed that wheat brain reduced the number of both adenomas and carcinomas arising in the colon in rats who had been given DMH. Fleiszer et al. (11) fed varying amounts of dietary fiber to rats receiving DMH. They found that the numbers of tumors induced was inversely related to stool bulk and to the amount of fiber given. Freeman et al. (12) showed that adding cellulose to a fiber-free diet given to rats who had been treated with DMH reduced the prevalence of colonic tumors. They concluded that "this study supports the hypothesis that fiber is an important protective agent against colonic neoplasia development." Cruse et al. (8) claimed to demonstrate that fiber was not protective against tumor formation in rats given DMH. Their findings were, however, challenged by Newcombe (23) who did not consider tests using injected carcinogens as a suitable model for demonstrating the effect of diet in the human situation. They were also criticized by Thome (27) who pointed out that all rats treated in this way died within a year, irrespective of bran content, whereas none of the controls died. The amounts of DMH were considered to be so large that any protective effects that bran might have could not operate. Lowenfels (17) commented that fiber may have acted by reducing the early deaths which were associated with the administration of the DMH, and that the prolonged life gave these rats at least the chance of developing tumors.

Although these studies suggest that the addition of fiber to the diet significantly reduces the number of both benign and malignant tumors in the large intestine in experimental animals, it has been questioned whether a carcinogen injected subcutaneously is a model relevant to the human situation. Crofts (7) pointed out that "unless it can be shown that DMH or its metabolic products actually enter the gastrointestinal tract in an active carcinogenic form and that the ability of DMH to produce neoplastic change from the systemic side of the colonic mucosa is negligible as compared with the luminal side, then giving fiber in whatever form or quantity would have no logical connection with proving or disproving Burkitt's hypothesis."

POSTULATED PROTECTIVE EFFECT OF FIBER

A number of complementary mechanisms have been postulated whereby adequate dietary fiber intake may confer protection against the development of colorectal cancer. It has now been well substantiated that fiber increases fecal volume with resultant dilution of its contents. Thus fiber dilutes the primary bile acids, which are degraded to potential carcinogens by the action of bacteria. The bacterial activity is reduced by this dilution of the substrate on which they act. Increased stool volume also dilutes any carcinogens or co-carcinogens formed in the gut. This consequently tends to reduce their activity. In addition, the reduced intestinal transit time associated with fiber-rich diets reduces the period of contact between fecal carcinogens and intestinal mucosa, presumably conferring further protection against colon cancer.

Colon Cancer and Fecal pH

MacDonald and Rao (19) have shown that dietary fiber consumed with milk can carry lactose into the colon and diminish the pH value of the stool. Fiber may also have a further protective action lowering fecal pH in other ways, and pH values have been shown to be directly related to colon cancer risk. Over a long period low pH values decrease the bacteriodes counts, and these organisms have been implicated most in the process of carcinogenesis. MacDonald et al. (20,21) have shown that increasing pH value *in vitro* greatly enhances the bacterial activity on bile acids, and that fecal pH increases as bowel cancer risk increases. pH values are higher in average Americans than they are in vegetarians and higher in American vegetarians than they are in Africans. This is in inverse ratio to their colorectal cancer risk. Fiber in the form of wheat bran has also been shown to actually reduce the bacterial decomposition of bile acids (25).

Walker et al. (31) lowered fecal pH by replacing maize meal by white bread in the diet of school children and by adding oranges to their diet. Altering the fat and sugar in their diet had no effect.

It would appear from these studies that fiber has an important function in lowering fecal pH and that this may protect against colon cancer.

Fecal Bile Acids

Antonis and Bersohn (2) in South Africa showed that both reducing the fat in a low fiber diet and increasing the fiber in a high fat diet resulted in decreases in fecal bile acid concentration. The reduction in concentration from increasing fiber (from 5 to 15 g crude fiber a day) was more than that from reducing fat (from 40 to 15% of calories). Walker (28) reduced fecal bile acid concentration in African children by 46% by adding five to seven oranges a day to their diet. Eastwood et al. (9) reduced the concentration of bile acids by 36% by supplementing diet with wheat bran 16 g/day.

N-Nitroso Compounds

Land and Bruce (16) have identified *N*-nitroso compounds in stools that may have carcinogenic properties and have been able to reduce the mutagens in stools by nearly half either by reducing fat intake by 50% or by adding about 30 g of wheat bran to the diet daily. They pointed out that mutagenic activity was more frequently observed in feces of patients with colorectal cancer than in laboratory personnel.

Other Protective Actions of Fiber

Another mechanism whereby fiber may protect against bowel cancer could be by adsorbing potentially carcinogenic particles in the manner in which it has been shown to protect against various toxic substances in rats (10). In addition to all these specific functions, Heaton (14) has pointed out that increased calorie intake tends to increase the risk of developing cancer in general, and adding nonenergy-providing bulk in the form of fiber to the diet tends to reduce overall calorie intake. Yet a further factor that might be mentioned is that increasing the proportion of energy desired from fiber-rich diets reduces that from fat-rich diets which would be beneficial with regard to removing possible causes of colorectal cancer.

CONCLUSION

Since bile acids and neutral sterols yield pre- or actual carcinogens on degradation, it is obviously important to reduce their concentration in the feces. This can be accomplished either by increasing fiber or by reducing fat in the diet, both of which would be nutritionally beneficial changes. These changes also reduce the amount of *N*-nitroso compounds in the feces. It is, however, much easier to increase fiber than to reduce fat, but attempts should be made to achieve both of these changes.

REFERENCES

1. Anderson, J. W. (1976): Beneficial effects from high carbohydrate, high-fibre diet on hyperglycemic diabetic men. *Am. J. Clin. Nutr.,* 29:895–899.
2. Antonis, A., and Bersohn, I. (1962): The influence of diet on faecal lipids in South African white and Bantu prisoners. *Am. J. Clin. Nutr.,* 11:142–155.
3. Burkitt, D. P. (1975): Appendicitis. In: *Refined Carbohydrate Foods and Disease,* edited by D. P. Burkitt and H. C. Trowell, pp. 87–98. Academic Press, London.
4. Burkitt, D. P. (1975): Hiatus hernia. In: *Refined Carbohydrate Foods and Disease,* edited by D. P. Burkitt and H. C. Trowell, pp. 161–172. Academic Press, London.
5. Burkitt, D. P. (1975): Haemorrhoids, varicose veins and deep vein thrombosis. *Can. J. Surg.,* 18:2912–2917.
6. Chen, W., Patchefsky, A. H., and Goldsmith, H. (1978): Colonic protection from dimethylhydrazine by a high fibre diet. *Surgery,* 147:503–506.
7. Crofts, T. J. (1979): Bran and experimental colon cancer. *Lancet,* 1:108.
8. Cruse, J. P., Lewin, M. R., and Clarke, G. C. (1979): Failure of bran to protect against experimental colon cancer in rats. *Lancet,* 2:1278–1279.
9. Eastwood, M. A., Kilpatrick, J. R., Mitchell, W. D., Bone, A., and Hamilton, T. (1973): Effects of dietary supplements of wheat bran and cellulose on faeces and bowel function. *Br. Med. J.,* 4:392–394.
10. Ershoff, B. A. (1974): Antitoxic effects of plant fibre. *Am. J. Clin. Nutr.,* 27:1395–1398.
11. Fleiszer, D., Murray, D., MacFarlane, J., and Brown, R. A. (1978): Protective effect of dietary fibre against chemically induced bowel tumours in rats. *Lancet,* 1:552–553.
12. Freeman, H. J., Spiller, G. A., and Kim, Y. S. (1978): A double blind study on the effect of purified cellulose dietary fibre on 1,2/dimethylhydrazine induced rat colonic neoplasia. *Cancer Res.,* 38:2912–2917.
13. Heaton, K. W. (1978): Are gallstones preventible? *World Med.,* 13:21–23.
14. Heaton, K. W. (1979): Dietary factors in large bowel cancer. In: *Tropics and Gastroenterology, Vol. 5,* edited by S. C. Truelove and E. Lee, pp. 29–44. Blackwell, Oxford.
15. Jenkins, D. J. A., Wolever, T. M. S., and Leeds, A. R. (1978): Dietary fibre, fibre analogues and glucose tolerance: Importance of viscosity. *Br. Med. J.,* 1, p. 1392–1394.
16. Land, P. C., and Bruce, W. R. (1976): *Origins of Human Cancer.* Cold Spring Harbor Laboratory, Cold Spring Harbor, N.Y.
17. Lowenfels, A. B. (1979): Bran and experimental colon cancer. *Lancet,* 1:108.
18. Lyon, J. L. (1975): Cancer incidence in Mormons and non-Mormons. *N. Engl. J. Med.,* 294:129–132.
19. MacDonald, I. A., and Rao, B. G. (1979): Diet, bacteria in the origin of bowel cancer. *Mod. Med. Can.,* 34:136–140.
20. MacDonald, I. A., Singh, G., Mahoney, D. E., and Mier, C. G. (1978): Effect of pH on bile salt degradation by mixed faecal cultures. *Steroids,* 32:245–256.
21. MacDonald, I. A., Webb, G. R., and Mahoney, D. E. (1978): Faecal hydroxysteroid dehydrogenase activities in vegetarians, Seventh-Day-Adventists controlled subjects and bowel cancer patients. *Am. J. Clin. Nutr.,* S.223–238.
22. McLennan, R., Jensen, O. M., Mosbech, J., and Vuori, H. (1978): Diet, transit time, stool weight, and colon cancer in two Scandinavian populations. *Am. J. Clin. Nutr.,* 31:S.239–242.
23. Newcombe, R. R. Q. (1979): Bran and experimental colon cancer. *Lancet,* 1:108.
24. Painter, N. S., and Burkitt, D. P. (1971): Diverticular disease of the colon. A deficiency disease of Western civilization. *Br. Med. J.,* 2:450–454.
25. Pomare, E. W., and Heaton, K. W. (1973): Alteration of bile salt metabolism by dietary fibre. *Br. Med. J.,* 4:262–264.
26. Reddy, B. C., Hedges, R., Laakso, K., and Wynder, E. L. (1978): Metabolic epidemiology of

large bowel cancer. Faecal bulk and constituents of high risk North American and low risk Finnish population. *Cancer,* 22:2832–2838.

27. Thome, M. C. (1979): Bran and experimental colon cancer. *Lancet,* 1:108.
28. Walker, A. R. P. (1975): Effect of high crude fibre intake on transit time and the absorption of nutrients in South African negro schoolchildren. *Am. J. Clin. Nutr.,* 28:1161–1169.
29. Walker, A. R. P. (1976): Gastrointestinal disease and fibre intake with special reference to South African populations. In: *Fibre in Human Nutrition,* edited by G. A. Spiller and R. J. Amen, pp. 242–261. Plenum Press, New York.
30. Walker, A. R. P., and Burkitt, D. P. (1976): Colonic cancer: Hypothesis of causation, dietary prophylaxis and future research. *Am. J. Clin. Nutr.,* 21:910–917.
31. Walker, A. R. P., Walker, B. F., and Segal. I. (1979): Faecal pH value and its modification by dietary means in South African black and white schoolchildren. *South Afr. Med. J.,* 55:495–498.
32. Wynder, E. L., and Shigematsu, T. (1967): Environmental factors of cancer of the colon and rectum. *Cancer,* 20:1520–1561.

Colorectal Cancer: Prevention, Epidemiology, and Screening, edited by S. Winawer, D. Schottenfeld, and P. Sherlock. Raven Press, New York © 1980.

Current Views on the Mechanisms Involved in the Etiology of Colorectal Cancer

John H. Weisburger, Bandaru S. Reddy, Ncil E. Spingarn, and Ernst L. Wynder

Naylor Dana Institute for Disease Prevention, American Health Foundation, Valhalla, New York 10595

In the last 30 years, an understanding of some of the key events during the development of cancer has been achieved even at the molecular level. Many elements of the progress made are reviewed in this volume. Careful recording of environmental influences favoring the development of specific types of cancer, or, in reverse, inquiries as to the reasons for a lower rate when a high rate might have been expected have furnished a reasonably satisfactory set of data points and arguments bearing on the etiology of many of the major types of cancer. In relation to two of the most important types of cancer in man around the world, namely, cancer of the stomach and cancer of the large bowel, there is an adequate, sound basis of facts on causative and modifying factors, and the underlying relevant mechanisms for these types of cancer, to begin making recommendations to the public aimed at a reduction of the risk for these neoplasms (48,56).

The data base was obtained not by a single observer utilizing a single instrument, but by multidisciplinary efforts on an international scale. It is this teamwork of epidemiologists, studying high and low risk populations, not only as to incidence parameters but also by laboratory scientists on metabolic indicators through controlled studies in man, in experimental animals, and in *in vitro* systems which has strengthened the arguments and interpretations developed in this paper.

Current concepts of etiology are based on three major approaches and lines of evidence (Doll, Burkitt, *this volume;* 56,59). The first is the variation in incidence of a specific type of cancer as a function of area of residence and in migrant populations. The second depends on changes of incidence as a function of time. The third consists of detailed laboratory studies in animal models or in *in vitro* systems.

When a carcinogen is introduced into the human environment, there is a change in incidence as a function of time (Doll, Burkitt, *this volume;* 5;12,49,52). This is seen most readily in the small population groups presenting with occupational cancers. A more striking case involving large numbers of people is that of cigarette smoking, which became popular in men about World War I, and in women about World War II. Twenty to thirty years later there was a pronounced upward change in the incidence of lung cancer. Thus introduction of carcinogens in cigarette smoke on a large scale results in a striking appearance of neoplastic disease. On the other hand, in the United States, cancer of the stomach has declined considerably over the last 50 years. The obvious conclusion is that the carcinogenic stimulus has diminished, or that a protective agent was introduced. A decline in stomach cancer is now being seen in other parts of the world also, where stomach cancer still has a high incidence, for example, Japan, Central and Western Latin America, and Northern and Eastern Europe.

EPIDEMIOLOGY AND METABOLIC EPIDEMIOLOGY OF LARGE BOWEL CANCER

In the United States, except for easily detectable and curable skin cancer, large bowel cancer ranks highest in incidence of neoplastic diseases in men and women, affecting 112,000 persons in 1979 (12,16,48,56). Within the United States, almost all socioeconomic groups have equal risk, although historically, the rate was somewhat lower in the South than in the North. This distinction is attributed mainly to the fact that the lower socioeconomic groups in the South, particularly Black individuals, had a lower risk (50). Because of changes ("improvements") in living conditions, even this gradient is now disappearing.

That colon cancer is judged to be an environmental "man-made" disease is deduced from the incidence patterns around the world. Japan, parts of Central and South America, and Africa exhibit a low incidence of colon cancer, and the Anglo-Saxon countries and parts of Western Europe, a high incidence. Within Scandinavia, Denmark has a high incidence of colon cancer, but Finland has a low incidence.

In the past, rectal cancer was often considered together with colon cancer as "colorectal" or "large bowel" cancer. There begins to be a realization that these may be two separate diseases. Current evidence indicates that a distinction needs to be made between colonic cancer and rectal cancer (50). The definition of rectal cancer has been standardized as disease within 8 cm from the anus. The difference in incidence of colonic cancer between a high risk country like the United States and a low risk country like Japan is 4 to 1, but for rectal cancer, this difference is merely of the order of 1.1 to 1, thus suggesting that the etiologies for colonic and for rectal cancer may be different. In the Western world, more cancer is seen along the sigmoid and descending colon, with relatively less in the ascending and transverse colon. In low-incidence countries, the disease appears more on the right side or the transverse colon. Colon cancer thus defined has a sex ratio of approximate unity, whereas rectal cancer occurs in excess in males, with a factor of 1.4:1 over females. Etiologic factors for rectal cancer remain to be defined. The following discussion will bear on factors related to colon cancer.

COLON CANCER

On the basis of variations in incidence for different regions of the world and in view of the altered risk of migrant populations, it has been accepted that diet is a major etiologic factor in colon cancer (48). Further epidemiologic evaluation has implicated a high intake of dietary fat (29,58,59), protein (1), and beef (17), and dietary fiber deficiency (Burkitt, *this volume*) as strongly associated with large bowel carcinogenesis. A major portion of the dietary fat in high risk areas is derived from meat, in particular, beef. Also, diets high in fat are often low in fiber. On the basis of epidemiologic and laboratory evidence, we have emphasized dietary fat and fiber, but new efforts are under way to round out knowledge on other dietary components suspected of playing a role in large bowel carcinogenesis.

Wynder and Hirayama (57) compared the dietary patterns of the United States white and Japanese populations in terms of calories, specific nutrients, and per capita yearly intake. About 40% of the total caloric intake in the United States stems from fat, mostly saturated, largely from dairy and animal products. In contrast, the Japanese derive only 10 to 20% of their caloric intake from fat, of which 35% is unsaturated. Their basic food is rice, which accounts for 41% of total calories (Table 1).

Despite the difficulties inherent in describing a representative diet for a given population, differences between the American and the traditional Japanese diets are so great that fairly accurate generalizations can be made. It is clear that there is no average daily American diet. Intake of particular foods is seasonal and varied. On the other hand, the traditional Japanese diet includes three daily servings of rice and one or two servings of soybean products per day. Meat is rarely eaten, except mainly by upper socioeconomic groups, although fish is consumed one or two times a week. Only small amounts of milk and other dairy products are part of the regimen. Eggs are also a luxury item. It is obvious that differences in dietary habits between the United States and Japan were much more pronounced four decades ago, although some differences have remained, as evidenced by a 33% greater calorie intake by United States whites than by Japanese, as well as by the significantly greater consumption of fats and fat-related nutrients in the United States. Soy products are the second most important source of unsaturated fat, next to vegetable oil, in the Japanese diet, whereas intake of this product is negligible in the United States. Although meats, poultry, and eggs contribute 30% of the total fat intake by the Japanese, they contribute almost 45% of fat in the United States diet. The daily total fat intake is 152 g in the United States and 46 g in Japan (Table 1).

The daily cholesterol intake differs between the two countries with the Japanese consuming 304 mg and United States whites consuming 556 mg. However, intake of cholesterol in the United States appears to be decreasing.

The mechanism whereby dietary fat translates to high risk has been investigated in a number of laboratories. One finding was that populations with a

TABLE 1. *Net food and fat supply per capita: 1968*

Food	Country	Food g/day	Fat g/day
Cereals	United States	177	2.3
	Japan	379	3.4
Potatoes, etc.[a]	United States	124	0.3
	Japan	181	—
Sugars and sweets	United States	135	—
	Japan	58	—
Pulses, nuts and seeds	United States	22	6.9
	Japan	46	4.8
Vegetables	United States	310	0.7
	Japan	361	0.6
Fruits	United States	223	0.8
	Japan	127	0.3
Meat	United States	290	51.9
	Japan	36	4.7
Eggs	United States	50	5.2
	Japan	32	3.2
Fish	United States	17	1.2
	Japan	84	2.6
Milk	United States	669	20.8
	Japan	118	3.8
Fats and oils (fat content)	United States	62	61.7
	Japan	22	22.5
Total fat	United States	—	152
	Japan	—	46
Cholesterol	United States	—	0.56
	Japan	—	0.30

[a]Potatoes and other starchy foods.
From Wynder and Hirayama (57).

high risk for large bowel cancer have a higher amount of fecal bile acids and cholesterol metabolites (Table 2) (19,29,36) and increased concentration of intestinal anaerobic bacteria. There were no great changes in the bacterial flora between high risk and low risk populations (14). This difference stems from the metabolic activity of the flora rather than its composition (29). In addition, people on a high fat diet appear to have a slightly higher level of total fecal anaerobic bacteria and bacterial β-glucuronidase activity. In a similar study, in which the protein content was altered without changing the fat content, there was no great change in the fecal bacterial flora (18).

Hill et al. (19) have reported that 82% of colorectal cancer patients had fecal bile acid levels above an arbitrary cutoff level compared with only 17%

TABLE 2. Daily fecal excretion (mg/day) of neutral sterols and bile acids in different populations with varied risk for colon cancer

	North Americans on a mixed Western diet (40)	North American vegetarians (12)	North American Seventh Day Adventists (25)	Japanese (25)	Chinese (25)
Neutral sterols					
Cholesterol	45 ± 10[a]	67 ± 17	60 ± 20	90 ± 20	60 ± 18
Coprostanol	520 ± 75	231 ± 49[b]	201 ± 26[b]	140 ± 25[b]	129 ± 25[b]
Coprostanone	140 ± 79	20 ± 6[b]	20 ± 3[b]	24 ± 6[b]	25 ± 6[b]
Total neutral sterols	705 ± 104	318 ± 53[b]	281 ± 34[b]	254 ± 35[b]	214 ± 36[b]
Bile acids					
Cholic acid	12 ± 4	7 ± 6	8 ± 1	5 ± 2	10 ± 3
Chenodeoxycholic acid	10 ± 3	6 ± 2	6 ± 1	6 ± 2	12 ± 2
Deoxycholic acid	115 ± 18	32 ± 6[b]	30 ± 5[b]	45 ± 5[b]	40 ± 6[b]
Lithocholic acid	90 ± 10	23 ± 5[b]	29 ± 3[b]	32 ± 3[b]	38 ± 4[b]
Other bile acids	48 ± 9	65 ± 10	17 ± 3	10 ± 2	2 ± 1
Total bile acids	275 ±	133 ± 15[b]	90 ± 6[b]	98 ± 6[b]	102 ± 10[b]

[a] Averages ± SEM.
[b] Significantly different from North Americans on a mixed Western diet ($p < 0.05$).
From Reddy et al. (30).

of the patients serving as controls. Also, 82% of the cancer patients had fecal nuclear-dehydrogenating clostridia (NDC), compared with 43% of the controls, whereas 70% of the cancer patients had the combination of NDC and high fecal bile acid levels compared with only 9% of the control patients. In a similar study, Reddy et al. (36) have shown that the concentration of the bile acids (deoxycholic acid and lithocholic acid) and cholesterol metabolites (cholesterol, coprostanol, and cholestan-3β,5α,6β-triol) in colon cancer patients and patients with adenomatous polyps was higher than in controls, as was the fecal 7α-dehydroxylase and cholesterol dehydrogenase activity. The area of specific endogenous metabolites deserves additional study to uncover other such characteristics of high risk groups.

Fat, rather than protein, appears to be the dietary ingredient associated with colon cancer, inasmuch as one highly controlled study in a metabolic ward in which the fat level was held constant and the protein varied yielded no difference in fecal bile acid patterns (18).

Patients with familial polyposis are at a high risk of developing colon cancer (Lipkin, Utsunomiya, *this volume*). This condition, for the most part, is under genetic rather than environmental control, as patients even in a low colon cancer risk country, as Japan, do develop colon cancer at approximately the same age as do Americans with familial polyposis. Characteristically, patients with familial polyposis excrete more undegraded cholesterol than controls (36).

Patients with familial polyposis, ulcerative colitis, and adenomatous polyps, who are at increased risk of developing carcinoma of the colon, fall into three distinct groups with regard to fecal bile acid and cholesterol metabolite profile (29). The patients with adenomatous polyps excrete high levels of both cholesterol metabolites and bile acids compared with controls; patients with ulcerative colitis excrete high levels of neutral sterols but similar levels of bile acids compared with controls. In these high risk patients, the common denominator is always found in the cholesterol metabolites. There appear to be some elements of genetic control, inasmuch as Wilkins et al. (53) have reported two distinct patterns of cholesterol metabolism.

With the collaboration of Dr. Lipkin of the Memorial Sloan-Kettering Cancer Center in New York, we found that the stools of individuals at high risk for colon cancer, and those of some of their family members, contain appreciable amounts of cholesterol, but interestingly not of the bacterial metabolites of cholesterol, namely, cholestanol and cholestanone. This finding parallels that found in some of the high risk groups such as those with adenomatous polyps or ulcerative colitis. We believe that these results are consistent with the concept that the mucosal cells in the lower large bowel of high risk people synthesize cholesterol. Were such cholesterol to originate in the liver, it would be likely to be metabolized by gut bacterial enzymes. Since the metabolites are not elevated and cholesterol is, it would seem that intestinal mucosa is involved in the biosynthesis of the amount present. The significance of this finding in relation to high risk for colon cancer remains to be defined.

ANIMAL MODELS FOR COLON CANCER

Chemicals Known to Induce Colon Cancer and Their Mode of Action

Research on the mechanisms of cancer causation in the large bowel has been assisted by the discovery over the last 20 years of several animal models that relatively faithfully mirror the type of lesions seen in man. These models are (7): (a) induction of large bowel cancer in rats through chemicals of the type 3-methyl-4-aminobiphenyl or 3-methyl-2-naphthylamine; (b) derivatives and analogues of cycasin and methylazoxymethanol (MAM), such as azoxymethane (AOM) and 1,2-dimethylhydrazine (DMH), which work well in rats and mice of select strains; (c) intrarectal administration of direct-acting carcinogens such as MAM acetate or alkylnitrosoureas such as methylnitrosourea (MNU) or methyl-N'-nitro-N-nitrosoguanidine (MNNG), which lead to cancer of the descending large bowel in every species tested so far; and (d) oral administration of large doses of 3-methylcholanthrene, which leads to large bowel cancer in select strains of hamsters.

Recently, a group at the U.S. National Cancer Institute in Bethesda (6) and one at the Krebsforschungszentrum in Heidelberg (15) demonstrated that even a single intraperitoneal injection of methyl(acetoxymethyl)nitrosamine induced epithelial cancers along the gastrointestinal tract. This powerful direct-acting carcinogen may be absorbed directly into the bloodstream in the tissues bathed by the peritoneal fluid, and thus acts locally (15). It is significant that this synthetic derivative of the putative hydroxymethyl metabolite should be so powerful a carcinogen in the intestine when intrarectal infusions of dimethylnitrosamine do not cause intestinal cancer. This finding indicates that the intestine cannot metabolize dimethylnitrosamine to the proximate carcinogen, the hydroxymethyl derivative.

In occupational carcinogenesis, where specific chemicals have induced specific kinds of cancer in man, these diseases have been reproduced relatively faithfully in animal models. If this condition also holds true for colon cancer, it is likely that chemicals responsible for large bowel disease may fall into one or more of the classes discussed above.

The possible role of dietary fat in the induction of human cancer of the large bowel has received validation support from carefully controlled experimental studies in the animal models described. Inasmuch as humans in various populations usually follow comparable dietary regimens over generations, we have designed our experiments so that animals are exposed to a given regimen for two generations prior to treatment with a carcinogen. Virgin female rats fed diets containing 5% corn oil, 20% corn oil, 5% lard, or 20% lard were bred, and the litters were weaned to the same diet consumed by the mothers (33). At 50 days of age, all second generation animals except controls received 20 weekly subcutaneous doses of 10 mg/kg of DMH.

More colon cancers were induced in a larger proportion of the rats at risk on the high fat diet than the low fat regimen. With the high fat level, the type of fat was immaterial, an important point since this level mimics the dietary fat intake in high risk Western people for colon cancer. Similar data were obtained with a combination of high beef protein (40%) and high beef fat (20%), or high soybean protein (40%) and high corn oil (20%) (34). More colon tumors appeared in rats given such high fat diets than control diets of beef protein (20%) and low beef fat (6%), or soybean protein (20%) and low corn oil content (6%) (Table 3).

A number of other investigators have likewise demonstrated that the level of dietary fat controls the eventual development of colon cancer in comparative experiments (3,8,9,23,28). Most investigators in such comparative tests killed all animals at a given time, and thus the variables studied, such as dietary fat or cholesterol, result in a specific incidence and multiplicity of colon tumors at the stated time point. In one case, the animals were allowed to survive, in which case the incidence of tumors was similarly high, but the time of death was somewhat earlier in animals on a high fat diet (37). The latter experimental approach is somewhat more difficult to interpret inasmuch as competing tumor sites are also affected and the situation is not as clear-cut.

As noted, the type of fat appears to yield identical effects at the 20% level. However, at the 5% fat level, there is a suggestion that unsaturated fat predisposes to more DMH-induced colon tumors than saturated fat. The animals on a high fat diet excreted more bile acids and neutral sterols than comparable animals on a low fat diet (32) (Table 4).

TABLE 3. *Colon tumor incidence in rats fed diets high in fat and treated with carcinogens*

Diet fat (%)	Protein (%)	Carcinogen	% Rats with colon tumors
5% lard	25% casein	DMH[a]	17
20% lard	"	"	67
5% corn oil	"	"	36
20% corn oil	"	"	64
20% beef fat	22% casein	DMH[b]	60
5% beef fat	"	"	27
20% beef fat	"	MNU[c]	73
5% beef fat	"	"	33
20% beef fat	"	MAM acetate[d]	80
5% beef fat	"	"	45

[a]Female F344 rats, at 7 weeks of age, were given weekly s.c. DMH at a dose rate of 10 mg/kg body wt. for 20 weeks and autopsied 10 weeks later.

[b]Male F344 rats, at 7 weeks of age, were given a single dose of s.c. DMH, 150 mg/kg body wt. and autopsied 30 weeks later.

[c]Male F344 rats, at 7 weeks of age, were given i.r. MNU, 2.5 mg/rat twice in 1 week and autopsied 30 weeks later.

[d]Male F344 rats, at 7 weeks of age, were given i.p. MAM acetate, 35 mg/kg body wt. once and autopsied 30 weeks later.

From Reddy et al. (30).

TABLE 4. *Effect of type and amount of dietary fat on some fecal bile acids in rats*

	5% Corn oil control (8)	20% Corn oil control (8)	5% Lard control (8)	20% Lard control (8)
		mg/day/kg body wt		
Cholic acid	0.68 ± 0.08[a,b,1]	0.64 ± 0.07[1]	0.74 ± 0.06[1]	0.86 ± 0.10[1]
Deoxycholic acid	2.53 ± 0.18[1]	4.80 ± 0.23[2]	2.61 ± 0.20[1]	4.54 ± 0.30[2]
Lithocholic acid	0.83 ± 0.11[1]	1.98 ± 0.16[2]	1.00 ± 0.10[1]	2.84 ± 0.13[2]
12-Ketolithocholic acid	0.44 ± 0.03[1]	0.77 ± 0.07[2]	0.51 ± 0.18[1]	0.77 ± 0.02[2]
Total bile acids[c]	10.5 ± 0.20[1]	14.9 ± 0.41[2]	11.2 ± 0.49[1]	14.9 ± 0.62[2]

[a] Mean $\pm$ SEM.
[b] Means with a common number (i.e., 1 and 1; 2 and 2), superscript between groups in a horizontal row are not significant, $p > 0.05$.
[c] Total includes other bile acids not mentioned here (see 30).

Western people and animals on a high fat diet excrete more total bile acids, and specific secondary bile acids in the stools, than low risk Japanese or African people or rats on a 5% fat level. Bile acids require priority consideration, since tests in germfree and conventional rats show that they have an appreciable promoting action in large bowel carcinogenesis (but not on mouse skin) (45). Contrary to a recent hypothesis (11), cholesterol and neutral sterols are not promoters (35) (Tables 5 and 6). However, in the animal model, bile acids can serve as promoters, and it seems that secondary bacterially produced bile acids are more potent than primary bile acids. These compounds are present in human stools in relatively high concentrations. Nigro, Chomchai [see Bull et al. (9)], and Asano et al. (2) observed that an increase of bile salts in the colon of rats, induced either by feeding cholestyramine or by surgically diverting bile to the middle of the small intestine, enhanced colon tumor formation.

On the other hand, removal of the gut contents, including bile acid flow, by colostomy has served to strongly suppress colon carcinogenesis (22,55). In some cases with a low dose or limited treatment of colon carcinogens, no colon cancer was observed when the promotional stimulus from the luminal contents was removed. This suggests that, in conventional unoperated animals, an important part of the carcinogenic process in the colon rests on promotion by bile acids. Considering the great differences in colon cancer incidence between the low risk Japanese people and the much higher risk Western population, it may be that the dietary fat and cholesterol intake exerts a crucial promoting role in colon cancer formation in man, through metabolic production of bile acids which, in turn, exert a disease-rate controlling effect by promotion.

Specific fibers such as wheat bran and pectin have an inhibiting effect in large bowel carcinogenesis in animals (47,54). In part, especially for bran, the mechanism may be simply dilution of intestinal bile acids. However, the phenomenon is clearly more complex and more research is necessary (Burkitt, *this volume*). For example, with pectin there is a considerable effect with azoymeth-

TABLE 5. Colon tumor incidence in germfree rats treated with intrarectal MNNG and/or bile acids or neutral sterols

Series[a]	Group[b]	No. of rats	Animals with tumors (%)	Tumors/rat			
				Total	Adenoma	Adenocarcinoma	
I	CA	10	0	0	0	0	
	CDC	10	0	0	0	0	
	MNNG	22	27	0.27	0.13	0.14	
	MNNG + CA	24	50	0.63	0.34	0.29	
	MNNG + CDC	24	54	1.08	0.79	0.29	
II	LC	12	0	0	0	0	
	MNNG	24	38	0.67	0.42	0.25	
	MNNG + LC	24	79	1.42	1.00	0.42	
III	Cholesterol	15	0	0	0	0	
	Epoxide	21	0	0	0	0	
	Triol	15	0	0	0	0	
	MNNG	24	46	0.63	0.50	0.13	
	MNNG + cholesterol	24	46	0.67	0.42	0.25	
	MNNG + epoxide	24	58	0.71	0.54	0.17	
	MNNG + triol	24	46	0.54	0.46	0.08	

[a] In series I, the CA or CDC group received intrarectally 20 mg of sodium salt of respective bile acids 3× weekly for 48 weeks; MNNG group received i.r. 2 mg of MNNG twice a week for 2 weeks, followed by vehicle for 46 weeks; MNNG + CA or MNNG + CDC group received i.r. MNNG for 2 weeks and bile acids thereafter for 46 weeks. In series II and III, the MNNG group received 2.5 mg MNNG twice a week for 2 weeks and the vehicle thereafter for ≤6 weeks. The experimental protocol for the bile acids and cholesterol metabolite administration is the same as described for series I.
[b] CA, cholic acid; CDC, chenodeoxycholic acid; LC, lithocholic acid; Epoxide, cholesterol-α-epoxide; Triol, cholestane-3,5,6-triol; MNNG, N-methyl-N'-nitro-N-nitrosoguanidine.
From Reddy et al. (35,47).

TABLE 6. Colon tumor incidence in conventional rats treated with intrarectal MNNG and/or bile acids or neutral sterols[a]

Series	Group	No. of rats	% Animals with tumors	Tumors/rat		
				Total	Adenoma	Adenocarcinoma
I	CA	12	0	0	0	0
	CDC	12	0	0	0	0
	MNNG	30	37	0.55	0.23	0.32
	MNNG + CA	30	67	0.87	0.24	0.63
	MNNG + CDC	30	70	1.23	0.27	0.96
II	LC	12	0	0	0	0
	MNNG	24	54	1.00	0.75	0.25
	MNNG + LC	24	83	1.83	1.50	0.33
III	Cholesterol	15	0	0	0	0
	Epoxide	21	0	0	0	0
	Triol	15	0	0	0	0
	MNNG	24	71	1.29	0.96	0.33
	MNNG + cholesterol	24	71	1.04	0.67	0.38
	MNNG + epoxide	24	58	1.08	0.71	0.38
	MNNG + triol	24	58	0.96	0.75	0.21

[a] The experimental protocols and abbreviations are the same as described for Table 5. From Reddy and Watanabe (35).

TABLE 7. *Colon tumor incidence in female F344 rats fed diets containing pectin, alfalfa, or wheat bran and treated with azoxymethane or methylnitrosourea*

| | % Animals with colon tumors | |
Diet	Azoxymethane treated	Methylnitrosourea treated
Control	57	69
Pectin	10[a]	59
Alfalfa	53	83[b]
Wheat bran	33[a]	60

[a]Significantly different from the groups fed the control diet or alfalfa diet by χ^2 test, $p < 0.05$.
[b]Significantly different from the other groups, $p < 0.05$.
From Reddy et al. (30).

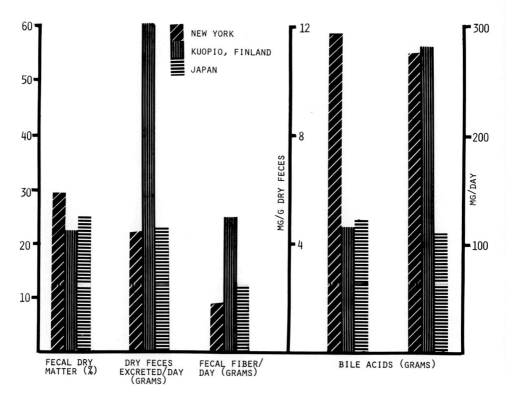

FIG. 1. Comparison of the fecal constituents in a group of New York people at high risk for colon cancer and groups of rural Finnish people (Kuopio) and Japanese at low risk for colon cancer. Note the larger amount of feces per day and fecal fiber per day in the Finnish group. At equal fat intake, the Finnish group excreted similar amounts of bile acids in feces but, because of the higher stool bulk, the concentration of bile acids in feces was similar to that of the Japanese. The Japanese have a low concentration and a low daily amount of bile acids excreted because of lower fat intake (32).

ane, but not much with methylnitrosourea. This suggests that digestive products from pectin may be absorbed and affect the metabolism of azoxymethane, a point currently under investigation. A similar inhibitory phenomenon has also been shown to occur in man. People from Finland and other areas, such as Utah, with high dietary fat and cholesterol intake have a high incidence of coronary heart disease, but interestingly a lower incidence of colon cancer (20, 31,48,56). In Finland it was demonstrated that the people eat diets high in fiber, mainly in the form of bread baked with whole wheat flour containing bran. This results in larger stool bulk which, in turn, lowers the concentration of bile acids in the intestinal tract and in the stools to levels which are similar to those of low risk Japanese people, who eat a diet much lower in fat, but not as high in complex fibers (Table 7, Fig. 1).

As described above, animal studies have confirmed that bran and pectin yield a lower colon cancer incidence through similar mechanisms. On the other hand, a high intake of carrageenan increased the incidence of colon cancer while increasing the intestinal and fecal bile acid levels (46). Animals in these studies also have a much lower serum cholesterol value, analogous to the situation with cholestyramine. With the latter drug, the situation may be more complex inasmuch as it may have an "irritating" effect on bowel mucosa, which may also be responsible for the higher colon carcinogenicity seen in rats on alfalfa diets (47). On the other hand, intake of tannic acid lowered colon carcinogenicity through unknown mechanisms.

CARCINOGENS IN COLON CANCER

Colon cancer, and also breast and prostate cancer, have shown only a slight upward trend in incidence in the United States in the last 40 years (12) (Fig. 2). It may be thus reasonable to conclude that the pronounced alterations in our environment—such as industrial pollution, intentional and inadvertent food additives, and food contaminants—are not directly or indirectly associated with the development of these three types of cancer in man, which are so important in the Western world. In Japan, where there is a high degree of industrialization like in the Western world, these three types of cancer have a low incidence. However, there has been a recent trend toward an increased incidence, associated with the progressive westernization of the Japanese dietary intake since 1945 (24,59). This alone is evidence that the dietary pattern, rather than industrial activity, is most important in relation to causative mechanisms for these types of human cancer.

Furthermore, industrial pollution often affects men in their workplace more than women who are not employed in such exposed situations. Yet colon cancer in the general public is seen equally in women and men. There are a number of instances in which occupation is possibly associated with an increased risk for large bowel cancer. High level intake of asbestos has increased the incidence of colon cancer (39,40). It is not known whether low level exposure, such as

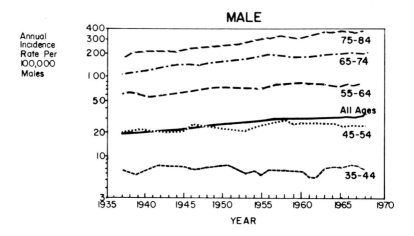

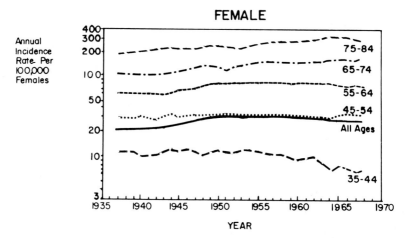

FIG. 2. Five-year moving averages in colon cancer incidence rates, by sex and age, in Connecticut, per 100,000 over a 35-year period. Note the small increase in males and the almost steady incidence in females. As noted in the text, this relatively constant incidence, despite many changes in food additives and preservatives, and industrial contamination, indicates that these elements have exhibited no effect. Rather, the causes and modifiers of colon cancer have been in the environment for a long time.

might have occurred years ago when certain foods or beverages such as beer were filtered through layers of asbestos and the resultant beverage possibly contained asbestos fibers, had any effect. A similar low level exposure situation may have existed when drinking water contained asbestos from various sources. On the basis of current concepts, it is not likely that such a low intake of fibers could play a role in colon carcinogenesis, but in reality there are no facts. Vobecky et al. (44) have noted a possible connection between employment in a carpet factory and large bowel cancer. Berg (4) has tabulated data from several occupational groups which suggest, but certainly do not prove, a relationship inasmuch as other causative factors for large bowel cancer in the general public relate mainly to diet, especially the mode of cooking and the fat content. This particular set of factors requires consideration even when evaluating certain occupational risks. For example, it is possible that workmen, for their own convenience, bring food from home along to their workplace on a daily basis which may include fried, high fat foods. Also, the workplace eating establishment may offer such foods on a daily basis to their employees. On the other hand, the possibility exists that there could be exposure to certain chemicals in the workplace which may be responsible for the disease. It is important not to lose any leads, but it is also essential not to chase a mirage. Pratt et al. (27) noted colorectal cancer in 13 patients, all under 20 years old, and he thought that exposure to agricultural chemicals might be a factor in the development of this cancer at such a young age. This is a potentially most important discovery which requires verification.

The main difference in diet characterizing low risk countries for cancer of the colon, breast, and prostate, versus high risk countries, is the amount of dietary fat. We have reviewed the mechanisms whereby dietary fat translates to promotional stimuli in the form of bile acids for colon cancer, and hormonal balances for cancer of the breast, and most likely for cancer of the prostate. Dietary fiber, increasing stool bulk, has a protective effect in colon cancer, although the nature of "fiber" requires study.

Promotion, as defined above, necessarily requires an antecedent gene change, either spontaneous or by action of a genotoxic agent, for the ultimate development of cancer (52). Hueper, many years ago, drew the realistic analogy to the photographic process. Film is exposed to light to impress an occult, permanent change. This is like the change in DNA from genotoxic carcinogens. Then the film is developed to reveal the photo, which in turn can be treated further by toners, etc. to obtain a final print with the desired features. This is like promotion of a latent cancer cell. Both steps, and in fact, more corollary events, are required for the final tumor formation.

Thus the problem of acquiring information on the carcinogenic stimulus for colon cancer as seen in the general public without obvious occupational chemical exposure is of high contemporary interest.

The question has been asked whether the dietary and body fat could act as a reservoir for environmental contaminants such as DDT, PCB, PBB, or TCDD. None of these contaminants has induced cancer in animal models in the colon. High dose levels of DDT and PCB yielded liver tumors in mice. This may occur by a promotion mechanism rather than by initiation (52). Some forms of PCB have produced liver tumors in rats. Trace contaminants in fat are not likely carcinogens in man since the type of fat, with distinct impurities, has not been found to exert a decisive influence in promoting cancer development.

An important clue as to the nature of carcinogens possibly associated with the diet-linked cancers came from the demonstration that charcoal broiling of meat or fish yielded mutagenic activity for *Salmonella typhimurium* (10,42,43). A significant feature with respect to structure was that the activity was detected more frequently in the strain TA 98, and required activation with a postmitochondrial fraction from induced rat liver. This suggested that the activity might relate to materials such as arylamines or certain polycyclic aromatic hydrocarbons, but not alkylnitrosamines.

A key finding was that a product from the pyrolysis of tryptophan was a γ-carboline derivative, an *o*-methylarylamine type of compound (7,43). Conceptually, this is important. Indeed, some arylamines induce liver or urinary bladder cancer in rodent models, but the corresponding *o*-methylarylamines often cause colon cancer in male rats and breast and colon cancer in female rats (7,48,52).

Preliminary tests of the carcinogenicity of the γ-carboline derived from the pyrolysis of tryptophan, namely, TRP-Pl, have been performed initially by subcutaneous injection. Under these conditions, local sarcoma production was noted (21). This is rather similar to the occurrence of subcutaneous tumors seen upon the feeding of simple analogues such as ortho-toluidine. Liver tumors were also observed in the treated rats. The Tokyo group, as well as we in this Institute, are currently planning additional tests of this new class of mutagens and carcinogens. The aim is to specifically determine whether this kind of chemical can induce cancer in epithelial tissues, such as colon or breast. This must remain an open question, despite the structural analogy to *o*-methylarylamines, in view of the developments described below.

In addition, we have established the conditions under which mutagenic activity is formed as a function of mode and temperature of cooking (42). When ground meat is placed in a preheated frying pan, the temperature curve shows a plateau at 100°C while the water is boiled off and initial browning occurs (Fig. 3).

During that period, virtually no mutagenic activity is seen. Subsequently, the temperature rises and mutagenic activity develops. Appreciable mutagenic activity is seen upon frying to a degree at which time the product is perfectly edible. Pariza et al. (25) have published similar results.

The temperature curve in broiling in an electric oven has a somewhat different shape since the heat input is mainly infrared radiation. Under these conditions, mutagenic activity does not develop for about 15 to 20 min when the temperature of the meat begins to rise above 100°C and mutagenic activity develops (Fig. 4).

Of considerable interest in relation to the mechanism of the formation of mutagenic activity is the fact that long boiling of a fat-free meat broth also develops mutagenic activity (10). The reaction is more rapid when the broth is allowed to boil in an open vessel, and thus is progressively more concentrated.

We are currently isolating by suitable fractionation and analytical techniques the compounds responsible for mutagenic activity as a function of mode of cooking. It is hoped that these experiments will provide information on the nature of the materials so that they in turn can be tested for mutagenicity and carcinogenicity.

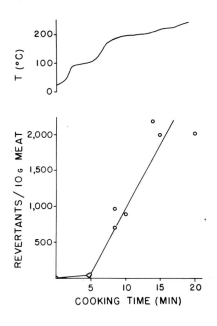

FIG. 3. Mutagenic activity in pan-fried beef as a function of temperature. A hamburger patty, 92 ± 3 g, was fried in an aluminum pan on a hot plate. The temperature was monitored by a thermocouple. Note rise in temperature to the boiling point of water without production of mutagens. When the surface water has boiled off, the temperature rises and mutagenic activity for *Salmonella typhimurium* TA 98 with liver S-9 fraction activation increases. The data are plotted as revertants per 10 g meat (42).

The structure of the mutagens to be outlined may stem not from the pyrolysis of amino acids or peptides but rather from the formation of heterocyclic compounds from starches and amino acids. Indeed, it was shown by Spingarn and Garvie (41) that when several kinds of simple sugars were refluxed with ammonium ions, mutagenic activity was obtained with mobilities, on high-pressure liquid chromatography systems, similar to those of mutagens obtained from

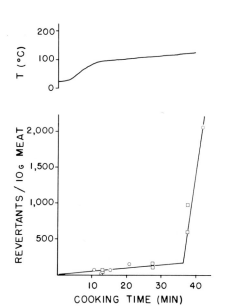

FIG. 4. Mutagenic activity in electric oven broiled *(circles)* or in charcoal broiled *(squares)* beef as a function of temperature. Note progressive rise in temperature with relatively little early development of mutagenic activity, followed by a sharp increase (42).

an extract of fried meat. Thus the reactions are akin to those which take place during the browning reactions.

Investigation of this system appears to be a sound lead. Indeed, as we have stated elsewhere (49,51), large bowel cancer has hardly increased over many decades, and we have noted that the conditions leading to large bowel cancer must have been in the human environment for decades, if not centuries. Whereas large bowel cancer has not increased much in the last 50 years, there was an apparent increase prior to that time. This may be due not to changing environmental conditions leading to the disease, but rather to improved means of diagnosis and record keeping. Another factor is no doubt the increase in longevity from the nineteenth to the twentieth century, which would be reflected in the statistics, since large bowel cancer is a disease presenting at an average age of 60.

Another specific factor, relevant on the basis of our data to large bowel cancer, but possibly not breast or prostate cancer, is the fact that during this century, many people ate bread and other cereals made with refined low-fiber flour, whereas in previous centuries, only the wealthy had access to white flour, and there were relatively few wealthy people. Thus most people ate food with more fiber and were perhaps at lower risk for this reason. Increasing the intake of fiber-containing bread or other cereals exerts a pronounced protective effect, as the data from Finland show clearly (20,31).

Bruce *(this volume),* Reddy at this Institute *(unpublished data),* and recently the group of T. Wilkins (13), have also demonstrated the occurrence of mutagenic activity in the stools of people at diverse risk for large bowel cancer. We have preliminary information that the mutagenic activity seen in the stools of people appears to be different from the mutagens found in fried meat. It may be that the mutagen in fried meat is metabolized with the production of materials present

TABLE 8. *Dietary intake of various nutrients and fecal excretion of various constituents in middle-aged male volunteers from Kuopio (Finland) and New York Metropolitan Area*

	Kuopio (15)	New York (40)
Dietary constituents	g/day	
Total protein	93 ± 4[a]	89 ± 2
Total fat	110 ± 4	115 ± 3
Saturated fat	59 ± 3	49 ± 2
Other fats	51 ± 3	66 ± 2
Carbohydrates	320 ± 4	285 ± 4
Total fiber	32 ± 3	14 ± 2
Fecal constituents		
Fresh feces excreted	277 ± 20	76 ± 12
Fiber	26 ± 2	9 ± 1
Fecal dry matter	61 ± 8	22 ± 1

[a] Averages $\pm$ SEM.
From Reddy et al. (31).

TABLE 9. *Current concepts on colon cancer causation and development*

Risk factors: Diets high in fat, cholesterol, fried foods, and low in fiber

Established mechanisms

High fat ―――→ High cholesterol biosynthesis ―――→ High gut bile acid levels
High dietary cholesterol ――↗

Low fiber ―――→ High concentration of gut bile acids
(low dilution through lack of bulk)

High bile acid concentration ―――――→ Promoting effect in colon carcinogenesis

Mechanisms under study

Fried food ―――→ Mutagens ―――――→ Colon carcinogens?

Role of micronutrients (vitamins and minerals) and different types of fiber in production and metabolism of carcinogens, bile acids, promoters?

Mechanisms of promotion?

in stool. On the other hand, it could also be that the fried meat mutagen does not appear in the stool at all and yet may affect the large bowel. We have some data demonstrating that the intestinal or fecal contents of animals given carcinogenic doses of the main colon carcinogens currently in use—specifically, 1,2-dimethylhydrazine or methylazoxymethanol and related compounds—are not mutagenic and do not contain appreciable amounts of those compounds or other metabolites. We have not yet tested whether the newly developed colon carcinogen in the rat, diketopropylnitrosamine (26), would lead to mutagenic activity in the intestinal contents. However, it seems already quite clear on the basis of experiments by Reddy with germ-free rats and other experiments, described above, involving surgical manipulation, that several kinds of carcinogens are active in the colon via the hematogenic route rather than by being present in the luminal contents of the gut. This does not mean that we need not continue the search for putative colon carcinogens in the stools. We need to be aware, though, that the carcinogens for colon cancer may reach the site via the blood. It is quite clear, however, that the promoting stimulus from bile acids plays an extraordinarily important role in large bowel cancer induction in man and in animals, and thus the luminal contents are important. In fact, they point to the possibility that the carcinogenic stimulus for large bowel cancer, although essential for initiation of the disease, is probably relatively weak, and therefore the concentration of the carcinogen is low and its total amount is small. This testifies to the difficulty of the task of finding and identifying these materials. Identical considerations are likely to appear in the search for carcinogens responsible for breast and prostate cancers, the other main nutritionally linked neoplasms.

We have not reviewed in this chapter moderating factors in this overall process which need consideration. These are micronutrients such as vitamins A, E, and C, or minerals such as selenium salts. These factors are considered in more detail elsewhere (29,38).

Current concepts suggest that the carcinogens for colon cancer may stem from the mode of cooking and, in particular, frying and broiling. The extent of the carcinogenic stress thus produced is probably rather weak. For that reason whether or not a given individual is at high risk for colon cancer may depend more on the rather important promoting stimulus from bile acids, themselves dependent on the amount of fat and cholesterol ingested. In this case fiber, and more specifically bran, has a protecting effect through dilution of the bile acids in presenting to the bowel mucosa a lower concentration of bile acids (Table 9).

ACKNOWLEDGMENTS

This investigation was supported in part by Contracts CP-33208 and CP-95604, and Grants CA-12376 and CA-17613, awarded by the National Cancer Institute, DHEW; and USPHS, National Cancer Institute Grants CA-15400,

CA-16382, and CA-24217, through the National Large Bowel Cancer Project. We are indebted to Mrs. C. Horn for editorial assistance and preparation of the manuscript.

REFERENCES

1. Armstrong, D., and Doll, R. (1975): Environmental factors and cancer incidence and mortality in different countries, with special reference to dietary practices. *Int. J. Cancer,* 15:617–631.
2. Asano, T., Pollard, M., and Madsen, D. C. (1975): Effects of cholestyramine on 1,2-dimethylhydrazine-induced enteric carcinoma in germfree rats. *Proc. Soc. Exp. Biol. Med.,* 150:780–785.
3. Bauer, H. G., Asp, N., Öste, R., Dahlqvist, A., and Fredlund, P. E. (1979): Effect of dietary fiber on the induction of colorectal tumors and fecal β-glucuronidase activity in the rat. *Cancer Res.,* 39:3752–3756.
4. Berg, J. W. (1975): Diet. In: *Persons at High Risk of Cancer,* edited by J. F. Fraumeni, Jr. (NCI), pp. 201–224. Academic Press, New York.
5. Berg, J. W. (1977): World-wide variations in cancer incidence as clues to cancer origins. In: *Origins of Human Cancer,* edited by H. H. Hiatt, J. D. Watson, and J. A. Winsten, pp. 15–19. Cold Spring Harbor Laboratory, Cold Spring Harbor, New York.
6. Berman, J. J., Rice, J. M., Wenk, M. L., and Roller, P. P. (1979): Dependence of tumor spectrum on route of administration in Sprague-Dawley rats as a result of single or multiple injections of methyl(acetoxymethyl)nitrosamine. *J. Natl. Cancer Inst.,* 63:93–100.
7. Bralow, S. P., and Weisburger, J. H. (1976): Experimental carcinogenesis. *Clin. Gastroenterol.,* 5:527–542.
8. Brockman, R. W., Shaddix, S. C., and Rose, L. M. (1977): Biochemical aspects of chemotherapy of mouse colon carcinoma: Fluoropyrimidines and pyrazofurin. *Cancer,* 40:2681–2691.
9. Bull, A. W., Soullier, B. K., Wilson, P. S., Hayden, M. T., and Nigro, N. D. (1979): The promotion of azoxymethane-induced intestinal cancer by high fat diet in rats. *Cancer Res.,* 39:4956–4959.
10. Commoner, B., Vithayathil, A. J., Dolara, P., Nair, S., Madyastha, P., and Cuca, G. C. (1978): Formation of mutagens in beef and beef extract during cooking. *Science,* 201:913–916.
11. Cruse, P., Lewin, M., and Clark, C. G. (1979): Dietary cholesterol is co-carcinogenic for human colon cancer. *Lancet,* i:752–755.
12. Cutler, S. J., and Young, J. L., Jr. (1975): Demographic patterns of cancer incidence in the United States. In: *Persons at High Risk of Cancer: An Approach to Cancer Etiology and Control,* edited by J. F. Fraumeni, Jr. (NCI), pp. 307–342. Academic Press, New York.
13. Ehrich, M., Aswell, J. E., Van Tassell, R. L., and Wilkins, T. D. (1979): Mutagens in the feces of 3 South-African populations at different levels of risk for colon cancer. *Mutat. Res.,* 64:231–240.
14. Finegold, S. M., Flora, D. J., Attebery, H. R., and Sutter, V. L. (1975): Fecal bacteriology of colonic polyp patients and control patients. *Cancer Res.,* 35:3407–3417.
15. Habs, M., Schmähl, D., and Wiessler, M. (1978): Carcinogencity of acetoxymethyl-methylnitrosamine after subcutaneous, intravenous and intrarectal applications in rats. *Z. Krebsforsch.,* 91:217–221.
16. Haenszel, W. (1975): Migrant studies. In: *Persons at High Risk of Cancer,* edited by J. F. Fraumeni, Jr. (NCI), pp. 361–372. Academic Press, New York.
17. Haenszel, W., Berg, J. W., Segi, M., Kurihara, M., and Locke, F. B. (1973): Large bowel cancer in Hawaiian Japanese. *J. Natl. Cancer Inst.,* 51:1765–1779.
18. Hentges, D. J., Maier, B. R., Burton, G. C., Flynn, M. A., and Tsutakawa, R. K. (1977): Effect of a high beef diet on the fecal bacterial flora of humans. *Cancer Res.,* 37:568–571.
19. Hill, M. J., Drasar, B. S., Williams, R. E. O., Meade, T. W., Cox, A. G., Simpson, J. E. P., and Morson, B. C. (1975): Faecal bile-acids and clostridia in patients with cancer of the large bowel. *Lancet,* i:535–538.
20. Jensen, O. M., and MacLennan, R. (1979): Dietary factors and colorectal cancer in Scandinavia. *Isr. J. Med. Sci.,* 15:329–334.
21. Kawachi, T., Nagao, M., Yahagi, T., Takahashi, Y., Mori, Y., Sugimura, T., and Takayama, S. (1979): Mutagens and carcinogens in food. In: *Proc. 12th International Cancer Congress.* Plenum Press, New York.

22. Narisawa, T., Reddy, B. S., and Weisburger, J. H. (1978): Effect of bile acids and dietary fat on large bowel carcinogenesis in animal models. *Gastroenterol. Jpn.,* 13(3):206–212.
23. Newberne, P. A., and Suphakarn, V. (1977): Preventive role of vitamin A in colon carcinogenesis in rats. *Cancer,* 40:2553–2556.
24. Oiso, T. (1975): Incidence of stomach cancer and its relation to dietary habits and nutrition in Japan between 1900 and 1975. *Cancer Res.,* 35:3254–3258.
25. Pariza, M. W., Ashoor, S. H., Chu, S. F., and Lund, D. B. (1979): Effects of temperature and time on mutagen formation in pan-fried hamburger. *Cancer Lett.,* 7:63–69.
26. Pour, P. (1978): A new and advantageous model for colorectal cancer. Its comparison with previous models for a common human disease. *Cancer Lett.,* 4:293–298.
27. Pratt, C. B., Rivera, G., Shanks, E., Johnson, W., Howarth, C., Terrell, W., and Kumar, A. P. M. (1977): Colorectal carcinoma in adolescents: Implications regarding etiology. *Cancer,* 40:2464–2472.
28. Raicht, R. F., Cohen, B. I., Fazzini, E., Sarwal, A., and Takahashi, M. (1980): Effect of cholic acid feeding on N-methyl-N-nitrosourea-induced colon tumors and cellular kinetics in rats. *J. Natl. Cancer Inst. (in press).*
29. Reddy, B. S. (1979): Nutrition and colon cancer, *Adv. Nutr. Res.,* 2:199–218.
30. Reddy, B. S., Cohen, L. A., McCoy, G. D., Hill, P., Weisburger, J. H., and Wynder, E. L. (1980): Nutrition and its relationship to cancer. *Adv. Cancer Res.,* 32:237–345.
31. Reddy, B. S., Hedges, A. R., Laakso, K., and Wynder, E. L. (1978): Metabolic epidemiology of large bowel cancer. *Cancer,* 42:2832–2838.
32. Reddy, B. S., Mangat, S., Scheinfeld, A., Weisburger, J. H., and Wynder, E. L. (1977): Effect of type and amount of dietary fat and 1,2-dimethylhydrazine on biliary bile acids, fecal bile acids, and neutral sterols in rats. *Cancer Res.,* 37:2132–2137.
33. Reddy, B. S., Narisawa, T., Vukusich, D., Weisburger, J. H., and Wynder, E. L. (1976): Effect of quality and quantity of dietary fat and dimethylhydrazine in colon carcinogenesis in rats. *Proc. Soc. Exp. Biol. Med.,* 151:237–239.
34. Reddy, B. S., Narisawa, T., and Weisburger, J. H. (1976): Effect of a diet with high levels of protein and fat on colon carcinogenesis in F344 rats treated with 1,2-dimethylhydrazine. *J. Natl. Cancer Inst.,* 57:567–569.
35. Reddy, B. S., and Watanabe, K. (1979): Effect of cholesterol metabolites and promoting effect of lithcholic acid in colon carcinogenesis in germfree and conventional F344 rats. *Cancer Res.,* 39:1521–1524.
36. Reddy, B. S., and Wynder, E. L. (1977): Metabolic epidemiology of colon cancer—Fecal bile acids and neutral sterols in colon cancer patients and patients with adenomatous polyps. *Cancer,* 39:2533–2539.
37. Schmähl, D., Danisman, A., Habs, M., and Diehl, B. (1979): Experimental investigation on the influence upon chemical carcinogenesis: 4th communication. *J. Cancer Res. Clin. Oncol.,* 93:57–66.
38. Schrauzer, G. N. (ed.) (1977): *Inorganic and Nutritional Aspects of Cancer.* Plenum Press, New York.
39. Selikoff, I. J., and Hammond, E. C. (1975): Multiple risk factors in environmental cancer. In: *Persons at High Risk of Cancer,* edited by J. F. Fraumeni (NCI), pp. 466–483. Academic Press, New York.
40. Selikoff, I. J., and Lee, D. (1978): *Asbestos and Disease.* Academic Press, New York.
41. Spingarn, N. E., and Garvie, C. T. (1979): Formation of mutagens in sugar-ammonia model systems. *J. Agric. Food,* 27:1319–1321.
42. Spingarn, N. E., and Weisburger, J. H. (1979): Formation of mutagens in cooked food. I. Beef. *Cancer Lett.,* 7:259–264.
43. Sugimura, T., Kawachi, T., Nagao, M., Takie, Y., Yuko, S., Toshihiko, O., Koichi, S., Takuo, K., Kuniro, T., Keiji, W., Yoichi, I., and Akiko, T. (1977): Mutagenic principles in tryptophan and phenylalanine pyrolysis products. *Proc. Jpn. Acad.,* 53:58.
44. Vobecky, J., Devroede, G., Lacaille, J., and Watier, A. (1978): An occupational group with a high risk of large bowel cancer. *Gastroenterol.,* 75:221–223.
45. Watanabe, K., Narisawa, T., Wong, C. Q., and Weisburger, J. H. (1978): Effect of bile acids and neutral sterols on benzo(*a*)pyrene-induced tumorigenesis in skin of mice. *J. Natl. Cancer Inst.,* 60:1501–1503.
46. Watanabe, K., Reddy, B. S., Wong, C. Q., and Weisburger, J. H. (1978): Effect of dietary

    undegraded carrageenan on colon carcinogenesis in F344 rats treated with azoxymethane or methylnitrosourea. *Cancer Res.,* 38:4427–4430.

47. Watanabe, K., Reddy, B. S., Weisburger, J. H., and Kritchevsky, D. (1979): Effect of dietary alfalfa, pectin and wheat bran on azoxymethane- or methylnitrosourea-induced colon carcinogenesis in F344 rats. *J. Natl. Cancer Inst.,* 63:141–145.
48. Weisburger, J. H. (1979): Mechanism of action of diet as a carcinogen. *Cancer,* 43:1987–1995.
49. Weisburger, J. H., Cohen, L. A., and Wynder, E. L. (1977): On the etiology and metabolic epidemiology of the main human cancer. In: *Origins of Human Cancer.* Cold Spring Harbor Laboratory, Cold Spring Harbor, New York.
50. Weisburger, J. H., Reddy, B. S., and Joftes, D. (eds.) (1975): Colo-rectal cancer. *UICC Technical Report Series, Vol. 19,* pp. 1–143. UICC, Geneva, Switzerland.
51. Weisburger, J. H., and Spingarn, N. E. (1979): Mutagens as a function of mode of cooking of meats. In: *Naturally Occurring Carcinogens-Mutagens and Modulators of Carcinogenesis,* edited by I. Hirono, E. C. Miller, J. A. Miller, T. A. Sugimura, and S. Takayama. University of Tokyo Press, Tokyo, and University Park Press, Baltimore.
52. Weisburger, J. H., and Williams, G. M. (1980): Chemical carcinogenesis. In: *Cancer Medicine, 2nd Ed.,* edited by J. F. Holland and E. Frei, III. Lea and Febiger, Philadelphia.
53. Wilkins, T. D., and Hackman, A. S. (1974): Two patterns of neutral steroid conversion in the feces of normal North Americans. *Cancer Res.,* 34:2250–2254.
54. Wilson, R. B., Hutcheson, D. P., and Wideman, L. (1977): Dimethylhydrazine-induced colon tumors in rats fed diets containing beef rat or corn oil with and without wheat bran. *Am. J. Clin. Nutr.,* 30:176–181.
55. Wittig, G., Wildner, G. P., and Ziebarth, D. (1971): Der Einfluss der Ingesta auf Kanzerisierung des Rattandarms durch Dimethylhydrazine. *Arch. Geschwulstforsch.,* 37:105.
56. Wynder, E. L. (1979): Dietary habits and cancer epidemiology. *Cancer,* 43:1955–1961.
57. Wynder, E. L., and Hirayama, T. (1977): Comparative epidemiology of cancers in the United States and Japan. *Prev. Med.,* 6:567–594.
58. Wynder, E. L., Kajitani, T., Ishikawa, S., Dodo, H., and Takano, A. (1969): Environmental factors of cancer of the colon and rectum. *Cancer,* 23:1210–1220.
59. Wynder, E. L., and Shigematsu, T. (1967): Environmental factors of cancer of the colon and rectum. *Cancer,* 20:1520–1561.

Colorectal Cancer: Prevention, Epidemiology,
and Screening, edited by S. Winawer, D. Schottenfeld,
and P. Sherlock. Raven Press, New York © 1980.

The Role of Diet and Intestinal Flora in the Etiology of Large Bowel Cancer

Barry Goldin

Department of Medicine, New England Medical Center Hospital,
Boston, Massachusetts 02111

Geographic variations in the incidence of large bowel cancer (1,3) indicate that environmental factors such as diet (3,10) are important in its etiology. A positive correlation has been demonstrated between the incidence of colon cancer and a high dietary intake of beef (8) and fat (24). In contrast, colon cancer incidence is inversely related to consumption of dietary fiber (11). Other dietary factors which have been implicated in the induction of intestinal tumors include nonnutritive substances in foods such as bacterial or fungal metabolites (13), food additives, nitrosamines and nitrosamides, and by-products arising from the frying or barbecueing of fish and meat (14). Although epidemiological studies do not provide definitive evidence for a particular food category, they do suggest strongly that diet plays a major role in the etiology of cancer.

There have been a number of explanations given for the effects of diet on the development of intestinal tumors. As cited above, it has been suggested that carcinogens may exist in food. Indirect effects of diet have also been cited as important in intestinal carcinogenesis (9). Diet can alter the metabolism of the intestinal microflora. An altered bacterial metabolic pattern can lead to either an increased or decreased conversion of procarcinogens to proximal carcinogens (5). The bacterial deactivation of procarcinogens or proximal carcinogens may also be changed by diet. In addition, specific dietary components may affect the levels of intestinal epithelial microsomal enzyme systems involved in the activation of carcinogens (21).

Several studies have shown that diet does influence enzyme activity of the intestinal microflora. Hill et al. (9) reported on an extensive study of intestinal bile acid metabolism among populations eating different diets. Fecal steroid metabolism and steroid concentrations were studied in the United States and Britain where the incidence of colon cancer is high, and in Uganda, Southern India, or Japan, where the incidence of this disease is low. Steroids were found in higher concentrations in the feces of Americans and British and the steroids were more extensively degraded. This observation was true for neutral sterols as well as bile acids. Neutral steroid reactions such as steroid 5-nuclear hydroge-

43

nase and 3-dehydrogenase were elevated in the groups with a high risk of colon cancer.

The bile acid-converting enzymes that were elevated in the Western populations included cholanylhydrolase, which deconjugates bile salts, and 7α-steroid dehydroxylase, which removes 7α-hydroxyl groups from cholic acid and chenodeoxycholic acid, giving deoxycholic acid and lithocholic acid, respectively.

The secondary bile acids derived from the action of these two enzymes may be important in the etiology of large bowel cancer. Investigators have found that secondary bile acids act as promoters in enhancing tumor induction in the presence of a carcinogen (15,18) and are co-mutagenic in a bacterial tester system (20).

Reddy and Wynder (19) compared bile acid and steroid levels in the feces of Americans on a mixed Western diet, American vegetarians, American Seventh Day Adventists (Western diet low in meat and animal fat), Japanese (Japanese diet), and Chinese (Chinese diet). The daily excretion of coprostanol and coprostanone (microbially degraded products of cholesterol) and total neutral sterols was higher in Americans eating a mixed diet than in other groups: these subjects had less than 5% of the total fecal sterols in the form of cholesterol and more than 90% as coprostanol and coprostanone. The other subjects in this study including vegetarians and individuals on conventional Asian diets had more than 30% of their fecal sterols in the form of cholesterol. Americans who ate a Western-type diet excreted higher levels of bile acids and microbially degraded bile acids than did others.

Mastromarino et al. (12) have observed that patients with adenomatous polyps and colorectal cancer have a significantly higher level of 7α-dehydroxylase and cholesterol dehydrogenase activity in their fecal bacteria.

In our laboratory, experiments using animals and volunteers have been performed, and are currently in progress, to further elucidate the relationship among diet, the metabolic activity of the intestinal flora, and the induction of colon cancer (4–7).

Bacterial enzymes have been used as markers to monitor the effect of diet on the intestinal microflora's ability to convert procarcinogens into proximal carcinogens. Bacterial β-glucuronidase activity has been measured because the enzyme has a wide substrate specificity and, consequently, can hydrolyze a large number of different glucuronides. These reactions are potentially important in the generation of toxic and carcinogenic substances inasmuch as many compounds are detoxified by glucuronide formation in the liver and subsequently enter the bowel via the bile. In this manner, toxic compounds can be regenerated in the bowel by bacterial β-glucuronidase. The hydrolytic reaction is predominantly carried out by bacteria rather than intestinal tissue β-glucuronidase because the pH optimum for the mammalian enzyme is 4.5 and is virtually inactive at the neutral pH in the lumen of the bowel. The bacterial enzyme has a pH optimum of 6.8.

The levels of fecal β-glucuronidase have been measured in rats fed a diet high in grain content and low in animal fat and meat protein and in the same animals after being shifted to a diet containing 70% hamburger by weight (5). There was a rapid and highly significant increase in fecal β-glucuronidase activity after the changeover to a beef diet. It required between 2 and 3 weeks after being placed on the new diet to reach optimum activity. A similar experiment was done measuring the fecal enzyme activity of nitroreductase and azoreductase. The enzyme levels also significantly increased in the meat-fed rats 15–20 days after the dietary shift (Table 1). The importance of this finding derives from the ability of nitroreductase and azoreductase to generate aromatic amines from the corresponding nitro and azo compounds. The end-product amines, as well as the highly reactive intermediates, are well-known mutagens and carcinogens. Studies with germfree rats indicate that bacteria are largely responsible for these reduction reactions in the host (16,23). Azoreductase can reduce food dyes (17) which cause the release of phenyl- and naphthyl-substituted amines. These compounds have been implicated as chemical carcinogens (22). Nitroreductase causes the formation of reactive nitroso and N-hydroxy intermediates in the course of converting aromatic nitro compounds to amines (2). The precursor aromatic nitro compounds are found in factory effluents as industrial chemical pollutants.

Studies conducted in our laboratory on human populations have revealed that American vegetarians have significantly lower fecal β-glucuronidase and nitroreductase activity when compared to omnivores (Table 2). Two groups of vegetarians were studied. The vegans or very strict vegetarians also had lower azoreductase activity (Table 2). The lactovegetarians, subjects eating butter and other dairy products, had decreased azoreductase activity but the difference was not statistically significant. As previously noted, the lactovegetarians also had lower activity of steroid-7α-dehydroxylase, an enzyme that converts primary to secondary bile acids. The levels of this enzyme were not measured in our vegetarian subjects.

The addition of a 30 g fiber supplement to a standard Western diet did not significantly reduce fecal β-glucuronidase, nitroreductase, or azoreductase activity (Table 3) (7). The fiber supplement did cause a reduction in steroid-7α-dehydroxylase activity. It is possible that the bile acid sequestering ability of fiber may be responsible for lowering the free substrate concentration for the dehydroxylase, subsequently causing a drop in enzyme activity.

TABLE 1. *Effect of diet on fecal bacterial enzyme activity in rats*

Diet	β-Glucuronidase	Nitroreductase	Azoreductase
Grain	2.41 ± 0.28[a]	3.63 ± 0.37	4.65 ± 0.62
Meat	6.05 ± 0.43	7.24 ± 0.49	9.68 ± 1.15

[a] Mean $\pm$ SE (units/mg fecal protein)—see Table 3. Enzymes significantly higher on meat diet ($p < 0.001$).

TABLE 2. *Effect of diet on fecal enzyme activity in omnivors, lactovegetarians, and vegan vegetarians*

Diet group	β-Glucuronidase	Nitroreductase	Azoreductase	7 α-Dehydroxylase
I. Omnivore (N = 15)	1.79 ± 0.18	6.03 ± 0.56	3.70 ± 0.27	1.30 ± 0.17
II. Lactovegetarian (N = 13)	0.93 ± 0.9[a]	3.57 ± 0.16[b]	3.28 ± 0.23	0.50 ± 0.11[d]
III. Vegan vegetarian (N = 7)	1.07 ± 0.12[a]	3.94 ± 0.39	2.59 ± 0.13[c]	N.D.
IV. Omnivore—L. acidophilus supplement (N = 7)	1.11 ± 0.11[a]	4.39 ± 0.09[c]	2.90 ± 0.25	N.D.

Mean ± SE; enzyme units see Table 3.
[a] β-Glucuronidase significantly different at $p < 0.001$ (I vs. II) and $p < 0.01$ (I vs. III or IV).
[b] Nitroreductase significantly different at $p < 0.01$ (I vs. II) and $p < 0.05$ (I vs. III or IV).
[c] Azoreductase significantly different at $p < 0.01$ (I vs. III). Azoreductase not significantly different I vs. II or IV.
[d] Steroid 7 α-Dehydroxylase significantly different at $p < 0.02$ (I vs. II).
N.D., not determined.

TABLE 3. *Effect of dietary fiber supplements on fecal enzyme activities among 9 omnivore subjects*

Status	β-Glucuronidase	Nitroreductase	Azoreductase	7α-Dehydroxylase
Baseline (N = 9)	2.32 ± 0.21	4.90 ± 0.32	3.97 ± 0.34	0.83 ± 0.08
Fiber supp.[a] (N = 9)	2.20 ± 0.19	4.91 ± 0.49	3.29 ± 0.31	0.45 ± 0.09[b]
Wheat germ (N = 5)	2.31 ± 0.19	5.02 ± 0.66	3.74 ± 0.24	0.49 ± 0.09
Bran (N = 4)	2.07 ± 0.16	4.77 ± 0.58	2.71 ± 0.51	0.40 ± 0.11

Mean ± SE. Units: μg product formed/hr/mg fecal protein; β-glucuronidase—μg product formed/min/mg fecal protein.
[a] Combined results for subjects taking wheat germ or bran.
[b] Significantly different from baseline; $p < 0.05$.

TABLE 4. *Effect of shifting to a non-red meat diet on fecal enzyme activity among 15 omnivore subjects*

Status	β-Glucuronidase	Nitroreductase	Azoreductase	7α-Dehydroxylase
Baseline I	1.79 ± 0.18	6.03 ± 0.56	3.71 ± 0.27	1.30 ± 0.17
Non-red meat	1.37 ± 0.16	4.75 ± 0.55	3.36 ± 0.33	0.41 ± 0.16[a]
Baseline II	1.43 ± 0.11	4.62 ± 0.39	3.24 ± 0.26	0.95 ± 0.46

Mean $\pm$ SE; $N = 15$; units: see Table 2.

[a] 7α-Dehydroxylase is significantly lower ($p < 0.02$). β-Glucuronidase, nitroreductase, and azoreductase are not significantly different.

The elimination of red meat from the diet for 30 days similarly had no effect on fecal bacterial enzyme activities, with the exception of 7α-dehydroxylase activity (Table 4) (7). These studies indicate that major long-term changes in diet are required to have an effect on the metabolism of bacterial flora.

Using another approach to achieve a rapid change in bacterial enzyme activity, investigators gave *Lactobacillus acidophilus* supplements to animals and human subjects (6,7). The bacterial supplements were added in high concentrations (10^{10}) daily to the diet. The vials containing the Lactobacillus were stored at $-80°C$, and the preparations were never refrozen and used a second time. Table 5 shows the effect of the Lactobacillus supplement on rat fecal enzyme activities. The animals were maintained on a high meat diet (70% hamburger). The bacterial supplements caused a decrease in the three fecal enzymes assayed. Feeding supplements for 2 to 3 weeks were sufficient to cause the maximum result.

In Fig. 1, the effect of the addition of *Lactobacillus acidophilus* supplements on human fecal bacterial enzyme activity is shown. In a 4-week period prior to the addition of the supplement, baseline enzyme values were obtained by collecting and assaying fecal specimens weekly (baseline I). The bacterial supplement was administered at the beginning of the second month of the study and assays were again performed each week. The supplement was then removed from the diet and the fecal enzyme activities of the subjects were measured for an additional month (baseline II).

The seven omnivores fed viable *L. acidophilus* for 1 month had a significantly reduced fecal β-glucuronidase and nitroreductase activity (Fig. 1). After the

TABLE 5. *Effect of* L. acidophilus *supplements on fecal β-glucuronidase, nitroreductase, and azoreductase activities*

Group	β-Glucuronidase	Nitroreductase	Azoreductase
Beef-fed rats	9.36 ± 1.04[a]	8.23 ± 1.43	9.97 ± 2.04
Beef-fed rats plus *L. acidophilus*	6.08 ± 1.12	4.28 ± 0.84	4.16 ± 1.32

Mean values $\pm$ SE. Ten rats in each group.

[a] β-Glucuronidase, nitroreductase, and azoreductase significantly lower at $p < 0.05$.

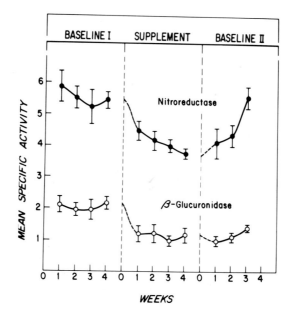

FIG. 1. Mean fecal nitroreductase and β-glucuronidase activities for 7 subjects are shown prior to, during, and after *L. acidophilus* feeding.

lactobacilli supplements were discontinued (baseline II), fecal enzymatic activities showed a progressive increase in activity. An analysis of variance done on the last 2 weeks of the supplement period and last 2 weeks of baseline II revealed a significant rise in β-glucuronidase activity ($p < 0.05$) and an increase in nitroreductase activity ($p = 0.06$). It is likely from these data that sampling during subsequent weeks would have shown a complete return to baseline I levels. The lactobacillus experiment indicates that rapid perturbation in human intestinal microflora metabolism is possible; however, the microflora appear to return to their normal state after removal of the perturbant.

CONCLUSIONS

There is a growing body of experimental evidence suggesting that diet can alter the metabolic activity of the microflora in the large bowel. The altered microbial metabolism, in turn, can affect the concentration of proximal and ultimate carcinogens in the large bowel. In this chapter the effects of diet on the chemical induction of large bowel tumors in animals were reviewed. These data tend to further confirm the concept that high fat, high animal protein, and low fiber diets are more conducive to the induction of large bowel tumors. The mechanism involved in this increased tumorigenesis is not known; however, the intestinal microflora may also be important in potentiating the action of exogenously administered chemical carcinogens.

The evidence for a relationship between diet, microbial metabolism, and carcinogenesis is neither direct nor definitive, it is only suggestive. The mechanisms by which diet influences carcinogenesis are complex, involving changes in tissue enzyme level, concentrations of endogenous substances, and the biochemical metabolism of the animal. In addition to these factors, the metabolic activity of the intestinal flora must be taken into account when evaluating the causes of large bowel cancer.

REFERENCES

1. Armstrong, B., and Doll, R. (1975): Environmental factors and cancer incidence and mortality in different countries with special reference to dietary factors. *Int. J. Cancer,* 15:617–631.
2. Billette, J. R., Kamm, J. J., and Sasame, H. A. (1968): Mechanisms of P-nitrobenzoate reduction in liver: The possible role of cytochrome P-450 in liver microsomes. *Mod. Pharmacol.,* 4:541–548.
3. Drasar, B. S., and Irving, D. (1973): Environmental factors and cancer of the colon and breast. *Br. J. Cancer,* 27:167–172.
4. Goldin, B. R., Dwyer, J., Gorbach, S. L., Gordon, W., and Swenson, L. (1978): Influence of diet and age on fecal bacterial enzymes. *Am. J. Clin. Nutr.,* 31:S136–S140.
5. Goldin, B. R., and Gorbach, S. L. (1976): The relationship between diet and rat fecal bacterial enzymes implicated in colon cancer. *J. Natl. Cancer Inst.,* 57:371–375.
6. Goldin, B. R., and Gorbach, S. L. (1977): Alterations in fecal microflora enzymes related to diet, age, lactobacillus supplements, and dimethylhydrazine. *Cancer,* 40:2421–2426.
7. Goldin, B. R., Swenson, L., Dwyer, J., Sexton, M., and Gorbach, S. L. (1979): Effect of diet and lactobacillus supplements on human fecal bacterial enzymes. *J. Natl. Cancer Inst. (in press).*
8. Haenszel, W., Berg, J. W., Segi, J., Kurihara, M., and Locke, P. B. (1973): Large-bowel cancer in Hawaiian Japanese. *J. Natl. Cancer Inst.,* 51:1765–1779.
9. Hill, M. S., Draser, B. S., and Aries, V. (1971): Bacteria and etiology of cancer of the large bowel. *Lancet,* 1:95–100.
10. Howell, M. A. (1975): Diet and etiological factors in the development of cancer of the colon and rectum. *J. Chronic Dis.,* 28:67–80.
11. Irving, D., and Drasar, B. S. (1973): Fibre and cancer of the colon. *Br. J. Cancer,* 28:462–463.
12. Mastromarino, A., Reddy, B. S., and Wynder, E. L. (1976): Metabolic epidemiology of colon cancer: Enzyme activity of fecal flora. *Am. J. Clin. Nutr.,* 29:1455–1460.
13. Miller, J. A., and Miller, E. C. (1976): Carcinogens occurring naturally in foods. *Fed. Proc.,* 35:1316–1321.
14. Nagao, M., Honda, M., Seino, Y., Yahazi, R., and Sugimura, R. (1977): Mutagenicities of smoke condensates and the charred surface of fish and meat. *Cancer Lett.,* 2:221–226.
15. Narisawa, T., Magodia, N. E., Weisburger, J. N., and Wynder E. L. (1974): Promoting effect of bile acids on colon carcinogenesis after intrarectal installation of N-methyl-N'-nitro-N-nitrosoguanidine in rats. *J. Natl. Cancer Inst.,* 55:1093–1097.
16. Peppercorn, M. A., and Goldman, P. (1972): The role of intestinal bacteria in the metabolism of salicylazosulfapyridine. *J. Exp. Pharmacol.,* 181:555–562.
17. Radomski, J. L., and Mellinger, T. J. (1962): The absorption and rates of excretion in rats of the water-soluble azo dyes. *J. Pharmacol. Exp. Ther.,* 136:259–266.
18. Reddy, B. S., Watanabe, K., Weisburger, J. H., and Wynder, E. L. (1977): Promoting effect of bile acids in colon carcinogenesis in germ-free and conventional F344 rats. *Cancer Res.,* 37:3238–3242.
19. Reddy, B. S., and Wynder, E. L. (1973): Large-bowel carcinogenesis: Fecal constituents of populations with diverse incidence rates of colon cancer. *J. Natl. Cancer Inst.,* 50:1437–1442.
20. Silverman, S. J., and Andrews, A. W. (1977): Bile acids: Co-mutagenic activity in the Salmonella-mammalian-microsome mutagenesis test. *J. Natl. Cancer Inst.,* 59:1557–1559.
21. Wattenberg, L. W. (1971): Studies of polycyclic hydrocarbon hydroxylases of the intestine possibly related to cancer. *Cancer,* 28:99–102.

22. Weisburger, J. J., and Weisburger, E. W. (1973): Biochemical formation and pharmacological, toxicological, and pathological properties of hydroxylamines and hydroxamine acids. *Pharmacol. Rev.,* 25:1–66.
23. Wheeler, L. A., Soderberg, F., and Goldman, P. (1975): The *in vivo* reduction of compounds containing the nitro group: Its relation to the character of the intestinal microflora. *Fed. Proc.,* 34:2959.
24. Wynder, E. L., and Reddy, B. S. (1975): Dietary fat and colon cancer. *J. Natl. Cancer Inst.,* 54:7–10.

Colorectal Cancer: Prevention, Epidemiology, and Screening, edited by S. Winawer, D. Schottenfeld, and P. Sherlock. Raven Press, New York © 1980.

Studies of Factors Relevant to Human Colorectal Carcinogenesis in Animal Models

Morris S. Zedeck

Memorial Sloan-Kettering Cancer Center, New York, New York 10021

The study of colon carcinogenesis was greatly enhanced with the introduction of several compounds having marked potency and selectivity for induction of colon tumors in laboratory animals. Single or relatively few doses of methylazoxymethanol (MAM) acetate, dimethylhydrazine (DMH) or azoxymethane (AOM) can induce large numbers of colon tumors in most of the treated animals in a relatively short period of time.

In 1965, Laqueur (25) reported on the carcinogenicity of MAM and of cycasin, methylazoxymethanol-β-D-glucoside. Cycasin, found in Cycad plants, has no effect when given parenterally or when given orally to germ free rats. This is because the intestinal flora are required to cleave the glucoside moiety of cycasin and liberate MAM; the aglycone MAM can induce tumors by any route of administration (26). MAM degrades spontaneously and the synthesis of MAM acetate (28) provides a form of the carcinogen that is stable and effective parenterally. These findings prompted Druckrey (13) to study the carcinogenic activities of dialkylhydrazines and azo- and azoxyalkanes, and these studies led to the development of DMH and AOM. These two agents can be administered either orally or parenterally and both are metabolized in the liver to MAM (see Fiala et al., 15). Many animal model systems using MAM, DMH, and AOM for study of colon carcinogenesis have been cited (46), and the literature pertinent to the field of experimental colon carcinogenesis has been reviewed (43).

The distribution of the intestinal tumors induced in animals and the histological characteristics of the tumors are similar to that found in humans. In the small intestine, the tumors are generally found within the duodenum and, in the large intestine, they occur mostly in the distal two-thirds of the colon. These animal systems serve as excellent models for the study of colon cancer and have been found useful for study of the many factors that may play a role in the induction and in the prevention of colon tumors.

Numerous studies of the etiology of human colon cancer have led investigators to strongly suggest dietary animal and vegetable fat as agents playing a role in the causation of this disease. The modifying effects of vegetable fiber content, the colonic flora, and fecal bile acids have also been studied. Much of the

51

early work has been published in *Cancer Research,* Vol. 35, No. 11, Part 2: Nutrition in the Causation of Cancer (1975). More recently, there are interesting results related to the preventive effects of trace elements. This review will summarize the studies pertinent to each of these modifying factors in an attempt to present a clearer understanding of the processes involved in colon tumorigenesis.

Prior to beginning this review, it might be of value to understand the mechanism that accounts for the marked organotropism exhibited by the carcinogens discussed above.

ORGANOTROPY OF COLON CARCINOGENS

Since MAM degrades spontaneously to liberate an alkylating moiety (30), the organotropism exhibited by this carcinogen is surprising. Gennaro et al. (19) have shown that segments of colon transposed to mid-small intestine develop tumors following treatment of rats with AOM, whereas in the same animals segments of small intestine transposed to the colon are not affected. Such results suggest that the colon is inherently more sensitive to the tumor-inducing effects of these agents than is the small intestine.

We supposed that the differences observed could be due to selective enhancement of the metabolism of these agents to their ultimate reactive form. In this regard, Schoental (37) had suggested that MAM, the product of DMH and AOM metabolism, might be further metabolized by alcohol dehydrogenase to the aldehydic derivative. We found that the NAD^+-dependent alcohol dehydrogenase activity of $169,000 \times g$ supernatant fractions of rat tissues was highest in colon, duodenum, and cecum, with little activity in jejunum and ileum. We also found that MAM, like ethanol, can act as substrate in NAD^+-dependent reactions and, under certain conditions, MAM, unlike ethanol, was also substrate for $NADP^+$-dependent reactions (20). The data suggest that NAD^+- and $NADP^+$-dependent enzymatic reactions may, in part, be responsible for the organ-specific effects of MAM.

When pyrazole, an inhibitor of NAD^+-dependent alcohol dehydrogenase, was given to rats 2 hr prior to their receiving carcinogen, the rats were prevented from the MAM-induced acute toxicity (20). On the other hand, the acute biologic effects of the carcinogen were potentiated in animals pretreated with disulfiram, an inhibitor of aldehyde dehydrogenase (12), suggesting that the biologically active metabolite of MAM is the corresponding aldehyde formed via metabolism by NAD^+-dependent dehydrogenases (44). Preliminary data (47) indicate that rats given pyrazole prior to MAM acetate do not develop intestinal tumors. It appears that the selective effects of MAM on colonic and duodenal tissue are due to the presence in these intestinal segments of NAD^+-dependent dehydrogenase enzymes able to metabolize MAM to its aldehydic derivative; such enzyme activity is absent in organs resistant to the effects of these carcinogens. It remains to be determined whether human colon has similar enzymatic activity and how the aldehydic derivative interacts with and alters a normal cell to become cancerous.

DIETARY FAT

There are a number of studies indicating that the incidence of colon cancer in a given country is related to the amount of animal fat consumed by that population (10). Many studies have been performed in both animals and humans to test the hypothesis that diets rich in animal fat play a role in colon carcinogenesis and in tumorigenesis in general (22). The hypothesis related to colon carcinogenesis states that a diet rich in fat results in an enhanced excretion of bile into the intestinal lumen which can then be acted on by intestinal flora to form carcinogens or other agents playing a role in the carcinogenic process.

To evaluate this proposal properly, we must consider that there are two steps in carcinogenesis, an initiation step in which the carcinogen has interacted with and, in some way, altered the cell, and a promotional step where the cell is now stimulated to replicate its genetic material and divide, at which time it has the opportunity to translate the previously induced alteration into abnormalities which can be expressed. This two-stage mechanism was first described by Berenblum (4) studying mouse skin carcinogenesis.

Results from animal studies clearly indicate that tumor initiation is not dependent on the presence of either bile acids or intestinal bacteria. Induction of colon tumors in germ-free rats is possible with MAM (26) and with DMH (1,33,35); although less effective than in conventional rats, MAM and DMH are still carcinogenic. Also, MAM, AOM, and DMH can induce tumors in that portion of the colon remaining after colostomy (8,27,42), even though there is no bile-containing fecal stream in contact with the colonic epithelium. The fact that these carcinogens are active under these conditions also suggests that their excretion in bile and their subsequent modification by the intestinal flora do not play a significant role in colon carcinogenesis.

The role of bile acids in promotion of tumor development has also been investigated, and methods that result in greater flow of bile through the colon increase the incidence of tumors in carcinogen-treated rats (9). Studies by Asano et al. (2) indicate that this promoting activity is due to the biliary substances themselves rather than to bacterial products of these materials since cholestyramine administration enhanced tumor incidence in DMH-treated germ free animals.

There are several reports of the increase in tumor incidence in carcinogen-treated rats given a diet rich in animal fat (31,34), and these results support the epidemiological findings (10,24). There are some reports, however, of an enhanced tumor incidence in rats given diets containing large amounts of vegetable fat (32). These data suggested a re-evaluation of the role of vegetable fats, and recently Enig et al. (14) have reviewed the evidence and present striking arguments for a role of vegetable *trans*-fatty acid components. Interestingly, the use of vegetable fat has risen considerably since 1909 while animal fat consumption remains constant. The authors carefully review the amount of vegetable saturated fats consumed per year and reconsider the incidence of colon cancer in countries using high and low amounts of dietary fat. They present an interesting case for reconsidering the roles of beef and vegetable fat in colon tumorigenesis. Reddy et al. (32) have shown that feeding high fat diets to animals increases the amount of total bile acid excreted and that there was no difference between diets containing 20% corn oil or lard.

To summarize the role of fats and bile acids, it appears that both dietary animal and vegetable fat increase tumor incidence, increase the excretion of total bile acids, and that some component of bile acid metabolism—other than that involving the bacterial flora and secondary bile acids—may play a role in promoting colon tumor development, and thus in the total incidence of colon cancer. The precise mechanism, however, remains to be determined.

DIETARY FIBER

The amount of fiber consumed in the diet has been implicated as having a role in the incidence of colon cancer. Burkitt (6,7) suggested that diets rich in fiber would shorten fecal transit time and reduce contact between the intestinal mucosa and carcinogens in the feces. The available epidemiologic data indicate that, in populations consuming large amounts of fiber, the fecal transit time is short and the incidence of colon cancer in these populations is lower than in groups of people consuming less fiber (29).

The effect of fiber-rich diets on colon tumor induction in experimental animals was studied. Rats given diets containing about 20% bran (3,17,41) or 4.5% cellulose (18) had significantly fewer colon tumors after being treated with DMH than did rats on a control diet. The groups receiving bran excreted greater amounts of feces and the fecal transit times were decreased relative to control groups.

Whether the tumor-inhibitory effect of diets rich in fiber is, in fact, due to an effect on fecal transit time and dilution of carcinogen is uncertain. Fiber is a complex mixture of substances, each varying in amounts in different cereals, vegetables, and fruits, and the extent of bacterial fermentation of the fiber within the colon depends on the composition of the material ingested (40). Rubio et al. (36) have reported that lignin can interact with and adsorb nitrosamines. They also suggest that lignin may exert its protective effects via its antioxidant properties. Since lignin content varies in different plant sources, the protective effect of dietary fiber may be dependent on the amount of lignin within the fiber consumed.

The role of fiber in inhibiting colon tumor development and its mechanism of action are worthy of further research. There are numerous reports indicating that colon carcinogens exert their effects on colonic epithelium via the circulation rather than by contact in the lumen, either from oral ingestion of carcinogen or following its excretion via the bile (16,21,45). Although it is possible that fiber-containing diets can prevent carcinogens from being absorbed in the intestine, it is unlikely that this is the mechanism for inhibition of tumorigenesis. There are two observations that suggest that fiber specifically inhibits colon tumor development by some other, albeit unexplained, mechanism. First, the incidence of duodenal tumors was not affected in animals whose incidence of colon tumors was decreased, and, second, in two studies (17,18) the DMH was given parenterally and could not have interacted with the fiber. Perhaps the fiber alters the promotional events in colon tumorigenesis rather than affecting the initiation reactions between carcinogen and cell.

SELENIUM

Results from a number of studies indicate that selenium can reduce the incidence of tumors in experimental animals; this effect was observed for spontaneous tumors as well as for those induced by chemicals (see ref. 23). In addition, there are several studies of the relationship between levels of selenium in human serum and the incidence of tumors (5,38), and it appears that in cancer patients, the serum level of selenium is lower than in non-cancer patients. The level of selenium in forage crops was determined for each state and the level was related to the human cancer mortality (39). The group of states in which the level of selenium in the crop was lower than in the other states had a higher rate of mortality from cancer. Analyses of the cancer death rate by site and sex in these states with varying levels of selenium in the crops indicated that there is an inverse relationship between the level of selenium and the incidence of gastrointestinal cancer, especially in males (39).

The effect of dietary selenium on the incidence of colon cancer in rats was studied by Jacobs et al. (23), and they found that selenium markedly reduced the incidence of tumors induced by DMH. Although the inhibitory effects were also observed against tumorigenesis induced by MAM, the effects were not as marked as against DMH. Daoud and Griffin (11) have found that selenium inhibits enzymes necessary for activation of acetylaminofluorene, and it is possible that alterations of those enzymes necessary for conversion of DMH to MAM are also inhibited. Clearly, additional studies of the inhibitory effects of selenium on colon carcinogenesis and on tumorigenesis in general are needed.

ACKNOWLEDGMENTS

The studies described herein that were conducted in the Laboratory of Pharmacology at Memorial Sloan-Kettering Cancer Center were supported in part by Public Health Service Grants CA 08748 from the National Cancer Institute and CA 15637 from the National Cancer Institute through the National Large Bowel Cancer Project.

REFERENCES

1. Asano, T., and Pollard, M. (1978): Strain susceptibility and resistance to 1,2-dimethylhydrazine-induced enteric tumors in germfree rats. *Proc. Soc. Exp. Biol. Med.,* 158:89–91.
2. Asano, T., Pollard, M., and Madsen, D. C. (1975): Effects of cholestyramine on 1,2-dimethylhydrazine-induced enteric carcinoma in germfree rats. *Proc. Soc. Exp. Biol. Med.,* 150:780–785.
3. Barbolt, T. A., and Abraham, R. (1978): The effect of bran on dimethylhydrazine-induced colon carcinogenesis in the rat. *Proc. Soc. Exp. Biol. Med.,* 157:656–659.
4. Berenblum, I. (1941): The mechanism of cocarcinogenesis: A study of significance of cocarcinogenic action and related phenomena. *Cancer Res.,* 1:807–814.
5. Broghamer, W. L., Jr., McConnell, K. P., and Blotcky, A. L. (1976): Relationship between serum selenium levels and patients with carcinoma. *Cancer,* 37:1384–1388.
6. Burkitt, D. P. (1971): Epidemiology of cancer of the colon and rectum. *Cancer,* 28:3–13.
7. Burkitt, D. P. (1978): The link between low-fiber diets and disease. *Human Nature,* 1(12):34–41.
8. Campbell, A. L., Singh, D. V., and Nigro, N. D. (1975): Importance of the fecal stream on the induction of colon tumors by azoxymethane in rats. *Cancer Res.,* 35:1369–1371.
9. Chomchai, C., Bhadrachari, N., and Nigro, N. D. (1974): The effect of bile on the induction of experimental intestinal tumors in rats. *Dis. Colon Rectum,* 17:310–312.
10. Correa, P., and Haenszel, W. (1978): The epidemiology of large-bowel cancer. *Adv. Cancer Res.,* 26:1–141.
11. Daoud, A. H., and Griffin, A. C. (1978): Effects of selenium and retinoic acid on the metabolism of N-acetylaminofluorene and N-hydroxyacetylaminofluorene. *Cancer Lett.,* 5:231–237.
12. Deitrich, R. A., and Hellerman, L. (1963): Diphosphopyridine nucleotide-linked aldehyde dehydrogenase. II. Inhibitors. *J. Biol. Chem.,* 238:1683–1689.
13. Druckrey, H. (1970): Production of colonic carcinomas by 1,2-dialkylhydrazines and azoxyalkanes. In: *Carcinoma of the Colon and Antecedent Epithelium,* edited by W. J. Burdette, pp. 267–279. Charles C Thomas, Springfield, Ill.
14. Enig, M. G., Munn, R. J., and Keeney, M. (1978): Dietary fat and cancer trends—A critique. *Fed. Proc.,* 37:2215–2220.
15. Fiala, E. S., Bobotas, G., Kulakis, C., Wattenberg, L. W., and Weisburger, J. H. (1977): Effects of disulfiram and related compounds in the metabolism *in vivo* of the colon carcinogen, 1,2-dimethylhydrazine. *Biochem. Pharmacol.,* 26:1763–1768.
16. Fiala, E. S., and Weisburger, J. H. (1975): On the metabolism of the carcinogen 1,2-dimethylhydrazine in rats. *Toxicol. Appl. Pharmacol.,* 33:178 (abst.).
17. Fleiszer, D., MacFarlane, J., Murray, D., and Brown, R. A. (1978): Protective effect of dietary fibre against chemically induced bowel tumours in rats. *Lancet,* 2:552–553.
18. Freeman, H. J., Spiller, G. A., and Kim, Y. S. (1978): A double-blind study on the effect of purified cellulose dietary fiber on 1,2-dimethylhydrazine-induced rat colonic neoplasia. *Cancer Res.,* 38:2912–2917.
19. Gennaro, A. R., Villanueva, R., Sukonthaman, Y., Vanthanophas, V., and Rosemond, G. P. (1973): Chemical carcinogenesis in transposed intestinal segments. *Cancer Res.,* 33:536–541.
20. Grab, D. J., and Zedeck, M. S. (1977): Organ-specific effects of the carcinogen methylazoxymethanol related to metabolism by nicotinamide adenine dinucleotide-dependent dehydrogenases. *Cancer Res.,* 37:4182–4190.
21. Hawks, A., and Magee, P. N. (1974): The alkylation of nucleic acids of rat and mouse *in vivo* by the carcinogen 1,2-dimethylhydrazine. *Br. J. Cancer,* 30:440–447.
22. Hopkins, G. J., and West, C. E. (1976): Possible roles of dietary fats in carcinogenesis. *Life Sci.,* 19:1103–1116.
23. Jacobs, M. M., Jansson, B., and Griffin, A. C. (1977): Inhibitory effects of selenium on 1,2-dimethylhydrazine and methylazoxymethanol acetate induction of colon tumors. *Cancer Lett.,* 2:133–138.
24. Kassira, E., Parent, L., and Vahouny, G. (1976): Colon cancer. An epidemiological survey. *Am. J. Dig. Dis.,* 21:205–214.
25. Laqueur, G. L. (1965): The induction of intestinal neoplasms in rats with the glycoside cycasin and its aglycone. *Virchows Arch. Pathol. Anat.,* 340:151–163.
26. Laqueur, G. L., McDaniel, E. G., and Matsumoto, H. (1967): Tumor induction in germfree rats with methylazoxymethanol (MAM) and synthetic MAM acetate. *J. Natl. Cancer Inst.,* 39:355–371.

27. Matsubara, N., Mori, H., and Hirono, I. (1978): Effect of colostomy on intestinal carcinogenesis by methylazoxymethanol acetate in rats. *J. Natl. Cancer Inst.,* 61:1161–1164.
28. Matsumoto, H., Nagahama, T., and Larson, H. O. (1965): Studies on methylazoxymethanol, the aglycone of cycasin: A synthesis of methylazoxymethyl acetate. *Biochem. J.,* 95:13c–14c.
29. Modan, B., Barell, V., Lubin, F., Modan, M., Greenberg, R. A., and Graham, S. (1975): Low-fiber intake as an etiologic factor in cancer of the colon. *J. Natl. Cancer Inst.,* 55:15–18.
30. Nagasawa, H. T., Shirota, F. N., and Matsumoto, H. (1972): Decomposition of methylazoxymethanol, the aglycone of cycasin, in D_2O. *Nature [New Biol.],* 236:234–235.
31. Nigro, N. D., Singh, D. V., Campbell, R. L., and Pak, M. S. (1975): Effect of dietary beef fat on intestinal tumor formation by azoxymethane in rats. *J. Natl. Cancer Inst.,* 54:439–442.
32. Reddy, B. S., Mangat, S., Sheinfil, A., Weisburger, J. H., and Wynder, E. L. (1977): Effect of type and amount of dietary fat and 1,2-dimethylhydrazine on biliary bile acids, fecal bile acids, and neutral sterols in rats. *Cancer Res.,* 37:2132–2137.
33. Reddy, B. S., Narisawa, T., Wright, P., Vukusich, D., Weisburger, J. H., and Wynder, E. L. (1975): Colon carcinogenesis with azoxymethane and dimethylhydrazine in germfree rats. *Cancer Res.,* 35:287–290.
34. Reddy, B. S., Watanabe, K., and Weisburger, J. H. (1977): Effect of high-fat diet on colon carcinogenesis in F344 rats treated with 1,2-dimethylhydrazine, methylazoxymethanol acetate, or methylnitrosourea. *Cancer Res.,* 37:4156–4159.
35. Reddy, B. S., Weisburger, J. H., Narisawa, T., and Wynder, E. L. (1974): Colon carcinogenesis in germ-free rats with 1,2-dimethylhydrazine and N-methyl-N'-nitro-N-nitrosoguanidine. *Cancer Res.,* 34:2368–2372.
36. Rubio, M. A., Pethica, B. A., Zuman, P., and Falkehag, S. I. (1979): The interactions of carcinogens and co-carcinogens with lignin and other components of dietary fiber. In: *Dietary Fibers Chemistry and Nutrition,* edited by G. E. Inglett and S. I. Falkehag, pp. 251–271. Academic Press, New York.
37. Schoental, R. (1973): The mechanisms of action of the carcinogenic nitroso and related compounds. *Br. J. Cancer,* 28:436–439.
38. Shamberger, R. J., Rukovena, E., Longfield, A. K., Tytko, S. A., Deodhar, S., and Willis, C. E. (1973): Antioxidants and cancer. I. Selenium in the blood of normals and cancer patients. *J. Natl. Cancer Inst.,* 50:863–870.
39. Shamberger, R. J., Tytko, S. A., and Willis, C. E. (1976): Antioxidants and cancer. VI. Selenium and age-adjusted human cancer mortality. *Arch. Environ. Health,* 31:231–235.
40. Van Soest, P. J., and Robertson, J. B. (1977): What is fibre and fibre in food? *Nutr. Rev.,* 35:12–22.
41. Wilson, R. B., Hutcheson, D. P., and Wideman, L. (1977): Dimethylhydrazine-induced colon tumors in rats fed diets containing beef fat or corn oil with and without wheat bran. *Am. J. Clin. Nutr.,* 30:176–181.
42. Wittig, V. G., Wildner, G. P., and Ziebarth, D. (1971): Der Einfluss der Ingesta auf die Kanzerisierung des Rattendarms durch Dimethylhydrazin. *Arch. Geschwulstforsch.,* 37:105–115.
43. Zedeck, M. S. (1978): Experimental colon carcinogenesis. In: *Gastrointestinal Tract Cancer,* edited by M. Lipkin and R. A. Good, pp. 343–360. Plenum Publishing Corp., New York.
44. Zedeck, M. S., Frank, N., and Wiessler, M. (1979): Metabolism of the colon carcinogen methylazoxymethanol acetate. *Front. Gastrointest. Res.,* 4:32–37.
45. Zedeck, M. S., Grab, D. J., and Sternberg, S. S. (1977): Differences in the acute response of the various segments of rat intestine to treatment with the intestinal carcinogen methylazoxymethanol acetate. *Cancer Res.,* 37:32–36.
46. Zedeck, M. S., and Sternberg, S. S. (1974): A model system for studies of colon carcinogenesis: Tumor induction by a single injection of methylazoxymethanol acetate. *J. Natl. Cancer Inst.,* 53:1419–1421.
47. Zedeck, M. S., and Tan, Q. H. (1978): Effect of pyrazole on tumor induction by methylazoxymethanol (MAM) acetate: Relationship to metabolism of MAM. *Pharmacologist,* 20:174.

Colorectal Cancer: Prevention, Epidemiology, and Screening, edited by S. Winawer, D. Schottenfeld, and P. Sherlock. Raven Press, New York © 1980.

Ascorbic Acid in Polyposis Coli

Jerome J. DeCosse, H. J. R. Bussey, James P. S. Thomson, Anthony A. Eyers, Sheila M. Ritchie, and Basil C. Morson

St. Mark's Hospital for Diseases of the Rectum and Colon, London, United Kingdom; and Memorial Sloan-Kettering Cancer Center, New York, New York 10021

It is possible to envision a spectrum of activities for cancer control, all of which are important. At the top of the list would be elimination of carcinogens from the environment. If, however, one accepts the premises that elimination of environmental carcinogens may not be possible scientifically or acceptable publically or that some carcinogens may be formed internally, particularly in the context of gastrointestinal cancer, a second approach, namely, nutritional blocking or chemoprevention, assumes importance.

Operative or endoscopic removal of large bowel adenomas is practiced widely to reduce the incidence of large bowel cancer. If the hypothesis is valid that destruction of adenomas of the large bowel can control large bowel cancer, then by extension of this view, prevention of adenomas may accomplish the same end. The concept also may have validity for other types of preneoplastic lesions, such as leukoplakia or cervical dysplasia, which precede most human cancer.

The underlying premises for chemopreventive studies in the large bowel are that metabolites of endogenously and exogenously derived sterols, modified by colonic microflora and exposed to the large bowel mucosa, are causal in development of large bowel neoplasms; that large bowel adenomas evolve into large bowel cancer; and that adenoma formation can be prevented, or even reverted, by pharmacologic agents which block this process of carcinogenesis.

Several antioxidants inhibit murine tumors in a variety of experimental settings. In particular, butylated hydroxyanisole (BHA), butylated hydroxytoluene (BHT), ethoxyquin, ascorbic acid, alpha-tocopherol, selenium, retinoids, and some sulfur-containing compounds demonstrate this activity. The subject has been reviewed (27,29).

In particular, experimental large bowel carcinogenesis can be altered. Dimethylhydrazine (DMH)-induced large bowel neoplasia in rodents has been inhibited by disulfiram, ethylene *bis*(dithiocarbamate), *bis*(ethyl)xanthogen, carbon disulfide, BHA, selenium, and 13,*cis*-retinoic acid (8,10,16,26,28,29).

Ascorbic acid has known antitumor effects in experimental animals, presumably from its antioxidant properties. Ascorbic acid inhibited experimental bladder tumor formation caused by 3-hydroxyanthranilic acid (20), DMBA-croton oil skin carcinogenesis (21,22), and growth of sarcoma 180 (30). Sodium ascorbate limited both carcinogenicity and mutagenicity of ethyl urea and sodium nitrite carcinogenesis in pregnant hamsters (19). Large doses of ascorbic acid protected rats against liver tumor production by aminotyrine and sodium nitrite (3). Addition of ascorbic acid to culture media protected against abnormal growth and malignant transformation in hamster lung cultures exposed to smoke from cigarettes (13). Recently, supplemental sodium ascorbate inhibited DMH-induced large bowel carcinogenesis in rats (17). Ascorbic acid also blocked formation of carcinogenic *n*-nitroso compounds and prevented formation of mutagenic activity in nitrite-treated fish (15). Ascorbic acid decreased both DNA synthesis and neoplastic cell proliferation of tumor cell lines in culture (1). In man, ascorbic acid administered orally reduced fecal mutagenesis as measured by the Ames test (12). However, a mutagenic action of vitamin C has been demonstrated in fibroblast cultures (23). Also, tumor-bearing guinea pigs required ascorbic acid for tumor growth (14).

Observations of laboratory animals and humans also suggest that tumors may regress either spontaneously or under certain experimental conditions. In human neoplasia, evidence that phenotypic reversion of lasting significance may be accomplished includes occasional reversion of human neuroblastoma to ganglioneuroma, stabilization or apparent regression of metastatic nonbeta islet cell tumors after total gastrectomy, and abundant evidence that human breast cancer can be responsive to the hormonal milieu of the host.

It is generally assumed that large bowel adenomas, once evident, gradually increase in size over a long period of time. Some ultimately develop into invasive cancer. However, there is evidence that growth of adenomas is not necessarily inexorable; adenomas sometimes recede or even disappear. Knoernschild (11) followed 213 patients with sporadic large bowel polyps and found that 18% of the polyps disappeared.

In particular, the spontaneous regression of adenomatous polyps in the remaining rectum of patients who have had total colectomy and ileorectal anastomosis for familial polyposis provides striking evidence of the capacity for reversion of adenomas. Spontaneous regression has been noted by many observers (4). In 1961 Cole et al. (5) suggested that exposure of the adenoma-containing rectum to ileal contents was required for spontaneous regression of rectal polyps. Rectal adenomas of a patient with polyposis coli exposed to ileal contents disappeared, whereas adenomas in the remaining defunctionalized colon persisted. It was speculated that the colonic luminal contents are essential for induction of neoplasia in the large bowel.

An increase in degraded fecal bile acids has been observed in patients with large bowel cancer (9,18). Presumably, some sterol metabolites are carcinogenic. However, fecal biochemical and microbiological findings seem different in patients with polyposis coli. Polyposis patients with an intact large bowel excrete an increased proportion of primary bile acids, cholic and chenodeoxycholic acid (2). Limited degradation of cholesterol has been noted in polyposis patients with an intact colon. Polyposis patients, even with an intact colon, have a shortened intestinal transit time, and diarrhea may be responsible for some of these biochemical differences (24).

METHODS AND RESULTS

In our initial study, ascorbic acid in a delayed release form, 3 g daily, was administered to nine patients who had active polyp formation in the remaining rectum after a total colectomy and ileorectal anastomosis for polyposis coli (7). A reduction in the number and size of rectal polyps was observed in some patients. At 18 months of follow-up, the mean polyp density (number of polyps/ cm of retained rectum) was 34% of baseline values, and at 34 months of follow-up, the polyp density averaged 36% of baseline levels. Three patients have had disappearance of rectal polyps at one or more examinations. Subsequently, confirmation of these results was obtained in another limited study (25).

Accordingly, a trial has been initiated at St. Mark's Hospital, London, U.K. The trial, which is randomized and double-blind, compares ascorbic acid to placebo. The main determinant is the effect of treatment on the number of adenomas in the rectum of polyposis patients who have had a colectomy and ileorectal anastomosis.

Of 50 consecutive patients who were approached, 49 entered the trial. By February 1979, 11 patients had been studied for 9 months, 15 for 6 months, 17 for 3 months, and 6 additional patients entered the trial at that examination session. Two of the patients have been withdrawn, one for noncompliance and the other because she became pregnant and proctoscopy might be hazardous.

The trial remains blind and an interim analysis is being deferred until an adequate follow-up has been achieved. Comparison of the number of adenomas at successive examination of the first 26 patients followed for 6 months or more showed little or no change in 11 and an increase in 4, but in 9 patients there has been a decrease in the number of adenomas. However, at this time, it is not known how these patients are distributed between the ascorbic acid group and the placebo group.

Of the 49 patients, 3 had no adenomas at the start of the trial. In the remaining 46 patients (Table 1), rectal polyps were enumerated and localized. The first 4 cm measured on the proctosigmoidoscope contains the distance from the anal verge to and beyond the dentate line, encompasses squamous and transitional epithelium, and is discounted. When the distribution of adenomas in the rectal mucosa is examined by a chi square test, goodness of fit uniformity is rejected ($X^2 = 301.4$; $p < 0.001$). Hence the distal or caudal one-third of rectal mucosa in patients with polyposis coli who have had a colectomy and ileorectal anastomosis is relatively spared of adenomas as compared to the more proximal or cephalad two-thirds of rectal mucosa.

TABLE 1. *Distribution of rectal polyps in 46 patients with polyposis coli*

Interval from anal verge (cm)	Polyps (no.)	Rectum at risk (cm)	Polyp density (no./cm)
4–5.9	57	92	0.620
6–7.9	54	92	0.587
8–9.9	140	91	1.538
10–11.9	136	89	1.528
12–13.9	127	85	1.494
14–15.9	83	54	1.537

DISCUSSION

The reduction or disappearance of rectal adenomas in some patients is indisputable and may indicate efficacy of an antioxidant as a chemopreventive agent. There is, however, a possible alternative explanation; namely, that long-term cyclical variation in adenoma formation may occur in patients with polyposis. The remote past history of several of our patients and a tendency of rectal adenomas to wax and wane in number during treatment suggest this possibility. Others have noted a tendency for slowing in the appearance of new adenomas and for stability of existing adenomas during long-term follow-up. Hence, outcome of the randomized trial must be awaited before any conclusions can be derived. The study should provide decisive information either by proving the value of ascorbic acid in the treatment group or by documenting cyclical variation of adenomas in both groups.

Further, if the study should demonstrate therapeutic effectiveness of an antioxidant in controlling adenomas, prevention of rectal cancer will be a different issue which will require many years of treatment and scrutiny before results can be obtained.

An explanation is not apparent for the differences in the distribution of adenomas in the retained rectum of polyposis patients. There is no discernible embryologic basis. This observation, however, in a strong inherited setting, correlates with similar differences in the distribution and frequency of sporadic rectal cancer between low risk populations who have proportionately more cancer in the distal rectum and high risk populations who have proportionately more cancer in the proximal rectum (6).

ACKNOWLEDGMENTS

Supported by Grant R26 CA 23760 from the National Institutes of Health. We thank the surgeons at St. Mark's Hospital for allowing patients under their care to be entered into the study.

REFERENCES

1. Bishun, N., Basu, T. K., Metcalfe, S., and Williams, D. C. (1978): The effect of ascorbic acid (vitamin C) on two tumor cell lines in culture. *Oncology,* 35:160–162.
2. Bone, E., Drasar, B. S., and Hill, M. J. (1975): Gut bacteria and their metabolic activities in familial polyposis. *Lancet,* 1:1117–1120.
3. Chan, W. C., and Fong, Y. Y. (1977): Ascorbic acid prevents liver tumor production by aminopyrine and nitrite in the rat. *Int. J. Cancer,* 20:268–270.
4. Cole, J. W., and Holden, W. D. (1959): Postcolectomy regression of adenomatous polyps of the rectum. *Arch. Surg.,* 79:385–392.
5. Cole, J. W., McKalen, A., and Powell, J. (1961): The role of ileal contents in the spontaneous regression of rectal adenomas. *Dis. Colon Rectum,* 4:413–418.
6. Correa, P. (1975): Comments on the epidemiology of large bowel cancer. *Cancer Res.,* 35:3395–3397.
7. DeCosse, J. J., Adams, M. B., Kuzma, J. F., and Condon, R. E. (1975): Effect of ascorbic acid on rectal polyps of patients with familial polyposis. *Surgery,* 78:608–612.
8. Fiala, E. S., Bobotas, G., and Kulakis, C. (1977): Effects of disulfiram and related compounds on the metabolism *in vivo* of the colon carcinogen, 1,2-dimethylhydrazine. *Biochem. Pharmacol.,* 26:1763–1768.
9. Hill, M. J., Drasar, B. S., Williams, R. E. O., Meade, T. W., Cox, A. G., Simpson, J. E. P., and Morson, B. C. (1975): Faecal bile-acids and clostridia in patients with cancer of the large bowel. *Lancet,* 1:535–538.
10. Jacobs, M. M. (1977): Inhibitory effects of selenium, 1,2-dimethylhydrazine and methylazoxymethanol on carcinogenesis. *Cancer,* 40:2557–2564.
11. Knoernschild, H. E. (1963): Growth rate and malignant potential of colonic polyps: Early results. *Surg. Forum,* 14:137–138.
12. Land, P. C., and Bruce, W. R. (1978): Fecal mutagens: A possible relationship with colorectal cancer. *Proc. Am. Assoc. Cancer Res.,* 19:167.
13. Leuchtenberger, C., and Leuchtenberger, R. (1977): Protection of hamster lung cultures by 1-cysteine or vitamin C against carcinogenic effects of fresh smoke from tobacco or marihuana cigarettes. *Br. J. Pathol.,* 58:625–633.
14. Migliozzi, J. A. (1977): Effect of ascorbic acid on tumor growth. *Br. J. Cancer,* 35:448–453.
15. Mirvish, S. S., Wallcave, L., Eagen, M., and Shubik, P. (1972): Ascorbate nitrite reactions: Possible means of blocking the formation of carcinogenic N-nitroso compounds. *Science,* 177:65–68.
16. Newberne, P. M., and Rogers, A. E. (1973): Rat colon carcinoma associated with aflatoxin and marginal vitamin A. *J. Natl. Cancer Inst.,* 50:439–448.
17. Reddy, B. S., and Hirota, N. (1979): Effect of dietary ascorbic acid on 1,2-dimethylhydrazine-induced colon cancer in rats. *Fed. Proc.,* 38:714.
18. Reddy, B. S., and Wynder, E. L. (1977): Metabolic epidemiology of colon cancer: Fecal bile acids and neutral sterols in colon cancer patients and patients with adenomatous polyps. *Cancer,* 39:2533–2539.
19. Rustia, M. (1975): Inhibitory effect of sodium ascorbate on ethylurea and sodium nitrite carcinogenesis and negative findings in progeny after intestinal inoculation of precursors into pregnant hamsters. *J. Natl. Cancer Inst.,* 44:1389–1393.
20. Schlegel, J. U., Pipkin, G. E., Michimura, R., and Schultz, G. N. (1970): The role of ascorbic acid in the prevention of bladder tumor formation. *J. Urol.,* 103:155–159.
21. Shamberger, R. J. (1972): Increase of peroxidation in carcinogenesis. *J. Natl. Cancer Inst.,* 48:1491–1497.
22. Shamberger, R. J., and Rudolph, G. (1966): Protection against cocarcinogenesis by antioxidants. *Experienta,* 22:116.
23. Stich, H. F., Karim, J., Koropatnick, J., and Lo, L. (1976): Mutagenic action of ascorbic acid. *Nature,* 260:722–724.
24. Watne, A. L., and Core, S. K. (1975): Rectal steroids in polyposis coli and ileorectostomy patients. *J. Surg. Res.,* 19:157–161.
25. Watne, A. L., Lai, H. Y. L., Mance, T., Carrier, J. C., and Coppula, W. (1977): The diagnosis and surgical treatment of patients with Gardner's syndrome. *Surgery,* 82:327–333.

26. Wattenberg, L. W. (1975): Inhibition of dimethylhydrazine-induced neoplasia of the large intestine by disulfiram. *J. Natl. Cancer Inst.,* 54:1005–1006.
27. Wattenberg, L. W. (1978): Inhibition of chemical carcinogenesis. *J. Natl. Cancer Inst.,* 60:11–18.
28. Wattenberg, L. W., and Fiala, E. S. (1978): Inhibition of 1,2 dimethylhydrazine-induced neoplasia of the large intestine in female CF_1 mice by carbondisulfide. *J. Natl. Cancer Inst.,* 60:1515–1517.
29. Wattenberg, L. W., Loub, W. D., Lam, L. K., and Speier, J. L. (1976): Dietary constituents altering the responses to chemical carcinogens. *Fed. Proc.,* 35:1327–1331.
30. Yamafuji, K., Kakamura, Y., and Omura, H. (1976): Antitumor potency of ascorbic, dehydroascorbic or 2,3-diketogluconic acid and their action of deoxyribonucleic acid. *Z. Krebsforsch.,* 76:1–7.

Colorectal Cancer: Prevention, Epidemiology, and Screening, edited by S. Winawer, D. Schottenfeld, and P. Sherlock. Raven Press, New York © 1980.

Introduction: Heredity Versus Environment in Colorectal Cancer

Paul Sherlock

Memorial Sloan-Kettering Cancer Center, New York, NY 10021

Colorectal cancer has been the subject of genetic inquiry since it has been observed that there is an increased familial aggregation of the disease. However, in order to invoke a genetic etiology, it must be determined that environmental factors are not responsible for the increased incidence of the disease, since environmental influences may simulate the action of genes. Environmental influences may be unknown, undetected, or subject to long periods of latency before exerting clinical expression of disease. In many diseases, including cancer, some presently unknown environmental influence, such as a virus or dietary component, may act early in life and result in disease later in life (1).

The proof that a single gene is involved is the demonstration that predicted mendelian ratios exist. However, most of the human diseases that appear to have some possible genetic predisposition resist analysis of specific gene difference. Manifest disease and genetic variability may be due to the combined action of a number of genes, the so-called polygenic or multifactorial inheritance. The presence or absence of clinically manifest disease may be all or none, but the underlying genetic basis may be characterized by a broad spectrum of variation in susceptibility which may reflect multifactorial inheritance. The resulting distribution of a disease in the population may therefore reflect both environmental and multifactorial genetic factors.

In certain families, the risk of developing cancer is much greater than in the general population. In familial polyposis and Gardner's syndrome, genetic factors have been clearly demonstrated to be responsible for the increased frequency of neoplastic disease. These are precisely defined autosomal dominant diseases. There is some indication of a familial tendency in patients with colorectal cancer, a tendency that is probably multifactorial. The risk of cancer of the colon in relatives of patients with colorectal cancer is probably about three times that expected in the general population. There is suggestive evidence that patients under age 40 who develop carcinoma of the colon or rectum are more likely to have a family history of colonic cancer than those over 40 who develop the neoplasm. There are families that have been considered cancer families because of their striking incidence of malignancy at multiple anatomic sites (most frequently endometrium and colon), multiple primary malignant neoplasms, and early age of onset. A multifactorial basis may explain the occurrence in such families. However, carcinomas that appear to have a genetic basis resist analytic efforts to prove a single gene difference except for the familial polyposis syndromes (2,3). In regard to cancers that have both hereditary and nonhereditary forms, Knudson et al. (4) offered the following hypothesis: The individual with the hereditary form already carries one mutation (germinal) that may lead to cancer but must acquire one more mutation (somatic) in order to develop the cancer. The patient with the nonhereditary form of cancer must acquire two or more new somatic mutations. As a result, nonhereditary cases are of later onset than hereditary ones.

Can individuals in families predisposed to develop gastrointestinal cancer be identified at an early stage of their disease, before evidence of malignancy appears? The main subject of this volume attempts to deal with this question. The improved identification of individuals and families at high risk for the development of colon cancer would mean better surveillance and probably earlier diagnosis, which are crucial for improved cure rates (5).

REFERENCES

1. Sherlock, P. (1976): Etiology of gastrointestinal cancer: Heredity vs. environmental (editorial). *Am. J. Dig. Dis.,* 21:68–70.
2. McKusick, V. A. (1974): Genetics and large bowel cancer. *Am. J. Dig. Dis.,* 19:954–957.
3. Lynch, H. T., and Krush, A. J. (1967): Heredity and adenocarcinoma of the colon. *Gastroenterology,* 53:517–527.
4. Knudson, A. G., Jr., Strong, L. C., and Anderson, D. E. (1973): Heredity and cancer in man. *Prog. Med. Genet.,* 9:113–158.
5. Sherlock, P., and Winawer, S. J. (1974): Modern approaches to early identification of large bowel cancer. *Am. J. Dig. Dis.,* 19:959–964.

Colorectal Cancer: Prevention, Epidemiology, and Screening, edited by S. Winawer, D. Schottenfeld, and P. Sherlock. Raven Press, New York © 1980.

Introduction: The Gardner Syndrome; Then and Now

Eldon J. Gardner

Department of Biology, Utah State University, Logan, Utah 84322; and University of Utah, Salt Lake City, Utah 84112

In 1947, eight closely related people (a grandmother, three of her children, and four of her grandchildren) had died with carcinoma of the colon at an average age of 39. Little or no medical attention had been obtained by the deceased in the early stages of the disease. Few if any medical records were available for most of the deceased. A brief hospital report on one victim indicated polyps in the colorectum. Proctoscopic examinations of all 51 living descendants of the deceased grandmother revealed multiple adenomas in six; two already had carcinoma of the colorectum (one died shortly after surgery, whereas the other survived the colostomy, lived for 21 years, and died from a heart attack). The four with benign adenomas were treated surgically and were in good health in 1979.

Abnormal growths other than colorectal polyps were observed in the six positive individuals. All six were shown clinically and pathologically to have multiple osteomas, fibromas, and epidermoid cysts. Data obtained from family members, photo albums, barbers, undertakers, and friends indicated that the deceased cancer victims also had extracolorectal lesions. The name "Gardner's syndrome" (GS) was suggested by W. G. Smith for this assemblage of abnormal growth that followed a dominant pattern of inheritance. This family group, designated as Kindred 109, has been followed with great interest over the past 30 years. A total of 29 kindred members now have or have had the syndrome. Seventeen of these are now living. Following the initial nine deaths from colorectal cancer, one patient died 12 years after subtotal colectomy from metastatic colon cancer in the brain arising from a neglected rectal adenoma, and two have died from desmoid tumors and uncontrolled mesenteric fibromatosis. Of the 29 affected members, 24 have or have had colorectal polyposis (5 are children under 16 who do not yet have polyps); 26 of 29, osteomas; 24, fibromas; 23, epidermoid cysts; 11, desmoid tumors or mesenteric fibromatosis; and 18, particular dental abnormalities, now associated with the syndrome. No primary cancer of the colon has occurred in Kindred 109 since the initial nine deaths.

The Gardner syndrome has now been reported from many locations around the world. An extensive bibliography has accumulated in the medical and scientific literature covering various aspects of the syndrome. People at risk for adenomatosis and colorectal cancer as well as their physicians have been alerted to the risk of carcinoma. Surgical technique for the removal of the involved colon has improved, and the young affected people have adjusted well to the surgery. Histology, pathology, and natural history of the benign adenomas and the adenocarcinoma are now well known. Investigations at the cellular and molecular (DNA) level are in progress; chromosome studies are being extended. A question still remains: whether GS is a clinical and genetic entity separate from familial polyposis coli (FPC) or a variant of FPC explained by differences in penetrance and expressivity of the FPC gene along with environmental factors.

The genetics of FPC have been established as a dominant pattern controlled by a single gene *(P)*. Many kindreds studied for years by Dukes, Bussey, Marston, and Veale at Saint Mark's Hospital, London, and those followed by several other investigators have not shown extracolorectal manifestations. It is therefore proposed that FPC and GS are separate genetic entities. Since multiple adenomatosis is basic to both diseases, an allele of P, P^G (superscript G for growth factor) is proposed to control the Gardner syndrome.

ACKNOWLEDGMENT

This research was supported by PHS Grant CA 21623.

Colorectal Cancer: Prevention, Epidemiology, and Screening, edited by S. Winawer, D. Schottenfeld, and P. Sherlock. Raven Press, New York © 1980.

Genetics of Familial Polyposis

Richard B. McConnell

Gastroenterology Unit, Broadgreen Hospital; and Department of Medicine, University of Liverpool Royal Liverpool Hospital, Liverpool, United Kingdom

Until this decade it was conventional to regard as distinct genetic entities the various familial polyposes with many colonic polyps, some of which have associated extracolonic lesions and all of which have an increased cancer risk. It was believed that each was inherited in a dominant manner due to the presence of its separate gene (2,5,8,13). These genes were not considered to be alleles sharing the same locus, but they were thought to be at separate loci, possibly even on different chromosomes. Any aspects of the family data which did not fit this theory were attributed to lack of penetrance or variable expression of the relevant gene.

Analysis of data completed during the past 10 years casts doubts on some of the previous genetic interpretations. In particular, the evidence now indicates that classic familial polyposis coli and Gardner's syndrome are not distinct genetic entities. In Sweden (1), in Baltimore (S. B. Cohen, *personal communication),* and in Japan (12), many families have been found in which all of the polyposis patients have been free of extracolonic manifestations with the exception of one or two patients with a few osteomata. Conversely, families in which there have been several cases of Gardner's syndrome have been found to contain an individual with polyposis but no extracolonic lesion.

To take another example, these recent surveys have reported polyposis families in which an individual has had a brain tumor. Often it has been a child with a medulloblastoma in whom polyposis has not developed. It thus seems probable that some polyposis syndromes based on one or two families, such as Turcot's syndrome, are also not distinct genetic entities. These recent analyses have lumped together several of the conditions in which large numbers of polyps occur in the colon with or without associated lesions.

GENETIC INTERPRETATION

The genetic theory which would best explain the family data so far collected is that there is one major pleotropic gene underlying the inheritance of all these syndromes. Without this gene neither the polyposis nor the extracolonic lesions will develop. What does develop in those individuals who have this gene depends on other parts of their genotype. In other words, other genes will determine whether or not extracolonic manifestations develop and also their type. Thus it would be theoretically possible for a polyposis patient to develop the full-blown syndrome with lesions in bones, connective tissues, sebaceous cysts, desmoids, tumors of central nervous system (11), and even polyposis of the stomach and duodenum.

In practice, the shared genotype of about half the polyposis families is such that only the colonic polyps develop with an occasional mandibular osteoma. In the other half, a variety of genes cause some or all of the polyposis patients to develop osteomata, fibromata, or sebaceous cysts but usually not all three. In an occasional family it is postulated that a gene is present which in the presence of the major polyposis gene leads to the development of medulloblastoma, often before the age at which the colonic polyps start to develop, or a gene which leads to gastroduodenal polyps in addition to the colonic polyps.

From the data so far published, it is not clear whether or not these modifying genes at other loci influence the age of development and thus, for the time being, Veale's hypothesis (13) of two alleles of the major polyposis gene remains an acceptable explanation. Genetic control of the number of polyps is possible but it is unlikely that it will be either demonstrated or disproved due to the evidence in large pedigrees being affected by early prophylactic colectomy. The implications of cell culture studies (3) are difficult to assess at present, but if they establish that there is increased tetraploidy in some families and not in others, a revision of the single major gene theory would have to be considered.

OTHER POLYPOSES

There are no new data which cast doubts on the theory that Peutz-Jeghers syndrome is determined by a pleotropic gene separate from that causing multiple adenomatous polyposis of the colon and rectum. The genetic basis of juvenile polyposis is uncertain, there being insufficient data on which to make worthwhile deductions. There is also the possibility that juvenile polyposis may be heterogeneous.

HERITABLE SOLITARY COLONIC POLYPS

Occasional discrete polyps of the colon and rectum were shown to be probably inherited in a large family more than 20 years ago (9). Half the members of the third generation had rectosigmoid polyps, and a third of the second generation had died of gastrointestinal cancer, mainly colonic. Since then there have been less convincing reports (10), but the numerous reports of "cancer families" involving particularly the colon and rectum (4) suggest the possibility that these cancers with dominant inheritance, as well as a proportion of the sporadic colorectal cancers with onset before 40 years of age, may also have genetically determined solitary polyps as their basis (6,7).

REFERENCES

1. Alm, T., and Licznerski, G. (1973): The intestinal polyposes. *Clin. Gastroenterol.,* 2:577–602.
2. Bussey, H. J. R. (1975): *Familial Polyposis Coli.* The Johns Hopkins Press, Baltimore.
3. Danes, B. D. (1978): Increased in vitro tetraploidy: Tissue specific within the heritable colo-rectal cancer syndromes with polyposis coli. *Cancer,* 41:2330–2334.
4. Lunch, H. T., Guirgis, H. A., Lynch, P. M., Lynch, J. F., and Harris, R. E. (1977): Familial cancer syndromes: A survey. *Cancer,* 39:1867–1881.
5. McConnell, R. B. (1966): *The Genetics of Gastro-intestinal Disorders.* Oxford University Press, London.
6. McConnell, R. B. (1978): Genetic aspects of colonic cancer. In: *Colon Cancer,* edited by E. Grundmann, pp. 51–60. Gustav Fischer Verlag, Stuttgart.
7. McConnell, R. B. (1978): Gastro-intestinal Cancer: Genetics and Genetic Markers. In: *Frontiers of Gastrointestinal Research, Vol. 4,* edited by P. Rozen, pp. 264–271. S. Karger, Basel.
8. McKusick, V. A. (1974): Genetics and large bowel cancer. *Dig. Dis.,* 19:954–958.
9. Richards, R. C., and Woolf, C. (1965): Solitary polyps of the colon and rectum; a study of inherited tendency. *Am. Surg.,* 22:287–294.
10. Smith, W. G. (1970): The cancer-family syndrome and heritable solitary colonic polyps. *Dis. Colon Rectum,* 13:362–367.
11. Smith, W. G., and Kern, B. B. (1973): The nature of the mutation in familial multiple polyposis. Papillary carcinoma of the thyroid, brain tumours, and familial multiple polyposis. *Dis. Colon Rectum,* 16:264–271.
12. Utsumoniya, J., and Nakamura, T. (1975): The occult osteomatous changes in the mandible in patients with familial polyposis coli. *Br. J. Surg.,* 62:45–51.
13. Veale, A. M. O. (1965): *Intestinal Polyposis.* Eugenic Laboratory Memoirs Series 40. Cambridge University Press, London.

Colorectal Cancer: Prevention, Epidemiology, and Screening, edited by S. Winawer, D. Schottenfeld, and P. Sherlock. Raven Press, New York © 1980.

Modifying Alleles in the Heritable Colorectal Cancer Syndromes with Polyps

*B. Shannon Danes, **T. Alm, and †A. M. O. Veale

*Laboratory for Cell Biology, Department of Medicine, Cornell University Medical College, New York, New York, 10021; **Department of Gastroenterology, St. Erik's Hospital, Stockholm, Sweden; and †Department of Community Medicine and Genetics, University of Auckland Medical School, Auckland, New Zealand*

On the basis of family studies, familial polyposis coli and the variant form, the Gardner syndrome, are each considered to be due to a dominant mutation which in familial polyposis coli is expressed solely as colonic polyps that become malignant, and in the Gardner syndrome as extracolonic connective tissue tumors and related neoplasms in addition to such colonic lesions (10). However, investigators (1,2,9,15,16) have been impressed by two contradictions to this statement: first, variable clinical expression in the colon, and second, variation of extracolonic lesions.

Description of the clinical phenotypes has established the common characteristics of the two syndromes but little understanding for the reason for such variability in gene expression. In order to explain such variability, Veale (16) postulated in 1965 a modifying allele which, when present, would enhance the expression of the main gene, P in familial polyposis coli and G in the Gardner syndrome. He estimated that 51% of the general population has this modifying gene (16).

Other family studies (12) have and have not (3) given supportive evidence for this hypothesis, perhaps due to the lack of an experimental approach to determine the presence of such a modifying allele. It is proposed that cell culture offers such a test system to study the influence of such modifying alleles in the expression of the dominant gene P in familial polyposis coli and G in the Gardner syndrome. *In vitro* studies done in several laboratories supported by the National Large Bowel Cancer Project in the past 5 years have demonstrated that cells cultured from families with both syndromes show cellular abnormalities presumably due to the *in vitro* expression of their mutation (4–8,11,14). One of these abnormalities is increased *in vitro* tetraploidy (4–8).

The following facts have been established concerning the occurrence of *in vitro* tetraploidy [that is, greater than 6% (4–8)]:

a. It is a cell culture phenomenon—not observed *in vivo,* that is, in the tissue from which the cultures are derived (4,5,7) (Fig. 1).

73

PRESENCE OF INCREASED IN VITRO TETRAPLOIDY[**]			
INDIVIDUALS STUDIED	WEEKS IN CULTURE		
	4-9	9-15	15-29
FPC AFFECTED			
2	+	+	+
3	-	+	+
15	-	-	-
NORMALS			
8	-	-	-

[**] RANGE OF TETRAPLOIDY IN CULTURES DERIVED FROM NORMALS NOT-AT-RISK 0-6%

INCREASED TETRAPLOIDY + = PRESENT - = ABSENT

FIG. 1. Occurrence of increased *in vitro* tetraploidy in cultures established from skin biopsies taken from 42 patients with familial polyposis coli and 8 normals not at risk for familial polyposis coli.

b. It occurs only in cultures containing epithelial cells as no increase is observed in pure cultures of fibroblasts (5,6) (Fig. 2).

c. It is tissue specific, occurring only in cultures derived from tissues, which, although appearing normal in the patient, are known to undergo malignant transformation *in vivo*. For example, colonic mucosa in familial polyposis coli and in the Gardner syndrome. Cultures established from tissues known not to show neoplastic growth or from benign tumors such as fibromas, cysts, and lipomas as in the Gardner syndrome do not show increased *in vitro* tetraploidy (6) (Table 1).

d. Within specific families this cellular abnormality can be traced *in vitro* through consecutive generations of affected members and normals at risk (Fig. 3) (7).

Based on these facts on the *in vitro* occurrence of increased tetraploidy (4–8,11,14), skin cultures from 40 families with either syndrome were studied. The majority of such family units showed concordance in the occurrence of *in vitro* tetraploidy in those affected in consecutive generations. In those families

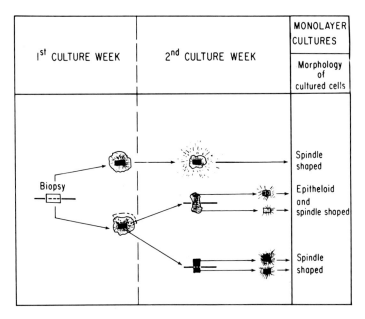

FIG. 2. Methodology used in the establishment of cultures composed of morphologically distinct cell types (epithelioid- and spindle-shaped) from human skin biopsies.

with the Gardner syndrome, increased tetraploidy was observed in skin cultures containing epithelium from affected members and some of the members at risk in each consecutive generation. In the majority of families with familial polyposis coli, no increased tetraploidy was observed in skin cultures. In seven of the familial polyposis coli families increased tetraploidy was observed.

For example, in one familial polyposis coli family, of the three affected offspring studied of an affected mother without increased *in vitro* tetraploidy, two showed increased tetraploidy whereas the other did not (Fig. 4). Repeat skin biopsies 6 months later yielded the same results.

In another classic familial polyposis coli family, the affected father had two similarily affected sons, one had increased *in vitro* tetraploidy as did his father and the other did not (Fig. 4). There are at least three possible explanations:

1. As the increased incidence of *in vitro* tetraploidy in a mixed cell population has been shown to depend on the presence of an epithelioid cell population (6), the absence of increased tetraploidy in any culture may be due to the absence or low number of such cells in the sample on which mitotic activity was determined.

Such a possibility was minimized by using culture techniques which maximize the initial migration of epithelium from the primary explant and their inclusion in the cell population from which the cell lines are established (Fig. 2) (5). In addition, biopsies from the same individual are taken at two different times to

TABLE 1. *Percentage of dividing cells showing tetraploidy in cultures derived from biopsies from 4 normals, 2 patients with familial polyposis coli, 8 with the Gardner syndrome, and 2 with a variant form of the Gardner syndrome (6)*

Individuals studied	Age (years)	Sex	Biopsy tissue cultured					
			Skin		Mesentery	Sigmoid colon		
			Epidermis	Dermis		Normal mucosa	Polyps	Colonic wall
			Dividing cells showing tetraploidy (%)[a]					
Normals								
1	20	F	1	0	0	2		2
2	32	M	1	1	2	3		0
3	40	F	2	3	1	1		4
4	59	M	0	2	0	2		0
Familial polyposis coli								
Family 1								
Pt. 1	31	M	0	2	1	20	18	1
Pt. 2	26	F	0	1	0	12	22	2
Gardner syndrome								
Family 2								
Pt. 1	44	F	11	3			12	
Pt. 2	25	M	22				18	
Pt. 3	23	M	20	0			20	
Pt. 4	21	M	29	0				
Pt. 5	13	F	17	0				
Pt. 6	54	F	14	1	0	14	16	2
Family 3								
Pt. 1	19	F	13	1		14		0
Family 4								
Pt. 1	33	F	18	4	1	26	32	2
Gardner syndrome variant								
Family 5								
Pt. 1	16	F	1	1		16	20	2
Pt. 2	22	M	0	0		10	15	1

[a] At least 50 mitoses were counted on each slide included in this study.
From Danes (6).

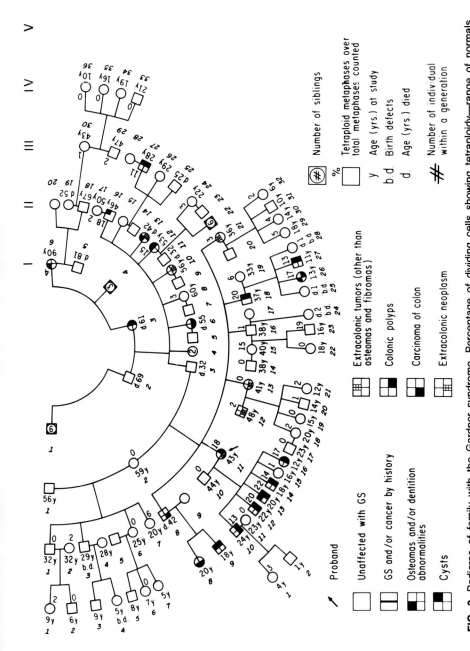

FIG. 3. Pedigree of family with the Gardner syndrome. Percentage of dividing cells showing tetraploidy—range of normals, 0–6%.

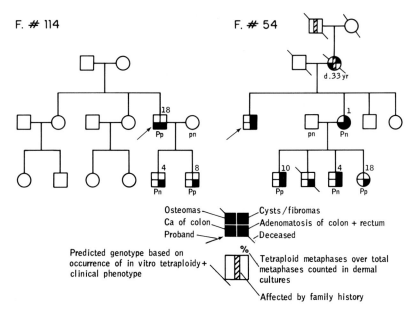

FIG. 4. Abbreviated pedigrees from two families with FPC (no. 114 and 54) from St. Erik's Hospital, Stockholm (appendix ref. 10) (1). FPC, adenomatosis of the colon and rectum. Genes: n = normal, P = major polyposis gene of FPC, p = modifying allele for FPC.
    From Danes (8).

establish cell lines to compare the occurrence of tetraploidy in such sublines from different biopsies from the same individual (Table 2) (4,6,7).

Until cultures composed solely of epithelial cells are available, the influence of the proportion of different cell types in the study cell population will always be of concern, especially as endoreduplication resulting in increased tetraploidy appears to occur solely in epithelium and not in other cell types such as fibroblasts.

2. The second possibility is that within these two clinically defined syndromes, there is a difference in the expression of the mutant gene in the cultured cell.

3. The third possibility is that increased *in vitro* tetraploidy reflects the *in vitro* interaction of a modifying allele with the major gene (Table 3).

It is proposed that increased *in vitro* tetraploidy identifies the presence of a modifying allele, designated *p* in familial polyposis coli and *g* in the Gardner syndrome, interacting with the major gene, *P* or *G*. As it has been postulated (16) that 51% of the general population has the *p* or *g* gene, and increased *in vitro* tetraploidy (that is greater than 6% of the dividing cells showing tetraploidy) (4,5,7,8), is observed rarely in dermal cultures derived from normals not at risk, it is assumed that *p* or *g* is not detected by increased *in vitro* tetraploidy unless a major gene such as *P* or *G* is present. Such gene interaction between the major gene and a modifying allele may enhance the genetic potential of

TABLE 2. *Percentage of dividing cells showing tetraploidy in cultures derived from separate skin biopsies taken over a 3-year period from a patient with familial polyposis coli, the Gardner syndrome, and not at risk for either syndrome*

		Skin biopsies			
			Dividing cells showing tetraploidy (%)[a]		
			Subculture no.		
Patient no.	Clinical status	No.	6	9	12
1	Gardner syndrome	First	11	14	12
		Second	18	18	20
		Third	16	12	11
2	Familial polyposis	First	2	0	2
		Second	3	4	4
		Third	1	4	2
3	Normal (not at risk for either GS or FPC)	First	3	3	5
		Second	2	3	3
		Third	4	4	0

[a] At least 50 mitoses were counted on each slide included in this study.

TABLE 3. *Proposed genotypes (16) in heritable colorectal cancer syndromes with polyps based on clinical features and occurrence of* in vitro *tetraploidy*

| | Phenotypes | | | |
| | Clinical | | Predicted culture increased tetraploidy | Predicted genotype |
Clinical diagnosis	Features	Onset		
FPC	Adenomatosis of colon and rectum	Late	−	Pn
		Early	+	Pp
Single or multiple polyps	Normal or <100 polyps	None or very late	−	pn
		Very late	+	pp
GS	Polyps, osteomas, cysts, fibromas	Late	−	Gn
		Early	+	Gg
	Normal or only some of the associated extracolonic lesions (osteomas)	None	−	gn
		Late	+	gg

FPC, adenomatosis of the colon and rectum; GS, Gardner syndrome. Genes: *n*, normal; *P*, major polyposis gene of FPC; *G*, major gene for GS; *p*, modifying allele for FPC; *g*, modifying allele for GS. Increased *in vitro* tetraploidy in dermal cultures: present (+), absent (−).
From Danes (8).

the major gene, in this case *P* or *G*, leading to an earlier clinical expression, that is, development of colonic adenomas,

With the concept of modifying alleles, the existence of homozygotes—that is, individuals having *pp* or *gg*, having inherited one *p* or *g* from each of their parents—should exist. The clinical expression in the homozygous state would be late onset, presence of a few polyps, and a family history of colonic adenocarcinomas with or without a few polyps (16). It is proposed that skin cultures established from such homozygotes will show increased tetraploidy.

As it has been postulated (16) that the proportion of the normal genotype, *nn* is 49%, of the heterozygous, *pn*, 42%, and of the homozygous, *pp*, is 9%, a major part of those individuals developing cancer of the colon after the age of 50 would be predicted to have the *pp* genotype. The potential clinical significance of this hypothesis is a possible genetic explanation for the occurrence of the majority of cases of colorectal cancer, especially those of early onset.

Neel and Schull (13) emphasized that the manner in which one gene modified the expression of another gene is no less important than the effect of environmental factors on the action of either gene. They pointed out that such gene interaction will be detected only if the expression of a few genes such as the *P* or *G* and its modifying allele, *p* or *g*, can be identified with the rest of the genetic background held relatively constant.

For this reason, it has rarely been possible in man to obtain evidence of the modification of one gene or genes by another. Identification of reliable characteristics of cultured cells with and without recognized mutant genotypes such as in familial polyposis coli and the Gardner syndrome may provide an *in vitro* model system to obtain such information on gene-gene and gene-gene-environment interactions.

SUMMARY

Based on *in vitro* studies on heritable colorectal cancer syndromes with polyps (adenomatosis of the colon and rectum, FPC), it is proposed that the presence/absence of specific abnormal culture phenotypes within and between such kindreds will demonstrate the interaction of a modifying allele with its proposed major polyposis gene, influencing expression of this major gene, at least *in vitro*. Such *in vitro* evidence suggests that the variability of clinical phenotype was due, at least in part, to such gene-gene interaction, and this should be considered as well as the influence of environmental agents on the development of both premalignant lesions and clinical cancer in such cancer-prone families.

ACKNOWLEDGMENTS

The research mentioned in this hypothesis was supported by Public Health Service Grant (CA-15973 from the National Cancer Institute through the National Large Bowel Cancer Project and in part by the International Cancer

Union, The Danes Medical Research Fund, Cornell University Medical College, the Zemurray Foundation, the *Riksforeningen mot Cancer,* Stockholm, Sweden, and the Medical Research Council of New Zealand. Portions of this hypothesis and supporting *in vitro* and family data presented in this chapter appear in (8).

REFERENCES

1. Alm, T. (1974): Hereditary adenomatosis of the colon and rectum. Stockholm, Thesis.
2. Alm, T., and Licznerski, G. (1973): The intestinal polyposes. *Clin. Gastroenterol.,* 2:577–602.
3. Berthon, B. (1959): Hérédite et pronostic de la polypose rectocolique généralisée. Bordeaux, Thesis.
4. Danes, B. S. (1975): The Gardner syndrome: A study in cell culture. *Cancer,* 36:2327–2333.
5. Danes, B. S. (1977): The Gardner syndrome: A study in cell culture. In: *Year Book of Cancer 1977,* edited by R. L. Clark and R. W. Cumley, pp. 361–364. Year Book Medical Publishers, Chicago.
6. Danes, B. S. (1978): Increased in vitro tetraploidy: Tissue specific within the heritable colorectal cancer syndromes with polyposis coli. *Cancer,* 41:2330–2334.
7. Danes, B. S., and Krush, A. J. (1977): The Gardner syndrome: A family study in cell culture. *J. Natl. Cancer Inst.,* 58:771–775.
8. Danes, B. S., Alm, T., and Veale, A. M. O. (1979): Role of modifying alleles in the heritable colorectal cancer syndromes with polyps. *Med. Hypotheses,* 5:1057–1064.
9. Dukes, C. E. (1952): Familial intestinal polyposis. *Ann. Eugencis,* 17:1–29.
10. Gardner, E. J. (1951): Genetic and clinical study of intestinal polyposis, a predisposing factor for carcinoma of the colon and rectum. *Am. J. Hum. Genet.,* 3:167–176.
11. Kopelovich, L. (1977): Phenotypic markers in human skin fibroblasts as possible diagnostic indices of hereditary adenomatosis of the colon and rectum. *Cancer,* 40:2534–2541.
12. Lovett, E. (1976): Family studies in cancer of the colon and rectum. *Br. J. Surg.,* 63:13–18.
13. Neel, J. V., and Schull, W. J. (1954): *Human Heredity,* pp. 17–29. University of Chicago Press, Chicago.
14. Pfeffer, L., Lipkin, M., Stutman, O., and Kopelovich, L. (1976): Growth abnormalities of cultured human skin fibroblasts derived from individuals with hereditary adenomatosis of the colon and rectum. *J. Cell. Physiol.,* 89:29–37.
15. Reed, T. E., and Neel, J. V. (1955): Genetic study of multiple polyposis of colon. *Am. J. Hum. Genet.,* 7:236–263.
16. Veale, A. M. O. (1965): *Intestinal Polyposis,* Eugenics Laboratory Memoirs Series 40. Cambridge University Press, Cambridge.

Colorectal Cancer: Prevention, Epidemiology, and Screening, edited by S. Winawer, D. Schottenfeld, and P. Sherlock. Raven Press, New York © 1980.

Adenomatosis Coli in Japan

J. Utsunomiya and T. Iwama

Second Department of Surgery and Polyposis Center, Tokyo Medical and Dental University, Tokyo, Japan

The biological and social characteristics of the Japanese, being a rather isolated race, with a long-established family register system and a well-developed academic system where information can be freely exchanged, have resulted in a significant contribution to the study of genetic diseases of man.

It has been suggested that comparison between Japan and Western countries could be a useful tool in the study of the epidemiology of cancer. The earliest trial of this type in which I was involved was in the epidemiology of breast cancer in 1964 (1).

Gastrointestinal polyposis in Japan also presents an attractive problem for study in genetic and environmental relationships in large bowel carcinogenesis.

This chapter summarizes the accumulated knowledge of adenomatosis coli in Japan.

DEFINITION, TERMINOLOGY, AND CLASSIFICATION

Definition and Terminology

A polyp is any localized elevation on the intestinal mucosal surface. "Polyposis" generally indicates a condition in which many polyps occur. Various types of polyposes were classified by histology and number of lesions according to Morson's method (2) (Table 1).

Adenomatosis coli is the general term for conditions in which more than 100 adenomas are detected in the large intestine regardless of whether it is familial or associated with extracolonic changes. It includes the following conditions: those not associated with extracolonic lesions, familial polyposis, those with osteomas and soft tissue tumors such as epidermoid cysts with or without fibrous tumors, Gardner's syndrome, and those with central nervous system involvement, Turcot's syndrome.

"Polyposis of the entire gastrointestinal tract," "polyposis coli with gastric polyps," and other expressions are not used in this text. The term "hereditary gastrointestinal polyposis" is used to include adenomatosis coli, Peutz-Jeghers syndrome, and juvenile polyposis coli.

TABLE 1. *Classification of polyposis coli*

Classification	Diseases
Neoplastic	Adenomatosis coli[a,b] Familial polyposis coli Gardner's syndrome Turcot's syndrome Multiple adenomas[c,d]
Hamartomatous	Peutz-Jegher's syndrome[a,e] Juvenile polyposis coli[a,e]
Inflammatory	Inflammatory polyposis Benign lymphofollicular hyperplasia
Unclassified	Metaplastic polyposis Cronkhite-Canada's syndrome

[a] Heredity proved.
[b] Extremely high tendency for production of cancer in the large bowel.
[c] Heredity not proved but sporadically observed.
[d] Some investigators do not classify this as polyposis.
[e] Higher incidence of large bowel cancer than the general population.

REGISTRATION SYSTEM

The first description of adenomatosis appeared in 1929 in one of the Japanese medical journals. Systematic studies, however, were not done until 1961. In that year, the first national survey was carried out by Komatsu (3). This was later developed into a government cancer research project by us. The Polyposis Center was organized in 1976 by the Tokyo Medical and Dental University.

In the Polyposis Center, information on the proband with hereditary gastrointestinal polyposis is being collected through the following sources: the Japan Large Intestinal Cancer Research Society, inquiry to hospital, published case reports, autopsy records, and voluntary referrals by physicians. The diagnoses were confirmed pathologically and classified according to the previously mentioned criteria. Working pedigrees of the probands were established using the "koseki" (the national family registration records). In order to identify families and members, we devised a system for establishing pedigrees, and a permanent coding was assigned to each individual (Fig. 1).

Individuals thus found to be at high risk for polyposis were placed under surveillance.

The information collected was computerized for analysis and storage. Individuals registered by different institutions were often found to belong to the same family as seen on 53 occasions; by this method, large unknown areas of pedigrees were clarified.

Currently, 534 cases and 397 families with adenomatosis coli have been regis-

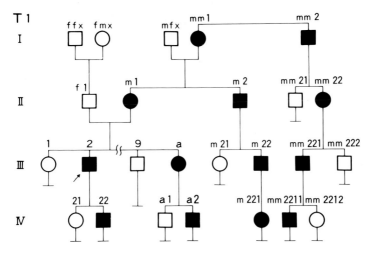

FIG. 1. A new coding system of "working pedigree."

tered (Table 2). Family surveys have been completed on 306 families with 4,535 members. The first-degree relatives of an affected individual were listed for survey. The surveys conducted up to this time have revealed the presence of 848 affected persons which include 383 probands, 173 "call-up cases," and 377 "survey cases" which were confirmed by indirect information such as death certificates or hospital records. The "possible polyposis carriers" were defined as the offsprings, siblings, and parents of the affected persons and numbered 3,424. They are the people at high risk of developing polyposis and large bowel cancers in an epidemiological sense.

The Polyposis Center sends the list of these high-risk people to the physicians who have registered their cases to promote local-level family examinations.

The number of registered patients has been increasing year after year. This trend was particularly marked in call-up cases. This suggests that the operations of the Polyposis Center have been successfully carried out.

GENETIC STUDIES

Population Genetics

Incidence

The incidence of adenomatosis coli among the Japanese population was estimated to be 1 per 10,000 (3). This was not much different from that of Caucasian populations previously reported (Table 3).

TABLE 2. *Number of registered cases (family) (through 12/78)*

Route of information	Adenomatosis coli	P-J syndrome	Multiple adenomas	Juvenile polyposis	Familial large bowel cancer
Society	79 (71)	13 (13)	62 (62)	2 (2)	11 (11)
Inquiry	184 (145)	70 (67)	91 (91)	2 (2)	41 (35)
Literature	50 (40)	7 (7)	7 (7)	0 (0)	1 (1)
Autopsy record	21 (19)	8 (8)	30 (30)	0 (0)	0 (0)
Voluntary	200 (122)	36 (27)	3 (3)	3 (3)	13 (8)
Total	534 (397)	134 (122)	193 (193)	7 (6)	66 (55)

TABLE 3. *Incidence of adenomatosis among the general population*

Country	Reference	Incidence
Japan	Komatsu (3)	1/9.467
U.S.A.	Reed and Neel (4)	1/7.437
U.S.A.	Pierce (5)	1/6.850
England	Veale (6)	1/23.930
Sweden	Alm and Licznerski (7)	1/7.646

Familial Cases and Sporadic Cases

In 46% of the families, no patient but the propositus was found (sporadic case). There was no difference between the familial and sporadic cases morphologically or clinically. The proportion of sporadic cases was found to decrease as the survey progressed (Table 4).

Assuming that all patients are the product of abnormal genes, the proportion of sporadic cases (0.46) is equivalent to the fresh mutation rate (M) plus the sporadic cases from nonpenetrant parents (N). M must be equivalent to the natural selection rate (Q). N was 0.07 and thus M was calculated to be 0.39. Q was calculated from relative fitness (F) (0.88) to be 0.12, which was significantly different from the value of M (8). The implication of data is under study.

Mode of Inheritance

Because both male and female members were affected, autosomal inheritance was apparently responsible. The sex ratio of the proband was 1.7 with females less frequently affected; however, there was no significant difference in patients other than the probands. The observed segregation ratio was calculated to be 0.377 in our series. Penetrance was 0.68. The corrected segregation ratio was 0.544, which closely approximates the theoretically expected value of 0.5 in dominant inheritance (8) (Table 5).

TABLE 4. *Adenomatosis coli: proportion of familial cases*

	No. of families	No. of familial cases	Proportion (%)
	58	21	36
1971.10	59	27	46
1972.10	157	72	46
1973.10	146	77	53
1974.10	166	86	52
1978.12	299	169	57

TABLE 5. *Genetic aspects of adenomatosis coli in Japanese and Caucasians*

	Japanese (authors)	British (Veale)	U.S.A. (Reed)
Familial cases	57%	67%	63%
Male/female ratio	1.61	1.31	1.48
Penetrance (m)	68%	80%	90%
Observed segregation ratio (s)	0.377	.361	0.400
Theoretical segregation ratio (p)[a]	0.543	.458	0.449

[a] $p = s \cdot (2 - m)/[m + 2s \cdot (1 - m)]$.

Cytogenetic and Cytologic Studies

The chromosomal constitution of the somatic cells showed no special karyotypic abnormalities. The number of CS-cells (cells with balanced rearrangement of chromosomes), however, was found to be significantly increased in the polyposis group (10).

A characteristic mode of proliferation in the culture of skin fibroblasts obtained from patients with polyposis has been found compared to normal cells. The former showed greater sensitivity to certain chemicals such as MMC (10), 4NQO (11), and MNNG (12) and to murine sarcoma virus (11).

The fact that the somatic cells of the patients with this disease exhibit "subclinical" abnormalities *in vitro* is of profound interest. It may explain the occurrence of various tumors in organs other than the large intestine such as fibrous tumors. It may also endorse the multihit theory of carcinogenesis. Efforts are being directed to studies along these lines.

PATHOLOGY

Lesions in the Large Intestine

The large bowel of patients with this disease is covered with relatively small polyps, giving a characteristic appearance (Fig. 2). The frequency distribution of patients with multiple polyps registered at our center according to the number of polyps revealed two distinct groups, those with less than 50 polyps and those with more than 100; the former was defined as multiple adenomas and the latter as adenomatosis. The patients with adenomatosis were further divided into two heterogeneous groups, the "dense type" and the "coarse type," depending on the number of adenomas. The criteria for delineating these clusters were macroscopically a count of 5,000 total polyps or a density of 10/cm² and, microscopically, two adenoma foci detected in a unit length of a histological section or adenoma estimated to occupy 20% of the total area of the section (adenoma percent) (11). In patients with the dense type, the onset of carcinoma had been

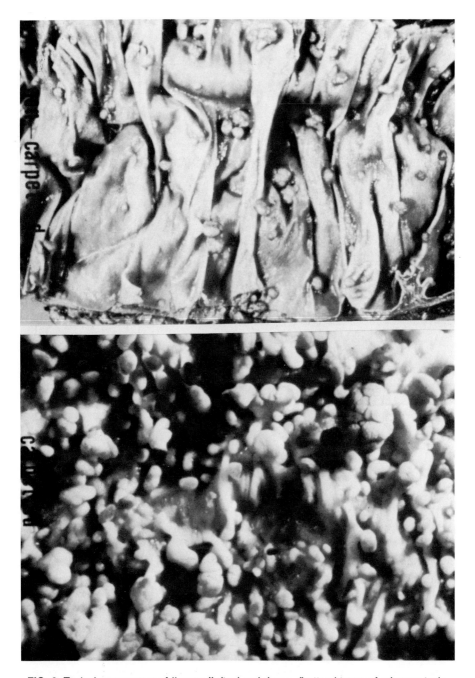

FIG. 2. Typical appearance of "coarse" *(top)* and dense *(bottom)* types of adenomatosis.

at an earlier age than that in patients with the coarse type. The distinction is thus clinically important.

The reason for the difference in manifestation remains unknown. It may be due to a difference in the penetrance of the abnormal single gene or the effect of an allelic modifier gene. Since the dense and coarse types appear to be genetically distinct, this suggests that the former appears to be more probable.

The density of the polyps was found to be distributed rather evenly throughout the large intestine. In 30 out of 32 cases we examined, sessile small polyps (diameter of less than 5 mm) accounted for 80% of the lesions.

Histologically, the majority of the lesions were tubular adenomas, although villous or tubulovillous types were found occasionally. The incidence of cancer in adenomas was 0.05% in adenomas less than 1 cm in diameter; 7% in 1 to 2 cm lesions; 44% in those 2 to 3 cm; and 71% in those over 3 cm. These figures were not significantly different from the figures for adenomas of the large intestine in the general population.

Using the ^{3}H-thymidine label method, DNA synthesizing cells were found only in the deeper two-thirds of the glandular crypts in the normal mucosa of the large intestine, whereas these cells were also found in the superficial layers in the adenomas. The mucosa between polyps in patients with adenomatosis coli was found to show an atypical pattern of DNA synthesizing cells despite the apparent normal morphology (12). In the mucosa of the large intestine of patients with this disease, a defect in the inhibitory mechanism of DNA synthesis was found to precede the occurrence of adenoma. Since such changes were found in children of those affected prior to the onset of the disease, this might be utilized in the future for the early detection of the carriers.

Extracolonic Lesions

Gardner's Syndrome

Among the recent registered cases of adenomatosis, 6.3% had all the stigmata of Gardner's syndrome and 13.3% had incomplete stigmata, whereas the remaining 73.4% had no stigmata or their status was unknown. If more careful observation were done, it is possible that more patients with adenomatosis might have been found to have stigmata of Gardner's syndrome. The above represents the incidence of detection of stigmata of Gardner's syndrome by routine clinical examination. Orthopantomography revealed multiple radiopaque lesions of the jaw representing occult osteomatous lesions in 94% of them (Fig. 3). In the control group, the incidence was 18% (13). The histologic examination at autopsy revealed that they were endosteomas (14). This finding was useful in understanding Gardner's syndrome and also in detecting patients through family surveys. From a clinical viewpoint, adenomatosis with Gardner's stigmata and that without did not show any significant difference in the large bowel manifestations with rare exceptions. The proband with apparent Gardner's stigmata had affected

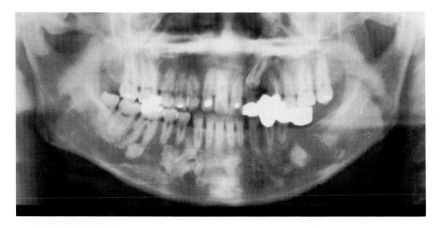

FIG. 3. Occult osteomatous changes and impacted teeth on orthopantomogram of the patient.

members with the stigmata in a significantly higher incidence than in probands without it (Table 6).

Thus I think a specific genotype for Gardner's stigmata may exist, but the penetrance is so weak that it is not able to produce any outstanding heterogeneous trait in the large bowel separately classifiable clinically or pathologically.

Lesions in the Upper Gastrointestinal Tract

We observed gastric polypoid lesions in 70% of the patients examined and in 100% of family members of those with it. Gastric polyps were thus considered to represent an essential trait of this disease (15). This finding was confirmed by others (16,17). The lesions were usually small and multiple, sometimes carpeting the stomach (Fig. 4).

Histologically, they were of two types: one with atypical cells which was found in the antrum and the other with nonatypical cells which was found in

TABLE 6. *Adenomatosis coli: correlation within family members with Gardner's stigmata*

	GS	Propositus		?
		+	−	
Other members	+	5 (2.7)[a]	6 (8.3)	2
	−	7 (9.2)	30 (27.8)	6
	?	2	7	7

$X^2 = 3.18$, $p = 0.1$.

[a] Numbers in parentheses indicate estimated value.

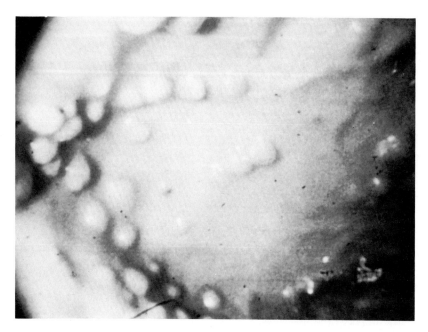

FIG. 4. Multiple polypoid lesions of the gastric body seen by fibergastroscopic study.

the fundic area. In some instances they disappeared after colectomy. No definite evidence of malignant transformation of these lesions was observed. However, gastric cancer seemed to occur more frequently in this disease than in the general population (17).

Polypoid lesions or adenomas were detected in the duodenum in almost 100% (16) and in the jejunum in 70% of the patients (18), if carefully examined.

The question is whether these findings are specific to the Japanese people.

CANCER OCCURRENCE

Malignant foci were detected in the large bowel in 64% of the registered patients.

The cancer in adenomatosis had no characteristic morphology compared to that of the general population other than the fact that the former was more frequently (54%) multiple than the latter (4%).

Distribution within the large bowel showed an increasing frequency in the lower segment which was a pattern similar to that seen in cancers in the general population (Fig. 5).

With the multihit theory of carcinogenesis, age-specific prevalence rate of colon cancer (p) is generally expressed as an exponential function of age (t), $P = At_r$, where r implies the number of mutations necessary for cancer to develop

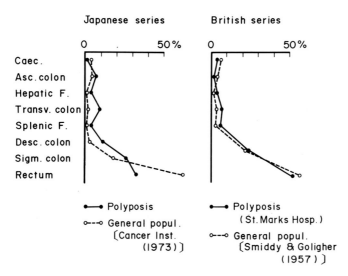

FIG. 5. Distribution of cancer in subsites of the large bowel; a comparison of adenomatosis patients and the general population.

(19). This is expressed as the slope of a straight line when plotted on a logarithmic scale. "A" is constant and indicates the probability of occurrence of the mutations. It is expressed by a shifting of the line in the logarithmic scale.

In colon cancer in the general population of Japan, r was 5.0 in both male and female. In colon cancer in adenomatosis (AC), r was 4.2 for males and 3.4 for females. This is one to two mutations less than that of the general population (20). Thus it is implied that the individual with AC has already received prezygotic mutations; therefore, cancer develops in response to a lesser number of mutations after birth. The age-specific prevalence of adenoma production was also shown as a straight line in full logarithmic scale, but with less slope than that of cancer. This indicates that adenoma production in adenomatosis may require some environmental factors, but the number of mutations must be less than that of cancer. These data were compared with those for Caucasian AC patients presented in Ashley's paper (21), which was mainly from St. Mark's Hospital (Fig. 6). It was unexpectedly observed that the age-specific prevalence curve in AC was quite similar in the two countries. The implications of this evidence should be evaluated further. The only conclusion that can be made thus far is that adenogenesis as well as carcinogenesis in adenomatosis in Caucasian people cannot be modified by changing their habits to those similar to Japanese people.

CONCLUDING REMARKS

According to Dukes (22), the three chief landmarks in the history of adenomatosis are (a) recognition of this condition as a separate disease, (b) recognition

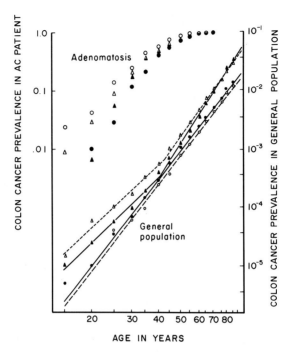

FIG. 6. Age-dependent prevalence of colon cancer in English and Japanese AC patients and the general population. ▲for males and △for females in English and ●for males and ○for females in Japanese. Theoretical curves with solid line for males and dotted line for females.

of its familial predisposition, and (c) understanding of its relation to cancer. We propose to add the fourth and fifth landmarks. They are the recognition of extracolonic manifestations such as Gardner's syndrome and polyps in the upper gastrointestinal tract, and acknowledgment of the "subclinical manifestation" of disease. Since the mode of inheritance is autosomal dominant, a single gene must be responsible for the manifestations of this characteristic condition.

There has now accumulated much knowledge of the phenotypic abnormality, but nothing is known of the interrelationship between genotypic and phenotypic abnormalities. The search for this process may provide the key to understanding carcinogenesis in general in the future.

REFERENCES

1. Bublbrook, R. D., Thomas, B. S., and Utsunomiya, J. (1964): Urinary 11-deoxy-17 oxosteroid in British and Japanese women with reference to the incidence of breast cancer. *Nature*, 201:1189.
2. Bussey, H. J. R. (1975): *Familial Polyposis Coli.* The John Hopkins University Press. Baltimore.
3. Komatsu, I. (1968): A clinical genetic study of multiple polyposis and allied condition. *Jpn. J. Hum. Genet.*, 12:246–297.
4. Reed, J. E., and Neel, J. V. (1955): A genetic study of multiple polyposis of the colon. *Am. J. Hum. Genet.*, 7:236–263.

5. Pierce, E. R. (1968): Some genetic aspects of familial multiple polyposis of the colon in a kindred of 1,422 members. *Dis. Colon Rectum,* 11:321–329.
6. Veale, A. M. O. (1965): *Intestinal Polyposis.* Eugenics Laboratory Memoirs Series 40. Cambridge University Press, London.
7. Alm, J., and Licznerski, G. (1973): The intestinal polyposes. *Clin. Gastroenterol.,* 2:577–602.
8. Utsunomiya, J., Iwama, T., Suzuki, H., et al. (1974): Polyposis coli and heredity. *Stomach Intestine,* 9:1146–1156 (in Japanese).
9. Utsunomiya, J., Iwama, T., Suzuki, H., et al. (1976): A clinical genetic study on familial polyposis coli. Sex ratio. *Jpn. J. Hum. Genet.,* 20:283–284.
10. Utsunomiya, J. (1977): Present status of adenomatosis coli in Japan. In: *Pathophysiology of Carcinogenesis in Digestive Organs,* edited by E. Farber et al., pp. 305–321. University of Tokyo Press, Tokyo, and University Park Press, Baltimore.
11. Iwama, T. (1978): A pathological study of adenomatosis coli. *Jpn. J. Surg.,* 79:10–24 (in Japanese).
12. Iwama, T., and Utsunomiya, J. (1977): The cytokinetic study on the intestinal mucosal epithelium of patients with familial polyposis coli. *Jap. J. Surg.,* 7:230–234.
13. Utsunomiya, J., and Nakamura, T. (1975): The occult osteomatous changes in the mandible in patients with familial polyposis coli. *Br. J. Surg.,* 62:45–51.
14. Ohya, K., Yamamoto, H., Lay, K. M., et al. (1976): The sclerotic changes in the mandible of an autopsy case in patients with familial polyposis coli. *J. Oral Pathol.,* 5:305–311.
15. Utsunomiya, J., Maki, T., Iwama, T., et al. (1974): Gastric lesions of familial polyposis coli. *Cancer,* 34:745–754.
16. Watanabe, H., Enjoji, M., Yao, T., et al. (1977): Accompanying gastro-enteric lesions in familial adenomatosis coli. *Acta Pathol. Jpn.,* 27:823–839.
17. Ohsato, K., Watanabe, H., Itoh, H., et al. (1974): Simultaneous occurrence of multiple gastric carcinomas and familial polyposis coli of the colon. *Jpn. J. Surg.,* 4:165–174.
18. Ohsato, K., Yao, T., Watanabe, H., et al. (1977): Small intestinal involvement in familial polyposis diagnosed by operative intestinal fiberscopy. *Dis. Colon Rectum,* 20:414–420.
19. Knudson, A. G. (1977): Genetic and environmental interaction in the origin of human cancer. In: *Genetics of Human Cancer,* edited by J. J. Mulvihill et al., pp. 391–399. Raven Press, New York.
20. Utsunomiya, J., and Murata, M. (1980): An analysis on the age distribution of colon cancer in adenomatosis coli. *Cancer,* 198–205.
21. Ashley, B. J. B. (1969): Colonic cancer arising in polyposis coli. *J. Med. Genet.,* 6:376–378.
22. Dukes, C. E. (1930): The hereditary factor in polyposis intestine or multiple adenomata. *Cancer Rev.,* 5:241–256.

Colorectal Cancer: Prevention, Epidemiology, and Screening, edited by S. Winawer, D. Schottenfeld, and P. Sherlock. Raven Press, New York © 1980.

Hereditary Adenomatosis of the Colon and Rectum: Recent Studies on the Nature of Cancer Promotion and Cancer Prognosis *in Vitro*

Levy Kopelovich

Memorial Sloan-Kettering Cancer Center, and Cornell University Graduate School of Medical Sciences, New York, New York 10021

Genetic susceptibility to cancer has often been recognized as a major contributor to cancer. Some forms of cancer are clearly hereditary (23,37), and individuals who are carriers are almost certain to develop cancer. Genetic disorders which predispose certain populations to an inordinate risk of cancer have been identified (23,37,53). Recently, another group with an apparent genetic predisposition to cancer has been recognized (4,5a,12,24,37,38). It consists of familial aggregates which show an excess of single or several apparently linked multiple primary cancers, which clearly comprise a nonrandom segment of the spectrum of all cancers. These occur in successive generations with an early age of onset, and at a frequency considerably higher than that found in the general population (4,5a,12,24,37,38). In many instances, members of a family at risk of cancer inherit the responsible trait in a dominant mendelian fashion (4,12,24,38). Presumably, genetic determinants which underlie such a variety of cancer syndromes are involved in the regulation of phenotypic expressions associated with oncogenesis. Further, the elucidation of genetic-environmental interaction could play a major role in the development of means for identifying conditions in individuals predisposed to cancer.

This chapter summarizes experiments on the *in vitro* characterization of human skin fibroblasts (SF) obtained from individuals with hereditary adenomatosis of the colon and rectum (ACR). The results show that although cutaneous biopsies of ACR patients and a portion of their F_1 progeny are histologically normal, the cultured fibroblasts are abnormal with regard to several aspects of *in vitro* growth control and cell architecture (25–34,44,45). The findings suggest a systemic disorder of stromal cells in ACR patients that might provide clues to carcinogenic mechanisms involving the large bowel and possibly other forms of internal cancer. The delineation of precursor states in this form of colorectal cancer may also help to clarify susceptibility mechanisms and identify high-risk individuals most likely to benefit from screening programs.

THE MODEL SYSTEM: EXPERIMENTAL APPROACHES AND
PROBLEMS

At present, it is seldom possible to detect persons at risk of developing any of the various forms of cancer before the appearance of a frank invasive or a metastatic growth. Two serious problems limit attempts to detect a preneoplastic state or a disposition to eventual neoplasia. They are the inherent low frequency of incidence of any single type of tumor and the difficulty of obtaining identical sample material from prospective or actual patients once they are located.

Our approach to the first of these two problems has been to study in detail an inherited form of cancer, adenomatosis of the colon and rectum, the ultimate manifestation of which is colonic neoplasia by the third decade of life. Because ACR is inherited as an autosomal dominant trait, patients can be expected to pass it on to one-half of their offspring. The other half have the same low probability of developing this cancer as do normal individuals. Thus, ACR families offer a chance to monitor children who have no oncological symptoms but who will certainly develop them.

Our approach to the second problem has been to concentrate on the *in vitro* properties of cells obtained by cutaneous biopsy from patients and their families rather than on cells grown from biopsy material of tissues at risk, or on biopsied tumor tissues. By using only cultured skin fibroblasts, we can examine a single cell type under reproducible conditions, for presumptive cellular differences between ACR^+ and ACR^- individuals.

Hereditary adenomatosis of the colon and rectum has been used in our laboratory during the past 6 years as an experimental model for the study of tumor promotion and tumor prognosis (26–28). It occurs in about 1 in 8,000 live births, and although it is inherited in an autosomal dominant pattern (3,13,41), it seems probable that additional genes may pleiotropically modify its expression (3,41; R. McConnell, *this volume*). The close association of ACR with neoplasia has been established in a large number of studies in which frank malignancy presumably develops from polyps, and carcinomas of the large bowel arise in virtually all untreated cases (3,41). A genetic variant called Gardner's syndrome combines ACR with bone tumors, especially osteomas, and lesions of the skin and soft tissues, such as sebaceous cysts and fibromas (13).

Fibroblastic cells are ubiquitous and provide the structural elements of all organs throughout the body. The cells used in our study were skin fibroblasts obtained as biopsies from normal-appearing skin on the lateral aspect of the forearm of affected and normal individuals. The skin fibroblasts were grown in culture and were monitored with respect to biological and biochemical parameters previously identified with the malignant state in experimental animals and in man (46,56,58). Parts of these studies, including all methods described here, have been published elsewhere (25,29–34,44,45), and the results are summarized in Table 1. In these studies no differences have ever been observed between SF derived from ACR patients and Gardner's syndrome patients.

TABLE 1. *Systemic manifestations associated with loss of regulatory control mechanisms and biochemical alterations in hereditary adenomatosis of the colon and rectum*

Human phenotypes	Phenotypic expressions in cultured human skin fibroblasts											
	Growth in nutrient-deprived environment	Loss of contact inhibition	Formation of cell aggregates	Increased proteolytic activity	Deformed actin cables	Increased agglutination by lectins	Increased 2-deoxy-glucose uptake	Decreased toxicity to TPA	Susceptibility to transformation by an oncogenic virus	Anchorage independence	Embryo-specific proteins	Ability to form palpable nodules
The preneoplastic phase (multiple steps presumably due to a single mutation)												
The neoplastic phase (multiple steps)												
Clinically symptomatic	+	+	+	+	+	+	+	+	+	+	+	+
Clinically asymptomatic progeny												
Positive	+	+	+	+	+	ND	ND	ND	+	+	+	+
Negative	−	−	−	−	−	ND	ND	ND	−	(+)	(+)	(+)
Normals	−	−	−	−	−	−	−	−	−	(+)	(+)	(+)

Vertical arrow indicates the transforming event; in this system the transforming agents were KiMSV and SV40, and possibly TPA as well. The efficacy of virus-transformation of cells from normal individuals (designated as +), and was considerably less than that from ACR individuals, but all transformed cells gave rise to the same phenotypic expressions. The clinically asymptomatic progeny has been subdivided into positive and negative according to our experimental findings (28).

CELL CULTURE STUDIES

Serum Requirements and Growth Properties

Fibroblast growth *in vitro* is regulated by at least three different environmental variables. In order for cell division to occur, the amount of serum present must be adequate, the cell density must not be too high, and the cells must be provided with a solid substrate on which to anchor and spread. Agents such as oncogenic viruses or chemical carcinogens may cause the loss of sensitivity to one or all of these variables (46,56,58). Some, but not all, of these transformations also confer a tumorigenic potential on the cells. For many transformants, the ability to grow without an anchoring substrate is the event most closely correlated with tumorigenicity (46,56). Certain cell populations that lack serum sensitivity but retain an anchorage requirement have been shown to be nontumorigenic. Apparently, selection for the loss of sensitivity to one regulatory constraint after transformation does not necessarily lead to the loss of sensitivity to any of the others (46,54,58).

SF from ACR individuals and from about one-half of their children, but not from normals, have partially lost serum- and density-sensitive growth control in culture (25,33,45). Their cloning efficiency is considerably higher, and their clonal morphology considerably tighter than those of normal cells (33,45). ACR skin fibroblasts are similar to normal SF in their failure to grow in the absence of anchorage and in their failure to form tumors *in vivo* (33). Recently, however, we have been able to show that anchorage sensitivity of ACR cells is not absolute and that growth in agar might occur spontaneously, albeit at low frequency.

Intracellular Proteases and Actin Matrices

Two major biochemical correlates of *in vivo* malignancy are increased production of plasminogen-dependent and plasminogen-independent proteases and deformed cytoskeletal structures (14,47). In the cytoplasm of well-spread cultured normal cells, actin is organized into a network of cables that run the length of the cell just inside the adherent cell membrane (14). A diffuse matrix replaces the cables in fibroblasts that have become tumorigenic as a result of chemical or viral transformation (14).

Using immunofluorescence with antibody to actin, we have found a similar disruption of actin organization in cultured SF from ACR individuals in about half of their children, while a distinct portion of the F_1 progeny showed a pattern identical to that found in normal SF (31). Apparently, this class of inherited colonic carcinoma is accompanied by a systemic aberration in the organization of fibroblast cytoskeleton (31). Elevated levels of intracellular plasminogen-dependent protease were also found in ACR, but not in normal cells (25).

Membrane-Related Parameters

In a related study we have been able to demonstrate that ACR cells, but not normal cells, show increased agglutination by concanavalin A (7; A. Braun and L. Kopelovich, *unpublished observations*) and increased uptake of 2-deoxyglucose (7). They were also considerably more resistant to the toxic effects of 12-*o*-tetradecanoyl phorbol-13-acetate (TPA), suggesting perhaps a decrease in the number of certain types of receptors and/or affinity, associated with the binding of TPA to the cell membrane (see below). The differential toxicity by TPA is currently being used in our laboratory as the most reliable single parameter to distinguish between normal and ACR individuals (L. Kopelovich, *in preparation*).

ACR cells were similar to normal SF in their ability to express intracellular LETS protein (S. Rennard and L. Kopelovich, *unpublished*). cholesterol feedback inhibition (25), and in their sensitivity to X-ray and UV-induced cell damage (L. Kopelovich, *unpublished*).

Differential Susceptibility to Transformation by Oncogenic Viruses

Virally induced cell transformation has been used to study variations in susceptibility of human mutant cells to neoplasia (1,22,44,55).

Infection of SF with the Kirsten murine sarcoma virus (KiMSV) showed that cell cultures derived from ACR individuals and a fraction of the clinically asymptomatic ACR progeny were considerably more susceptible to transformation by KiMSV than were normal subjects (44). These results are probably due to the transformation process and not to a type C virus replication step (44). In a separate study, we have shown that ACR cells are also more susceptible to an SV40-induced T antigen display and transformation (34). SF from several clinically asymptomatic ACR progeny were resistant to transformation by both these viruses. The virally transformed cells have become anchorage-independent and, in the case of KiMSV, formed transient nodules s.c. in athymic mice.

The susceptibility of ACR cells to transformation by KiMSV and SV40 appears to segregate among the ACR progeny in a fashion identical with our previous observation about the occurrence of abnormal phenotypic expression in these cells. It suggests that the ACR trait and its mode of inheritance are also responsible for the increased sensitivity to transformation by the viral probes. The apparent correlation between the results obtained with SV40 and those with KiMSV further suggests that genetic information residing within ACR cells, probably in the form of an ACR mutation, renders them more susceptible. In this respect, the oncogene postulate (18) and the DNA provirus hypothesis (54) are of interest. We are currently searching for putative gene products which may play a role in the malignant transformation of the ACR cell. These may be similar perhaps to the pp60 or the pp53 proteins, also known as sarc and "middle t" polypeptides, respectively (9,11,19,36,42,51).

Cancer-Related Antigens

The appearance of embryo-specific proteins in tumor cells suggests an association of cancer-related antigens with malignancy (2,8,52).

The occurrence of embryo-specific proteins in SF from ACR individuals during the preneoplastic state (26–28) and following transformation by KiMSV and SV40 was investigated. The results show that cancer-related antigens are expressed in the virally transformed cells, but not in mock infected SF (17). Apparently, the occurrence of embryo-specific proteins in ACR cells is not associated with the preneoplastic state, but is a consequence of viral transformation. It is of considerable interest that infection of these cells by the RNA oncogenic virus elicited the synthesis of fetal-like antigens, whereas that by the DNA oncogenic virus affected the appearance of placental-like antigens (17). How the type of viral nucleic acid and its mode of replication might affect the synthesis of specific host-cell neoantigens in the course of a virally-induced cell transformation remains to be established. In this respect, mock infected cells and both KiMSV and SV40 transformed normal or ACR cells were negative with regard to human choriogonadotropin, α-2 microglobulin, carcinoembryonic antigen, and α-fetoprotein (17).

ON THE QUESTION OF TUMOR PROMOTION

Malignant transformation is a multiphase process apparently caused by carcinogens and subject to the influence of promoters (5,6,16,39). A potent class of tumor promoting agents are the naturally occurring phorbol esters (15,57), such as TPA. Through the use of phorbol esters, a two-stage process of malignant transformation has been demonstrated in the mouse skin model (5,6,57) and more recently in cell culture systems (35,39a,40,59). Studies *in vitro* suggest that TPA reversibly affects terminal differentiation in certain model systems, and that its function is presumably to increase the probability of expression of the malignant phenotype (59)

To date, no specific biological feature has been identified with the process of cancer initiation (59). The ACR cell presumably represents an "initiated state" due to a dominant mutation, and therefore, for the first time provides a means for the characterization of the initiated state. Thus the possibility that ACR cells exist in a state which in the presence of a promoter(s) alone may become malignantly transformed has been a subject of considerable research in our laboratory. We have previously demonstrated an unusual biphasic dose response of cultured human SF to TPA (29). This may indicate that TPA affects at least two distinct processes of cell proliferation: one which is inhibitory to cell growth, but can be saturated at relatively low concentrations, and another at the higher concentration range which stimulates cell proliferation. Whether these results suggest the existence of at least two cell populations, each of which displays a distinct type of receptor for TPA, or a single cell population with at least two types of receptors for TPA, remains to be established. These seemingly diametrically opposed results may possibly be related to some, but not all, of the tumor promoting effects of TPA. The non-tumor promoter analogue of TPA, 4-*O*-methyl-12-*O*-tetradecanoyl-phorbol-13-acetate (15), gave a usual dose-response pattern characteristic of a drug with a single mode of action. In addition, the epithelial growth factor (EGF) showed a dose response different from that of TPA, suggesting that at least some receptor sites are not shared by these two growth stimulating factors (L. Kopelovich, *unpublished*). It is also of interest that the greatest toxicity due to TPA in our cell system (1 to 2 ng/ml) coincided almost exactly with the maximum of SCE induction by TPA in rodent cell lines (John B. Little, *personal communication*).

The chronic application of TPA has been shown to effect a partial loss of anchorage sensitivity of ACR cell cultures, and cells selected for anchorage independence through isolation from agar apparently respond primarily to the growth-stimulating ability of TPA (29). The agar-growing cells either plated in monolayer cultures or put through a second passage in agar cloned at an efficiency considerably higher than that of non-agar growers (29). They also showed a tighter clonal morphology, similar to that of transformed rodent cells *in vitro*. However, we have also found that growth in agar due to TPA cannot be serially sustained beyond two passages in agar; it is transient during consecutive passages in liquid culture and is variable for a given human cell strain during different periods of TPA application (29,30). The results indicate a high degree of heterogeneity during selection for the anchorage-independent phenotype.

Previous attempts to inoculate TPA-treated ACR cells s.c. in the nude mouse have failed to yield any tumors (29). Recently, the inoculation of these cells into the anterior chamber of the eye of a nude mouse apparently gave rise to a tumor which is characterized by uniformly appearing, highly basophilic, fibroblast-like cells (30). TPA has been shown to enhance the stable transformation of murine and, more recently, of human foreskin fibroblasts previously exposed to a carcinogen (35,39a,40). Thus our results may indicate that the ACR mutation is a complete one for tumor growth, representing an initiated state (28), and that the chronic application of TPA, in support of the two-stage "Berenblum hypothesis" (5) can precipitate the final oncogenic event. Alternatively, this cell mass growing *in vivo* may represent an intermediary state, similar perhaps to the TPA-induced stable papillomas in the mouse skin model (5,6) or to the clinical occurrence of polyps in the colon. The latter would suggest that an additional mutation(s) is necessary for the malignant transformation of ACR cells with certain promoters acting during all phases of oncogenesis to increase the probability of expression of the malignant phenotype.

Just how the presence of TPA in ACR cells effects a transition from the initiated state to the neoplastic state is still a matter of conjecture. SF from ACR individuals are karyollogically normal (45), and we are investigating the possibility that chromosomal restructuring and/or increased ploidy are associated with the promotion of tumorigenicity by TPA in our cell system. These might conceivably be consistent with a somatic mutation(s). In this respect, an elegant analysis of lymphoma development that proposes diversity of initiation followed by convergent cytogenetic evolution has been recently enunciated (21). If as has been suggested, the dominant cancer trait occurs in a class of tissue differentiating genes (24), the elucidation of their mechanism of action in response to tumor promoters *vis à vis* differentiation would be important not only for the problem of cancer but also for the understanding of normal development.

SYSTEMIC ABNORMALITIES

The abnormalities we found in the cancer-bearing and the cancer-prone ACR individuals appear to be systemic. They are expressed in the skin although the affected organ is primarily the colon. This is of particular importance since most malignant tumors in man are of epithelial origin. We have previously suggested that defects in fibroblast growth control and organization may be related to the development of adenocarcinomas (31). It is possible that one element of normal growth regulation of epithelial cells *in situ* may be provided by the fibroblasts residing beneath the basement membrane (21). Indeed, efficient *in vitro* culture of normal human keratinocytes requires the presence of irradiated fibroblasts (48). Moreover, a tight temporal relationship has been shown to exist between epithelial and stromal cells in the epitheliomesenchymal matrix of the colon during cell differentiation (20). Recent work also suggests that fibroblastic abnormalities detectable *in vitro* may be concomitant with certain nonhereditary tumors of epithelial origin (43,50).

Clearly, it is an easier task to scan cultured SF than it is to obtain epithelial cells from most tissues at high risk for malignancy. However, other cell types which might be accessible for tests similar to those indicated above should be considered, e.g., epithelial, endothelial, and lymphoid cells. We are currently studying epidermis-derived epithelial cells alone, and in the presence of fibroblasts as feeder layers, from normal and ACR individuals in all possible permutations. Preliminary experiments indicate that SF from ACR individuals enhance both the growth and differentiation of mouse epidermis-derived epithelial cells under physiological conditions *in vitro* (L. Kopelovich and N. Fusenig, *unpublished*). It is hoped that such a study will provide further insight into the nature of systemic expressions in individuals genetically predisposed to cancer. In this respect, a spontaneous increase in ploidy has been observed in epithelial cells derived from the skin and colon of Gardner individuals (10), but not in skin fibroblasts of ACR patients (45).

In the context of the preceding paragraphs, it should be noted that when the inherited gene in an individual predisposed to cancer supplies the event and/or information for more than one kind of tumor, the array of tumors seen in such individuals would depend not only on the spontaneous occurrence of further events in somatic cells (24), but also on epigenetic control mechanisms

(49), and on environmental factors (23,28,39). For example, a tentative explanation for the high specificity of colon cancer in ACR individuals might be that the colon is the major organ which is exposed to potential carcinogens and cancer promoters in large amounts and is highly sensitive to their action. The higher susceptibility to these compounds may also be due, in part, to its considerable proliferative and cell renewal activities.

ON THE QUESTION OF TUMOR PROGNOSIS

We propose that phenotypic expressions occurring systemically can be used together as diagnostic indices for individuals with latent ACR, and possibly for those who are at high risk of other forms of internal cancer. Among those of the clinically asymptomatic F_1 progeny who have been diagnosed by our criteria as potential carriers of the ACR trait, several have eventually shown the clinical manifestations of the disease, and the others are being monitored at regular time intervals for colonic and extracolonic abnormalities. A prospective study has thus been initiated on the predictive value of tests carried out on skin fibroblasts of ACR pedigrees (Table 1). In general, however, the scatter of values emphasizes that each test by itself cannot be used with absolute certainty as a marker of cancer risk for this or any other population at risk. The use of all tests together, and a large sample, may help define confidence limits for determining the probable risk of cancer in any individual with a certain value. In addition, the specificity of these tests with regard to malignancy should be ascertained in a large number of cancer syndromes. For example, persons from colon cancer-prone families without adenomatous polyposis showed no disturbance of actin-containing cables in SF (32).

Current efforts in our laboratory are directed at studying large population groups who develop multiple forms of cancer, and in which extensive familial aggregates of cancer occur. In such families, the gene carriers will have a high probability of cancer development, and as in ACR families, events that are necessary for cancer development may have a high probability of occurrence in any environment. However, we should anticipate that other genetically determined differences among people will become apparent with exposure to environmental agents.

We have recently identified apparently normal individuals in our control group whose skin fibroblasts display a pattern similar to that of the ACR cell phenotype. Whether the occurrence of such individuals in the control population indicates persons at risk of cancer or is coincidental with a "risk profile" of the ACR patient remains to be established. Clearly, the frequency at which such individuals occur in the general population should be determined.

Based on our current knowledge, it seems that the time is near for a major undertaking to screen for persons who are likely to be at an increased risk of cancer, perhaps through walk-in clinics. The identification of such "risk profiles" might provide invaluable information about cancer prognosis and cancer control.

SUMMARY

In the studies described here, we have proposed that the ACR cell exists in an *initiated state* due to a dominant mutation. We have demonstrated that these cells can be made to grow *in vivo* when exposed to TPA alone. This simple experimental model provides a novel system for the study of tumor promotion *in vitro*.

The apparent susceptibility of ACR cells to transformation by both KiMSV and SV40 indicates that genetic information residing within these cells, probably in the form of an ACR mutation, renders them more susceptible.

Our findings suggest a systemic disorder of stromal cells in ACR individuals that might provide insight about carcinogenic mechanisms involving the large bowel.

The ability to delineate precursor states through the identification of transformation-related phenotypic expressions may help identify high-risk groups most likely to benefit from screening programs.

ACKNOWLEDGMENTS

This work is dedicated to the memory of Dr. Aaron Bendich—scientist, teacher, friend. I wish to thank Ms. N. Bias, Ms. P. Monagham, Ms. R. Vuolo, and Ms. T. Shapiro for excellent technical assistance. This work was supported in part by Contract NO1 CP-43366 and Grant CA-08748 from the National Cancer Institute and by Grants CA-19259 and CA-21623 from the National Large Bowel Cancer Project.

REFERENCES

1. Aaronson, S., and Todaro, G. (1975): Transformation and virus growth by murine sarcoma viruses in human cells. *Nature,* 225:458–459.
2. Alexander, P. (1972): Foetal antigens in cancer. *Nature,* 235:137–141.
3. Alm, T., and Licznerski, G. (1973): The intestinal polyposes. *Clin. Gastroenterol.* 2:577–601.
4. Anderson, D. E., and Romsdahl. M. M. (1977): Family history: A criterion for selective screening. In: *Genetics of Human Cancer,* edited by J. J. Mulvihill, R. W. Miller, and J. F. Fraumeni, Jr., pp. 357–362. Raven Press, New York.
5. Berenblum, I. (1978): Established principles and unresolved problems in carcinogenesis. *J. Natl. Cancer Inst.,* 60:723–726.
5a. Blattner, W. A., McGuire, D. B., Mulvihill, J. J., Lampkin, B. C., Hananian, J., and Fraumeni, J. F., Jr. (1979): Genealogy of cancer in a family. *J.A.M.A.,* 241:259–261.
6. Boutwell, R. K. (1974): Some biological aspects of skin carcinogenesis. *Prog. Exp. Tumor Res.,* 4:207–250.
7. Chopan, M., and Kopelovich, L. (1980): The suppression of tumorigenicity in cell hybrids. II. The relationship between tumorigenicity and transformation-related parameters *in vitro. Exp. Cell Biol. (in press).*
8. Coggins, J. H., and Anderson, N. G. (1974): Cancer, differentiation and embryonic antigens: Some central problems. *Adv. Cancer Res.,* 19:105–165.
9. Collett, M. S., Erikson, E., Purchio, A. F., Brugge, J. S., and Erikson, R. L. (1979): A normal cell protein similar in structure and function to the avian sarcoma virus transforming gene product. *Proc. Natl. Acad. Sci. U.S.A.,* 76:3159–3163.
10. Danes, B. S. (1976): Increased tetraploidy: Cell-specific for the Gardner gene in the cultured cell. *Cancer,* 38:1983–1986.

11. Deleo, A. B., Jay, G., Appella, E., Dubois, G. C., Law, L. W., and Old, L. J. (1979): Detection of a transformation related antigen in chemically induced sarcomas and other transformed cells of the mouse. *Proc. Natl. Acad. Sci. U.S.A.*, 76:2420–2424.
12. Fraumeni, J. F., Jr. (1977): Clinical patterns of familial cancer. In: *Genetics of Human Cancer,* edited by J. J. Mulvihill, R. W. Miller, and J. F. Fraumeni, Jr., pp. 223–235. Raven Press, New York.
13. Gardner, E., and Richards, R. (1953): Multiple cutaneous and subcutaneous lesions occurring simultaneously with hereditary polyposis and osteomatosis. *Am. J. Hum. Genet.,* 5:139–148.
14. Goldman, R., Pollard, T., and Rosenbaum, J. (eds.) (1976): *Cell Motility, Vol. 1–3,* pp. 1–1373. Cold Spring Harbor Laboratory, Cold Spring Harbor, New York.
15. Hecker, E. (1971): Isolation and characterization of the cocarcinogenic principle from croton oil. *Methods Cancer Res.,* 6:439–484.
16. Heidelberger, C. (1975): Chemical carcinogenesis. *Annu. Rev. Biochem.,* 44:79–121.
17. Higgins, P., and Kopelovich, L. (1980): Expression of embryo-specific proteins in human skin fibroblasts transformed by an oncogenic virus. *(Submitted for publication).*
18. Huebner, R. J., and Todaro, G. J. (1969): Oncogenes of RNA tumor viruses as determinants of cancer. *Proc. Natl. Acad. Sci. U.S.A.,* 64:1087–1094.
19. Karess, R. E., Hayward, W. S., and Hanafusa, H. (1979): Cellular information in the genome of recovered avian sarcoma virus directs the synthesis of transforming protein. *Proc. Natl. Acad. Sci. U.S.A.,* 76:3154–3158.
20. Kaye, G. I., Lane, N., and Pascal, R. R. (1968): Colonic pericryptal fibroblasts sheath: Replication, migration, and cytodifferentiation of a mesenchymal cell system in adult tissue. *Gastroenterology,* 54:835–865.
21. Klein, G. (1979): Lymphoma development in mice and humans: Diversity of initiation is followed by convergent cytogenetic evolution. *Proc. Natl. Acad. Sci. U.S.A.,* 76:2442–2446.
22. Klement, V., Friedman, M., McAllister, R., Nelson-Rees, W., and Huebner, R. (1971): Differences in susceptibility of human cells to mouse sarcoma virus. *J. Natl. Cancer Inst.,* 47:65–73.
23. Knudson, A. G. (1977): Genetics and etiology of human cancer. In: *Advances in Human Genetics,* edited by H. Harris and K. Hirshhorn, pp. 1–66. Raven Press, New York.
24. Knudson, A. G. (1979): Hereditary cancer. *J.A.M.A.,* 241:279.
25. Kopelovich, L. (1977): Phenotypic markers in human skin fibroblasts as possible diagnostic indices of hereditary adenomatosis of the colon and rectum. *Cancer,* 40:2534–2541.
26. Kopelovich, L. (1977): Familial polyposis: A model of tumor progression. In: *Workshop on Cancer Invasion and Metastasis: Biologic Mechanisms and Therapy,* edited by S. Day, pp. 375–387. Raven Press, New York.
27. Kopelovich, L. (1978): Cutaneous manifestations occurring systemically in heritable forms of cancer. Proc. 1st Int. Symp. on Inborn Error of Metabolism in Man. *Monogr. Hum. Genet.,* 10:154–168.
28. Kopelovich, L. (1980): Familial polyposis: A model of tumor progression and tumor prognosis. *Surg. Rounds,* 3:30–34.
29. Kopelovich, L., and Bias, N. (1979): Tumor promoter induces loss of anchorage dependence in human skin fibroblasts from individuals genetically predisposed to cancer. *Exp. Cell Biol.,* 48:207–217.
30. Kopelovich, L., Bias, N., and Helson, L. (1979): Tumor promoter alone induces malignant transformation of human skin fibroblasts from individuals genetically predisposed to cancer. *Nature,* 282:619–261.
31. Kopelovich, L., Conlon, S., and Pollack, R. (1977): Defective organization of actin in cultured skin fibroblasts. *Proc. Natl. Acad. Sci. U.S.A.,* 74:3019–3022.
32. Kopelovich, L., Lipkin, M., Blattner, W. A., Fraumeni, J. F., Jr., Lynch, H. T., and Pollack, R. (1980): Organization of cytoskeletal actin in cultured skin fibroblasts from individuals at high risk of colon cancer. *J. Clin. Invest., (submitted).*
33. Kopelovich, L., Pfeffer, L., and Bias, N. (1979): Growth characteristics of human skin fibroblasts *in vitro.* A simple experimental approach for the identification of hereditary adenomatosis of the colon and rectum. *Cancer,* 43:218–223.
34. Kopelovich, L., and Sirlin, S. (1980): Human skin fibroblasts from individuals genetically predisposed to cancer are sensitive to an SV40-induced T antigen display and transformation. *Cancer,* 45:1108–1111.
35. Lasne, C., Gentil, A., and Chouroulinkov, I. (1974): Two-stage malignant transformation of rat fibroblasts in tissue culture. *Nature,* 247:490–491.

36. Linzer, H. I., and Levine, A. J. (1979): Characterization of a 54K dalton cellular SV40 tumor antigen present in SV40-transformed cells and uninfected embryonal carcinoma cells. *Cell,* 17:43–52.

37. Lynch, H. T. (1976): *Cancer Genetics,* pp. 1–639. Charles C Thomas, Springfield, Ill.

38. Lynch, H. T., Harris, R. E., Lynch, P. M., Guirgis, H. A., Lynch, J. P., and Bardawil, W. A. (1977): Role of heredity in multiple primary cancers. *Cancer,* 40:1845–1849.

39. Miller, E. C. (1978): Some current perspectives on chemical carcinogenesis in humans and experimental animals. *Cancer Res.,* 38:1479–1496.

39a. Milo, G. F., and Dipaolo, J. A. (1978): Neoplastic transformation of human diploid cells *in vitro* after chemical carcinogen treatment. *Nature,* 275:130–132.

40. Mondal, S., Brankow, D. W., and Heidelberger, C. (1976): Two-stage oncogenesis in cultures of C3H 1OT ½ cells. *Cancer Res.,* 36:2254–2260.

41. Morson, B., and Bussey, H. (1970): Predisposing causes of intestinal cancer. *Cur. Probl. Surg.,* 1–50.

42. Oppermann, H., Levinson, A. D., Varmus, H. E., Levintow, L., and Bishop, J. M. (1979): Uninfected vertebrate cells contain a protein that is closely related to the product of the avian sarcoma virus transforming gene (src). *Proc. Natl. Acad. Sci. U.S.A.,* 76:1804–1808.

43. Owens, R., Smith, H., Nelson-Rees, W., and Springer, E. (1976): Epithelial cell cultures from normal and cancerous tissues. *J. Natl. Cancer Inst.,* 56:843–849.

44. Pfeffer, L., and Kopelovich, L. (1977): Differential genetic susceptibility of cultured human skin fibroblasts to transformation by Kirsten murine sarcoma virus. *Cell,* 10:313–320.

45. Pfeffer, L., Lipkin, M., Stutman, O., and Kopelovich, L. (1976): Growth abnormalities of cultured human skin fibroblasts derived from individuals with hereditary adenomatosis of the colon and rectum. *J. Cell. Physiol.,* 80:29–38.

46. Pollack, R. (ed.) (1975): *Readings in Mammalian Cell Culture,* pp. 1–864. Cold Spring Harbor Laboratory, Cold Spring Harbor, New York.

47. Reich, E., Rifkin, D. B., and Shaw, E. (eds.) (1975): *Proteases and Biological Control,* pp. 1–1021. Cold Spring Harbor Laboratory, Cold Spring Harbor, New York.

48. Rheinwald, J., and Green, H. (1975): Serial cultivation of strains of human epidermal keratinocytes: The formation of keratinizing colonies from single cells. *Cell,* 6:331–344.

49. Riccardi, V. M. (1977): Cellular interaction as a limiting factor in the expression of oncogenic mutations: A hypothesis. In: *Genetics of Human Cancer,* edited by J. J. Mulvihill, R. W. Miller, and J. F. Fraumeni, Jr., pp. 383–385. Raven Press, New York.

50. Smith, H. S., Owens, R. B., Hiller, A. J., Nelson-Rees, W. A., and Johnston, J. O. (1976): The biology of human cells in tissue culture. I. Characterization of cell derived from osteogenetic sarcomas. *Int. J. Cancer,* 17:219–237.

51. Stehelin, D., Varmus, H. E., Bishop, J. M., and Vogt, P. K. (1976): DNA related to the transforming gene(s) of avian sarcoma viruses is present in normal avian DNA. *Nature,* 260:171–173.

52. Stonehill, E., and Bendich, A. (1970): Retrogenetic expression: The reappearance of embryonal antigens in cancer cells. *Nature,* 228:370–372.

53. Swift, M. (1976): Malignant disease in heterozygotes carriers. Cancer and genetics. *Birth Defects,* 12:133–144.

54. Temin, H. M. (1977): The relationship of tumor virology to an understanding of nonviral cancers. *Bioscience,* 27:170–176.

55. Todaro, G., and Martin, G. (1967): Increased susceptibility of Down syndrome fibroblasts to transformation by SV40. *Proc. Soc. Exp. Biol. Med.,* 124:1232–1236.

56. Tooze, J. (1973): *The Molecular Biology of Tumor Viruses,* pp. 1–743. Cold Spring Harbor Laboratory. Cold Spring Harbor, New York

57. Van Duuren, B. L. (1976): Tumor-promoting and cocarcinogenic agents in chemical carcinogenesis. In: *Chemical Carcinogens,* Monograph 173, edited by C. E. Searle, pp. 24–51. American Chemical Society, Washington, D.C.

58. Watson, J. (1979): *The Transformed Cell,* pp. 1–121. Cold Spring Harbor Laboratory, Cold Spring Harbor, New York.

59. Weinstein, I. B., Yamasaki, H., Wigler, M., Lee, L. S., Fisher, P. B., Jeffrey, A., and Grunberger, D. (1979): Molecular and cellular events associated with the action of initiating carcinogens and tumor promoters. In: *Carcinogens: Identification and Mechanisms of Action,* edited by A. Clark Griffin and Charles R. Shaw, pp. 399–418. Raven Press, New York.

Colorectal Cancer: Prevention, Epidemiology, and Screening, edited by S. Winawer, D. Schottenfeld, and P. Sherlock. Raven Press, New York © 1980.

Risk in Families of Patients with Colon Cancer

David E. Anderson

Department of Biology, The University of Texas System Cancer Center M. D. Anderson Hospital and Tumor Institute, Houston, Texas 77030

The large bowel is perhaps the site of more familial-occurring and heritable cancers than any other site. Large bowel cancer long has been divisible into a number of inherited types including familial polyposis, Gardner's syndrome, Peutz-Jeghers syndrome, discrete polyps, Turcot syndrome, diffuse gastrointestinal polyposis, juvenile polyposis, familial site-specific colon cancer, and the cancer family syndrome. This listing suggests that most cases of inherited large bowel cancer are associated with some type of polyposis. But this impression is erroneous because the inherited forms of polyposis account for only a minor fraction of all large bowel cancers (7). In the series of patients with cancer of the colon and rectum reported by Lovett (12), less than 1% had polyposis, whereas 26% had a family history of colon cancer not associated with polyposis. High frequencies of familial colon cancer not associated with polyposis have also been reported by Postlethwait et al. (18) and Anderson and Strong (7).

The present report will be concerned with the risks of large bowel cancer in families of patients with cancer of the colon developing independently of preexisting polyposis coli or other disease.

RETROSPECTIVE STUDIES

That cancer of the large bowel may involve a genetic component comes from two primary sources: retrospective and pedigree studies. Retrospective studies are concerned with the morbidity or mortality rates or both of large bowel cancer in relatives of patients compared with the rates in some type of control or with expected rates based on population statistics. An early example of this type of investigative approach applied to colon cancer was the study of Woolf (21). He compared mortality rates in the first-degree relatives of patients with the rates in controls, who matched the relatives in the year of death, county of residence, race, sex, and age. Of the 763 deaths among relatives, 26 had cancer of the large bowel compared with eight in the controls. The relatives of patients thus had a 3.2-fold higher mortality rate from large bowel cancer than controls. The number of deaths from other types of cancer was similar in the relative and control groups.

Macklin (16), in a later study, used a slightly different approach. She compared the frequency of large bowel cancer in deceased relatives of patients with large bowel cancer to the rate expected on the basis of age-specific proportionate death rates for the state of Ohio. She made a special attempt to exclude patients with multiple polyposis. Among 392 first-degree relatives, 31 had cancer of the large bowel, whereas only 9.7 were expected. This 3.2-fold excess was identical to the value obtained in Woolf's (21) study. Macklin was able to rule out biased ascertainment and environmental similarity as explanations of the increased risks for relatives of patients.

The most recent family study of colon cancer using the retrospective approach was by Lovett (12) in England. Her methodology was similar to that of Macklin (16), and particular care was again taken to exclude patients with multiple polyposis. In Lovett's series of patients, 26% had a family history of the malignancy, and this frequency was highest for those 40 years of age and younger. Among 352 deaths among the first-degree relatives, 41 were from cancer of the large bowel, whereas only 11.7 were expected, making the relatives' risk 3.5.

Clearly, therefore, cancer of the large bowel appears to occur three times more often in relatives of patients with this neoplasm than in the general population and independent of multiple polyposis.

HETEROGENEITY

These three studies by virtue of their design were based on the implicit assumption that large bowel cancer was a single, homogeneous disease. Boyd et al. (8) proposed on the basis of physiologic, clinical, and epidemiologic evidence the involvement of two separate diseases. Cancer of the rectum and the left side to the splenic flexure was proposed as one disease, and cancer of the remainder of the colon, the transverse, and the right side, as another. This proposal had validity since the epidemiologic studies of Correa and Llanos (10), Haenszel and Correa (11), and Correa and Haenszel (9) showed that high risk or high-incidence geographic areas were characterized by an excess of left-sided cancers and low-risk areas by a right-sided distribution involving the cecum and ascending colon. Also, in keeping with these observations, the changes in incidence in migrant populations related more to left- than right-sided sites (9).

Based on these epidemiologic findings of an environmental influence in left-sided sites, the right-sided sites would be expected to involve a genetic component; therefore, the risks for relatives would also be expected to be higher when the patient had right-sided rather than left-sided cancer. However, no retrospective studies utilizing this distinction have as yet been reported. Such a study would probably yield results similar to those obtained for breast cancer (2). For example, when breast cancer was assumed to be a single disease, the risks for relatives were twofold to threefold higher than those of women from the general population, the same as that now observed for colon cancer. But epidemiologic and clinical evidence pointed to two different disease processes, with premenopausal breast cancer differing from postmenopausal breast cancer. When a classification was made according to menopausal status based on the age at diagnosis, the relatives of patients with diagnoses occurring between ages 20 and 49 had a threefold higher risk than control relatives, whereas for ages after 49 years, the risk was only 1.5-fold higher than in controls. A classification was also made according to whether the patients had bilateral or unilateral disease. The rationale for this classification was based on the observation that inherited tumors in man and animal are characterized by tumor multiplicity (1). The risk for relatives of patients with bilateral disease increased to a 5.4 level, whereas the risk for relatives of unilateral patients was only 1.3-fold higher than controls. When the patients were classified according to both early diagnosis and bilaterality, the risks for their relatives then increased to an 8.8-fold level, whereas relatives of late-onset, unilateral patients manifested risks only 1.2-fold higher than controls (2).

For purposes of identifying groups of relatives at varying risks for large bowel cancer, therefore, a classification of patients according to right- and left-sided cancer would appear useful (3). A further classification according to age at diagnosis would also appear useful, because existing data indicate that human cancers with a genetic basis are characterized by an early average age at onset of diagnosis (3). In the study by Lovett (12), the percentage of patients with affected relatives was highest (62.5%) for those who were 40 years of age and younger and lowest for those older than 40 years of age. Another useful characteristic for identifying a high-risk group would be tumor multiplicity, since this, too, is a feature of heritable cancers (3). So individuals at high risk for large bowel cancer might be identified among the first-degree relatives of patients

TABLE 1. *Distribution (%) and average age at diagnosis (±SE) of large bowel cancer according to site in unselected patients and patients with inherited types of large bowel cancer not associated with polyposis*

Site	Inherited types[a]		Unselected[b]	
	% Site distribution	Av. age at diagnosis	% Site distribution	Av. age at diagnosis
Cecum	20.5 ⎤	42.3 ⎤	11.3 ⎤	61.9 ⎤
Ascending	18.6 ⎬ 65.0	46.6 ⎬ 45.3	4.9 ⎬ 23.7	59.9 ⎬ 60.4
Transverse	25.9 ⎦	46.6 ⎦ ±1.02	7.5 ⎦	58.6 ⎦ ±0.71
Descending	8.6 ⎤	43.9 ⎤	5.6 ⎤	59.1 ⎤
Rectosigmoid	16.8 ⎬ 35.0	50.4 ⎬ 49.2	37.3 ⎬ 76.3	59.5 ⎬ 60.3
Rectum	9.6 ⎦	51.9 ⎦ ±1.66	33.4 ⎦	61.4 ⎦ ±0.34
No. of patients	220		1,599	

[a] Includes pedigree patients summarized by Anderson (1,5), Anderson and Romsdahl (6), Anderson and Strong (7), and Lynch et al. (15).

[b] Consecutive series of patients admitted to M. D. Anderson Hospital and Tumor Institute.

with early occurring, multiple primaries, most often of the right side, because such patients should have a high probability of having a genetic basis of their disease.

That an early average age at diagnosis and a right-sided distribution do in fact characterize patients with inherited types of large bowel cancer is shown in Table 1. Unselected patients average about 60 years of age at diagnosis regardless of the site of origin, whereas patients with a genetic basis for their disease average about 46 years. The distribution of cancers also differs in that 76% of the cancers in unselected patients originate on the left side and only 24% on the right. But in patients with family histories of large bowel cancer (not associated with polyposis), almost the reverse is seen with some 65% of the cancers originating in the right side and 35% in the left side of the large bowel (6,7).

PEDIGREE STUDIES

The evaluation of single families or pedigrees is perhaps the most satisfactory and meaningful approach for demonstrating a genetic basis for susceptibility to colon cancer. The method helps bypass the problem of heterogeneity, and it provides data amenable to tests of genetic hypotheses. The method also provides relatively homogeneous data of basic and clinical interest, more so than those derived from series of patients whose disease may have heterogeneous etiologies. Pedigree studies have demonstrated clearly that colon cancer may indeed aggregate in families in the absence of polyposis, and that the segregation pattern of colon cancer in such families is consistent with a mendelian inheritance pattern. These inherited forms of colon cancer also have been shown to be characterized by an early average patient age at onset or diagnosis, tumor multiplicity, two characteristics of other inherited types of cancer, and a right-sided distribution pattern (6,15).

Families with impressive aggregations of colon cancer, summarized by Anderson (1), Anderson and Strong (7), and Lynch et al. (15), appear to be classifiable into four different inherited types of large bowel cancer based on the patients' average age at onset and the specific types of associated benign and malignant tumors (4). Probably the most frequent of these is the type first publicized by Warthin (20), his family G. This type has been primarily reported under the term "cancer family syndrome" by Lynch et al. (14). The term "hereditary adenocarcinomatosis" was also proposed for this entity by Anderson (1) to emphasize its hereditary potential and the occurrence of adenocarcinomas at multiple sites, primarily of the colon and uterus, but also of the stomach, ovaries, and possibly the breast. The neoplasms in this dominantly inherited disorder are generally first detected at about age 45 and are more frequent on the right than on the left side. Penetrance is about 75% (13), meaning that the risk of a member from such a family developing primarily a colon or uterine neoplasm or both is about 40%.

A second type, and seemingly the least frequent, is referred to as "hereditary gastrocolonic cancer." This type refers to the familial occurrence of adenocarcinoma of the large bowel and stomach either as double primaries in one individual or as a combination of single primaries among relatives. This type might be considered a variant or incomplete expression of hereditary adenocarcinomatosis, because both types follow a dominant inheritance pattern and are characterized by a right-sided distribution. The two types differ, however, in the patient's average age at diagnosis, about 40 years for gastrocolonic cancer and 45 years for adenocarcinomatosis. They also differ in their penetrance values, 90% versus 75%, respectively. The frequency of gastric cancer is also higher in gastrocolonic than in adenocarcinomatosis, 20% versus 5%, respectively (4,7). The high penetrance value indicates that the risk of a member from a family with gastrocolonic cancer developing one or both of the neoplasms is about 45%.

Another type with a limited range of phenotypic expressivity is hereditary colon cancer, in which cancer of the large bowel is the only malignancy occurring in a family. This type is also characterized by a right-sided distribution, an average patient age at diagnosis of approximately 40 years, and a penetrance of about 85% (4,7).

Torre's or Muir's syndrome is still another inherited type of large bowel cancer and perhaps the least recognized (5). Muir's syndrome would appear to be the preferred eponym, since Muir et al. (17) were the first to describe the clinical and pathologic features of the disorder and to provide a differential diagnosis, whereas Torre (19), a year later, provided a brief, one-paragraph case report. This disorder differs both quantitatively and qualitatively from the other types. It can be identified by (a) the occurrence of skin lesions, generally involving a sebaceous component; (b) diagnosis averaging about 50 years of age; (c) the occurrence of multiple adenocarcinomas of the large and small bowel and uterus, squamous cell carcinomas of the mucous membranes, and transitional cell carcinoma of the urinary system; (d) sporadic polyps of the intestinal tract and bladder; (e) diverticulosis; and (f) a low degree of malignancy as reflected by a relatively long survival following the occurrence of an internal malignancy. The syndrome follows a dominant inheritance pattern with high penetrance of about 80 to 85% (4,5). The risk of a family member developing the disorder is about 40%.

DISCUSSION

It is clear that cancer of the large bowel may indeed aggregate in families, and a family history of the neoplasm can increase a person's risk for developing that neoplasm, depending on the extent and type of family history. History of the disease in a first-degree relative, regardless of the age or site at which the neoplasm developed, is capable of increasing a person's risk about threefold. So if the lifetime probability of developing cancer of the large bowel is 5%, a family history of it in a first-degree relative would increase the probability to at least 15%.

However, neoplasms with a genetic basis are characterized by multiple primaries and an early average age at onset or diagnosis. And in the case of large bowel cancer, patients with a family history of the neoplasm are further characterized by a right-sided distribution, i.e., their neoplasms tend to originate in the cecum, ascending colon, and transverse colon. Based on these characteristics, it is conceivable that even higher risks, possibly eightfold higher than controls, would be obtained if a person were related to a patient with early onset of a malignancy who also developed a second primary and whose first malignancy originated primarily in the right side.

This estimate of an eightfold risk is based on the risk derived from families that are representative of one of four hereditary types of large bowel cancer. Large bowel cancer in such families is characterized by an early patient age at onset or diagnosis, a distinct tendency of developing at multiple sites, and a right-sided distribution. Since the neoplasm in these families is inherited in a dominant fashion with penetrance ranging from 75 to 90%, the risks for the neoplasm in the members of such families would range from 40 to 45%, risks that are eightfold to ninefold higher than those usually expected.

A family history of large bowel cancer can thus have important utility for identifying a high-risk group of individuals. The feasibility of using family history as a criterion of high risk and its utility in early detection and the institution of early therapy were demonstrated by Anderson and Romsdahl (6). The tendency for multiplicity in the familial form of the disease further means that patients should be closely followed for subsequent tumor development in the large bowel or elsewhere. The patients should also be counseled about the increased risk for tumor development in their children or other siblings and the need for these high-risk individuals to participate in a surveillance program. Primary prevention through prophylactic surgery may be possible for some of the inherited forms of polyposis but does not appear possible for the nonpolyposis types, because no biologic, tumor, or genetic markers have as yet been identified by which family members specifically at high risk to cancer of the large bowel can be identified. The only option for cancer control in these cases is the identification of high-risk families through pedigree studies coupled with a surveillance program of family members involving periodic combinations of fecal occult blood testing, colonoscopy, and air-contrast barium enema, as advocated elsewhere in this volume.

ACKNOWLEDGMENT

This research was supported in part by Grant GM 19513–C1 from the National Institutes of Health.

REFERENCES

1. Anderson, D. E. (1970): Genetic varieties of neoplasia. In: *Genetic Concepts and Neoplasia,* pp. 85–104. Williams & Wilkins Co., Baltimore.

2. Anderson, D. E. (1972): A genetic study of human breast cancer. *J. Natl. Cancer Inst.*, 48:1029–1034.
3. Anderson, D. E. (1975): Familial susceptibility. In: *Persons at High Risk of Cancer*, edited by J. F. Fraumeni, Jr., pp. 39–54. Academic Press, New York.
4. Anderson, D. E. (1978): Familial cancer and cancer families. *Semin. Oncol.*, 5:11–16.
5. Anderson, D. E. (1980): An inherited form of large bowel cancer: Muir's syndrome. *Cancer*, 45:1103 1107.
6. Anderson, D. E., and Romsdahl, M. D. (1977): Family history: A criterion for selective screening. In: *Genetics of Human Cancer*, edited by J. J. Mulvihill, R. W. Miller, and J. F. Fraumeni, Jr., pp. 257–262. Raven Press, New York.
7. Anderson, D. E., and Strong, L. C. (1974): Genetics of gastrointestinal tumors. *Proceedings of XIth International Cancer Congress*, Florence, Italy, pp. 267–271. Excerpta Medica, Series No. 351, Amsterdam.
8. Boyd, J., Langman, M., and Doll, R. (1964): The epidemiology of gastrointestinal cancer with special reference to causation. *Gut*, 5:196–200.
9. Correa, P., and Haenszel, W. (1975): Comparative international incidence and mortality. In: *Cancer Epidemiology and Prevention Current Concepts*, edited by D. Schottenfeld, pp. 386–403. Charles C Thomas, Springfield, Ill.
10. Correa, P., and Llanos, G. (1966): Morbidity and mortality from cancer in Cali, Colombia. *J. Natl. Cancer Inst.*, 36:717–745.
11. Haenszel, W., and Correa, P. (1973): Cancer of the large intestine: Epidemiologic findings. *Dis. Colon Rectum*, 16:371–377.
12. Lovett, E. (1976): Family studies in cancer of the colon and rectum. *Br. J. Surg.*, 63:13–18.
13. Lynch, H. T., and Kaplan, A. R. (1974): Cancer concordance and the hypothesis of autosomal dominant transmission of cancer diathesis in a remarkable kindred. *Oncology*, 30:210–216.
14. Lynch, H. T., Krush, A. J., Thomas, R. J., et al. (1976): Cancer family syndrome. In: *Cancer Genetics*, edited by H. T. Lynch, pp. 355–388. Charles C. Thomas, Springfield, Ill.
15. Lynch, P. M., Lynch, H. T., and Harris, R. E. (1977): Hereditary proximal colonic cancer. *Dis. Colon Rectum*, 20:661–668.
16. Macklin, M. T. (1960): Inheritance of cancer of the stomach and large intestine in man. *J. Natl. Cancer Inst.*, 24:551–571.
17. Muir, E. G., Yates-Bell, A. J., and Barlow, K. A. (1966): Multiple primary carcinomata of the colon, duodenum, and larynx associated with keratoacanthomata of the face. *Br. J. Surg.*, 54:191–195.
18. Postlethwait, R. W., Adamson, J. E., and Hart, D. (1958): Carcinoma of the colon and rectum. *Surg. Gynecol. Obstet.*, 106:257–270.
19. Torre, D. (1968): Multiple sebaceous tumors. *Arch. Dermatol.*, 98:549–551.
20. Warthin, A. S. (1913): Heredity with reference to carcinoma as shown by the study of the cases examined in the pathological laboratory of the University of Michigan, 1895–1913. *Arch. Intern. Med.*, 12:546–555.
21. Woolf, C. M. (1958): A genetic study of carcinoma of the large intestine. *Am. J. Hum. Genet.*, 10:42–52.

Colorectal Cancer: Prevention, Epidemiology, and Screening, edited by S. Winawer, D. Schottenfeld, and P. Sherlock. Raven Press, New York © 1980.

Analysis of Genetics of Inherited Colon Cancer

Henry T. Lynch, Patrick M. Lynch, and Jane F. Lynch

Department of Preventive Medicine and Public Health, Creighton University School of Medicine, Omaha, Nebraska 68178

Hereditary cancer may differ from its sporadically occurring counterpart in the following respects: (a) a much earlier average age of cancer onset (19), (b) a marked excess of multiple primary cancer (involving multifocality in certain organs, bilaterality in paired organs, and synchronous and metachronous occurrence in discrete organs) (16), (c) apparent differences in host tolerance of tumors, as evidenced by prolonged survival in certain hereditary cancer syndromes (10,12), (d) frequent premonitory signs of cancer risk, some of which may be recognized at birth (11,25), and (e) perhaps most importantly, highly predictable risk to certain classes of individuals, with or without preclinical markers (23). Yet, the variability of phenotypic expression in syndromes demands cautious interpretation of pedigree data. The hereditary colon cancer-predisposing syndromes serve as excellent models for the discussion of these issues.

That colon cancer is exceedingly heterogeneous is reflected by the diversity in expression from family to family. A fraction of colon cancer-prone families are characterized by multiple adenomatous polyps, with a varying spectrum of extracolonic signs, and early onset of predominantly distal colon cancer (30). Families lacking such signs exhibit a proximal predominance of colon cancer (24); in many such families, there is a proclivity to cancer of other anatomic sites, particularly of the endometrium, ovary, breast, and stomach, as in the cancer family syndrome (CFS) (16,19,20).

As in attempts to understand the genetic contribution to cancer generally, comprehension of genetic factors in colon cancer may be complicated by (a) a lack of reliable markers of the premalignant state; (b) competing mortality, i.e., early death of possible carriers who might have expressed cancer had they lived; (c) sporadic colon cancer non-gene carriers, coexisting with the genetic variety and sometimes indistinguishable from it; and (d) malignancy of other anatomic sites, whose presence in a family may or may not suggest the existence of a syndrome with a broader tumor spectrum.

In order to facilitate a better comprehension of hereditary factors in colon cancer-prone families, hereditary colon cancer syndromes may be classified operationally into two broad categories: (a) those with multiple gastrointestinal polyps, adenomatous or hamartomatous, with or without distinguishing extracolonic signs; and (b) those without multiple gastrointestinal polyps or other premonitory features which must be characterized according to peculiarities in clinical expression and pedigree transmission. Recent findings in the disorders comprising these classes will be reviewed.

FAMILIAL POLYPOSIS COLI

Few genetic diseases have been studied with as much intensity as has familial polyposis coli (FPC). According to Shiffman (29), the first recognition of diffuse polyposis coli was in 1847. The familial aspect of this disease was first described by Cripps in 1881 (2). More detailed description of the syndrome's natural history, including its autosomal dominant mode of genetic transmission, was reported by Lockhart-Mummery (1925) (8) and Dukes (1930) (5). Since these pioneering efforts, other features associated with polyps of the colon have suggested the existence of genetically distinct syndromes. Among the recent evidence of variability in phenotype was our observation of several FPC families having patients with virtually no polyps at the time of colon cancer diagnosis (22). Yet such patients were capable of transmitting the deleterious gene to offspring who showed the typical presentation of diffuse polyposis of the colon (Fig. 1).

HEREDITARY COLON CANCER IN THE ABSENCE OF MULTIPLE COLON POLYPS

Due to the lack of reliable precancer markers, genetic analysis of colon cancer syndromes not associated with multiple polyposis has been much more difficult, and perhaps as a consequence of this fact, they have unfortunately received less attention than the FPC syndromes. We will, therefore, devote greater attention to the discussion of these disorders.

The cumulative lifetime risk of colorectal/endometrial cancer to progeny of matings which involve an affected direct-line parent in the cancer family syndrome is presented in Fig. 2. The incidence curves for 581 progeny (307 males and 274 females) of affected parents are contrasted with a lifetime projection for a hypothetical sex/age matched sample. The lifetime risk for carcinoma of the two anatomic sites is approximately 55% in "at risk CFS relatives" compared to only 6 to 7% in the general population (14). The excess lifetime risk to progeny of affected parents is therefore approximately 50%, suggesting that one-half of these individuals received a deleterious cancer-predisposing gene from their direct-line parent. Figures 3 to 5 show representative pedigrees of CFS families [C-196 (17), C-113 (21), C-197 (18)].

Four pedigrees manifesting either hereditary site-specific colon cancer (HSCC) or the CFS have been subjected to the initial stages of segregation analysis according to methods developed by Elston and Stewart (6). In general, the method involves comparing three pedigree likelihoods: L_g = the likelihood under an autosomal dominant genetic model; L_e = the likelihood under the assumption

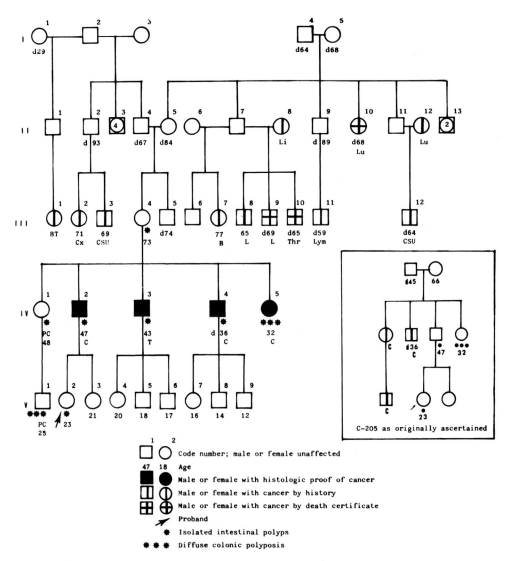

FIG. 1. Pedigree of a family presenting with diffuse polyposis of the colon and marked variation in this phenotype. From Lynch et al. (22). PC: prophylactic colectomy, B: breast, BT: brain tumor, C: colon, CSU: cancer site unknown, Cx: cervical, L: leukemia, Li: liver, Lu: lung, Lym: lymphoma, T: testicular, Thr: throat, D: died.

that phenotype is independent of genotype; and L_o = the likelihood of the pedigree when parameters of the genetic model are allowed to take on their maximizing values. The likelihoods are compared on the assumption that twice the difference in log-likelihoods has a Chi square distribution with degrees of

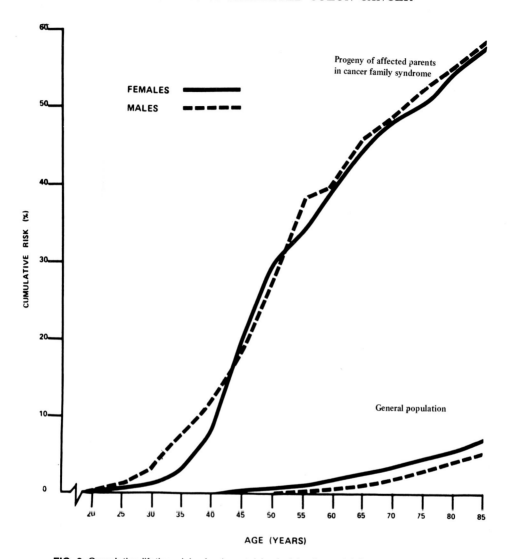

FIG. 2. Cumulative lifetime risk of colorectal (males)/endometrial (females) cancer to progeny of direct-line parents in the cancer family syndrome vs the general population. Rates for the general population are based on the Third National Cancer Survey. From Lynch, et al. (14).

freedom equal to the difference in the number of fixed parameters between models.

Results of segregation analysis from one of the CFS pedigrees (C-196) showed that the likelihood under the genetic model, L_g, corresponds with the likelihood under the free parameterized model, L_o, whereas the likelihood under the environmental model, L_e, deviates from L_o ($p < 0.007$) (17). Results are therefore supportive of autosomal dominant inheritance with gene carriers showing a lifetime susceptibility (penetrance) of 89% and a mean onset of 42.5 years of age.

An HSCC pedigree is depicted in Fig. 6. Segregation analysis under the maximum method described above yielded results in which the tumor expression pattern fit a single (autosomal dominant) gene model significantly better ($p < 0.01$) than either the L_o or L_e models.

Although the pedigree likelihood of these kindreds is consistent with a major gene hypothesis, proof of this assumption can be verified unequivocally only through the establishment of genetic linkage. Unfortunately, as already mentioned, reliable biochemical and/or immunological markers to date have not been identified in the CFS or in HSCC. Clinical features common to these families will be discussed briefly.

MULTIPLE PRIMARY CANCERS

Of 316 relatives with cancer in 12 CFS or HSCC families, 68 (21.5%) had two or more primary malignancies and 59 (86.8%) of these multiple primaries involved the colon and/ or endometrium (16). A pooled analysis of this resource revealed a consistent 3% annual risk for second primary cancer, with each year of survival following first onset. Interestingly, when a second primary cancer occurred, the risk for a third was extremely high (6.9% annual risk) but showed a nonlinear trend with increasing survival following second onset. No significant sex differences were noted in the risk for multiple primary cancer.

The average span of time between the occurrence of a first and second primary cancer was longer when the second tumor involved colon as opposed to other anatomic sites (8.1 versus 3.75 years). The biological significance of this difference is not clear, although it could be a function of differential growth rates of tumors of the colon, relative to those of other anatomic sites.

MANAGEMENT IMPLICATIONS

Since the remaining colon segment is at high risk for a second primary cancer, total or subtotal colectomy rather than partial colectomy for initial colon cancer is indicated. In the case of women with colon cancer from families with the CFS, the problem becomes more complex because of their high risk for endometrial and ovarian carcinoma. Thus such a patient should be considered for hysterectomy and bilateral salpingo-oophorectomy when the colon is resected, particularly if she has completed her family. However, this matter presents a dilemma. The earlier the colon cancer occurs (e.g., ages 25 to 35), the more likely it is to be of the genetic variety, and therefore indicative of cancer risk to the endometrium. Yet it is in this age interval that the affected woman is most likely to

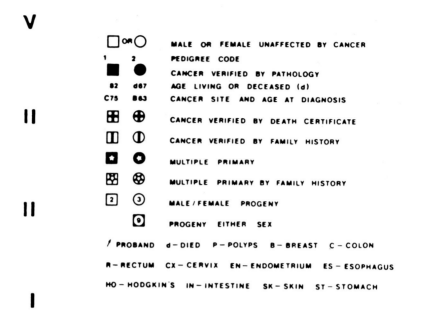

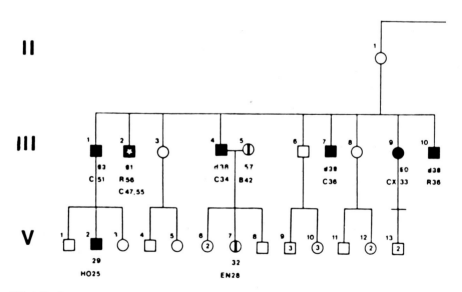

FIG. 3. Pedigree of a family representing the cancer family syndrome (CFS). Note the occurrence of cancer of the colon and/or endometrium through 4 generations. From Lynch et al. (17).

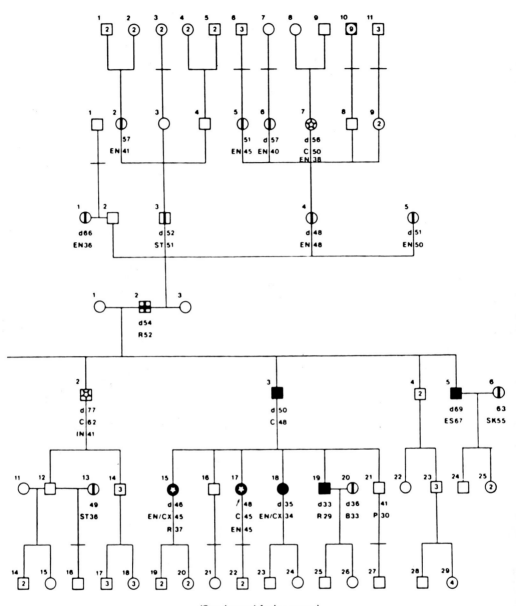

(See legend facing page.)

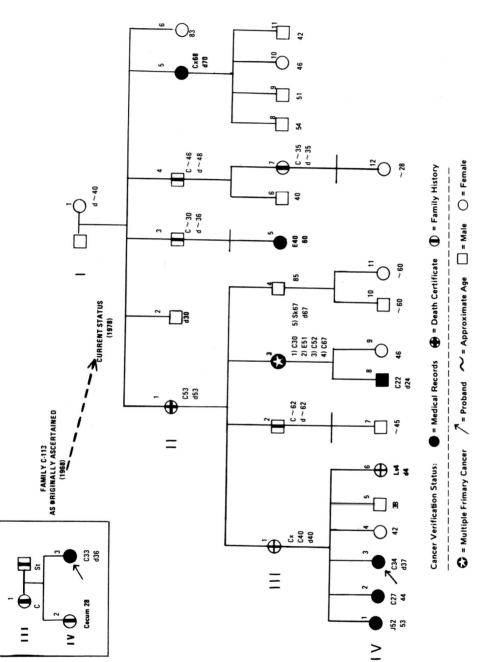

FIG. 4. Pedigree of a family with the cancer family syndrome. The insert represents the importance of extending the family for better evaluation of cancer risk and surveillance of high-risk patients. C: colon, Cx: cervix, E: endometrium, J: jejunum, Ls: lymphosarcoma, Sk: skin, St: stomach, d: died.

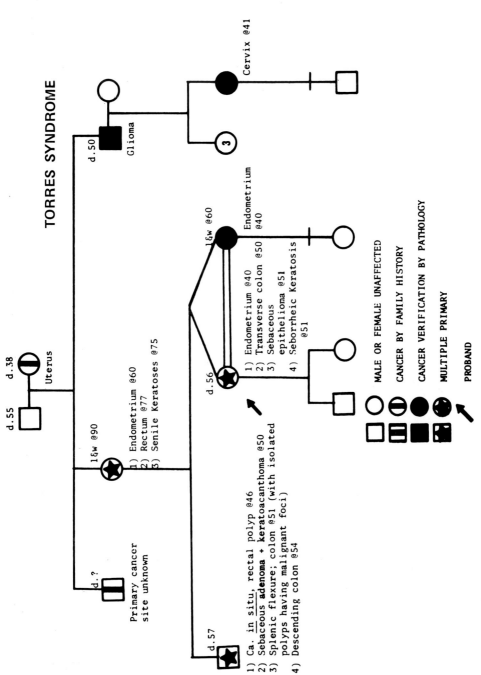

FIG. 5. Pedigree of a kindred showing the cancer family syndrome wherein cancer-affected siblings had cutaneous stigmata of Torre's syndrome.

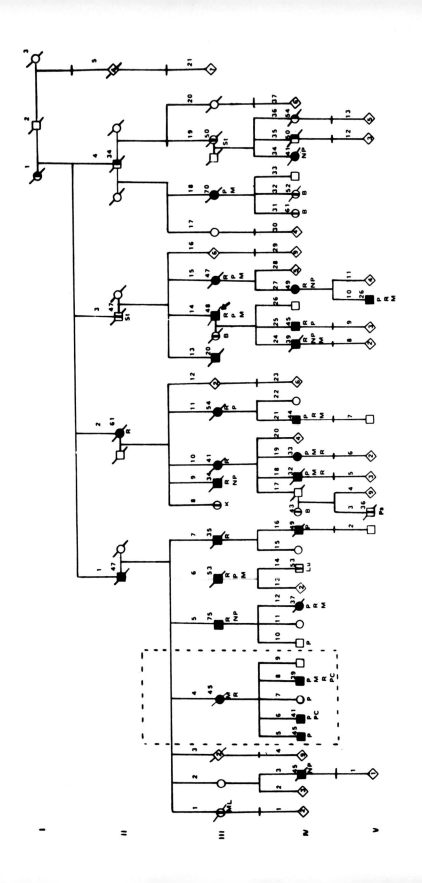

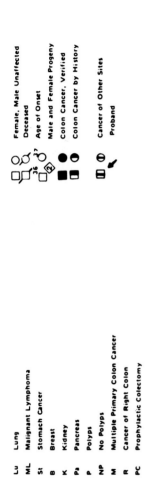

FIG. 6. Pedigree of a family with hereditary site-specific colon cancer in which the tumor expression pattern fit a single-gene model. From Lynch, et al. (15).

desire children. The later occurring colon cancer, less clearly associated with endometrial cancer risk, is also less likely to complicate family planning. Should the initial lesion involve the endometrium at an early age, then the patient should be considered a prime candidate for intensive surveillance versus prophylactic colon resection during the same operation.

PROLONGED SURVIVAL

Spontaneous regression of metastatic cancer and failure of invasive cancers to metastasize have been seen to occur with an increased frequency in the hereditary variety of certain cancers (10,12). Malignant melanoma associated with xeroderma pigmentosum (4) and the familial atypical multiple mole-melanoma syndrome (13) are excellent examples of this phenomenon. A colon cancer syndrome involving prolonged survival in patients with invasive or metastatic cancer is Torre's syndrome (28), which we feel may actually be a variant of the CFS (23a). [One kindred under investigation by our group (Fig. 5) includes colon cancer-affected siblings with cutaneous stigmata of the Torre's syndrome, namely, sebaceous epitheliomas and keratoacanthomas.]

We have reviewed the subject of prolonged survival in patients from families manifesting the CFS, and have described the details in one of these kindreds (10). In this particular family, the proband, her mother, and a cousin had early onset, multiple primary cancers. The proband and her mother manifested the same tumor combination (endometrial and colon cancers), but the mother had at least two other types of cancer, carcinoma of the ovary and eventual chronic myelogenous leukemia. Her cancer history began at the age of 46 years with a lesion that typically has a grave prognosis, namely, bilateral ovarian carcinoma. As long as 12 years before her death, there was histologic evidence of invasion, extension, and metastases of colonic cancer to regional lymph nodes. The patient seemingly tolerated these malignant neoplasms well; eventually, chronic myelogenous leukemia developed, which may have contributed to her death. It is possible that the leukemia was related to her prior radiation therapy.

We believe that host factors contribute significantly to the relationship between the early age of onset, multiple primary cancers, and prolonged survival seen in certain CFS families. Early onset of generally late occurring tumors apparently provides the initially cured patient many more years of life during which to be affected again. In addition, younger patients appear to have a greater fitness to withstand surgical procedures and adjuvant therapy, leading to their improved survival. An alternative hypothesis is that the residual genotype affords immunologic protection against the tumor, once it has occurred in the genetically predisposed patients. Over many generations, those patients who can "tolerate" cancer are selected over those who cannot. Since the age of onset is early, and the possibility for procreation thereafter is dependent on such survival, selection for a "cancer tolerance factor" may exist.

MARKER STUDIES

Because affected patients from a large fraction of colon cancer-prone families exhibit no apparent physical stigmata of the precancerous state, recent work has increasingly turned toward efforts to identify more subtle subclinical markers of the genetic trait. The identification of cytogenetic and other cellular or subcellular evidence of preneoplastic activity in young patients at risk for the polyposis coli syndromes (but prior to the onset of polyps or cutaneous stigmata) has provided a major contribution in this regard (4). Important laboratory findings have included but are not necessarily limited to the following: (a) the observation of an abnormally high rate of cellular proliferation in the upper compartments of colonic crypts (4,9), the possible precursor to clinically evident adenoma formation, (b) increased *in vitro* tetraploidy in epithelial cells from patients with Gardner's syndrome (but not familial polyposis) (3), (c) peculiar growth characteristics of cutaneous fibroblasts *in vitro,* including diminished serum requirement, decreased contact inhibition of proliferation as indicated by a high cell density plateau, and abnormal cytoskeletal (actin) structure (7), (d) an increased susceptibility to transformation by the Kirsten murine sarcoma virus (KiMSV) (26), and (e) a higher excretion of undegraded cholesterol in the feces (27).

Attempts to validate the relationship between the above markers and gene-carrier status has, of course, been greatly facilitated by the eventual expression of clinically evident polyposis (or in the case of Gardner's syndrome, extracolonic signs) in asymptomatic high-risk patients. Marker studies in families in which colon cancer expression lacks informative premonitory signs cannot be so readily interpreted, due primarily to the longer latent period between performance of a given assay and the manifestation of the cancers themselves, which constitute the most reliable qualitative measure of the deleterious gene-carrier status. Nevertheless, collaborative efforts are now being initiated to perform a battery of marker studies on affected as well as symptomatic high- and low-risk members of CFS and HSCC families. Although none of these tests have been definitively confirmed or excluded as markers of gene-carrier status in these hereditary cancer syndromes, there have been preliminary findings suggesting that failure to repress cell proliferation in the upper compartments of the colonic crypts may be a feature of both the CFS and HSCC (M. Lipkin, E. Deschner, and H. T. Lynch, *unpublished*). Because the CFS and its variants seem to be entities distinct from the multiple polyposis coli syndromes, it would indeed be unrealistic to anticipate that all promising marker systems in FPC will necessarily correlate with susceptibility in the CFS and related hereditary colon cancer syndromes.

A possible marker that holds particular promise in the CFS relates to cell-mediated immunity. Specifically, Berlinger et al. (1) have generated pilot data showing defective recognitive immunity in familial colon cancer aggregates in the absence of polyposis, expressed within families in patterns consistent with the segregation of an autosomal dominant gene. This and related assays will clearly require much more intense scrutiny in the context of some of the larger extended kindreds available for such study.

SUMMARY AND CONCLUSIONS

Genetic heterogeneity must be given primary consideration in any discussion of colon cancer genetics. The initial phase of hereditary colon cancer syndrome identification will be fostered by categorizing families into one of the two major categories, those with gastrointestinal polyps and those without. In the former, the frequency of distal colon cancer is comparable to that seen in the general population. In the latter, an excess of proximal colonic cancer involvement is encountered. These aspects of cancer distribution in the colon, as well as associated malignant neoplastic lesions in both categories, harbor important implications of surveillance, early diagnosis, and hence, cancer control. In both cases, careful family history evaluation is a necessity.

We have focused our major research attention on colon cancer-prone syndromes which are not associated with gastrointestinal polyps or any other recognizable markers of genotypic status. Therefore, precision in determining the mode of genetic transmission of colon cancer diathesis is difficult to achieve. Evidence supporting a dominant mode of genetic transmission includes the lifetime incidence of colorectal/endometrial carcinoma and pedigree likelihood analyses. Although genetic linkage studies will ultimately be required for definitive confirmation of the genetic mechanism in these diseases, a host of potential markers are being evaluated.

REFERENCES

1. Berlinger, N. T., Lopez, C., Lipkin, M., Vogel, J. E., Good, R. A. (1977): Defective recognitive immunity in family aggregates of colon carcinoma. *J. Clin. Invest.,* 59:761–769.
2. Cripps, H. (1881): Two cases of disseminated polyps of the rectum. *Trans. Pathol. Soc. Lond.,* 33:165–168.
3. Danes, B. S., and Gardner, E. J. (1978): The Gardner syndrome—A cell culture study on kindred 109. *J. Med. Genet.,* 15:346–351.
4. Deschner, E., and Lipkin, M. (1970): Study of human rectal epithelial cells *in vitro.* III. RNA, protein, and DNA synthesis in polyps and adjacent mucosa. *J. Natl. Cancer Inst.,* 44:175–185.
5. Dukes, C. (1930): The hereditary factor in polyposis intestini or multiple adenomata. *Cancer Rev.,* 5(4):241–256.
6. Elston, R. C., and Stewart, J. (1971): A general model for the genetic analysis of pedigree data. *Hum. Hered.,* 21:523–542.
7. Kopelovich, L. (1977): Phenotypic markers in human skin fibroblasts as possible diagnostic indices of hereditary adenomatosis of the colon and rectum. *Cancer,* 40:2534–2541.
8. Lockhart-Mummery, P. (1925): Cancer and heredity. *Lancet,* 1:427–429.
9. Lipkin, M. (1977): The identification of individuals at high risk for large bowel cancer. *Cancer,* 40:2523–2530.
10. Lynch, H. T., Bardawil, W. A., Harris, R. E., Lynch, P. M., Guirgis, H. A., and Lynch, J. F. (1978): Multiple primary cancers and prolonged survival: Familial colonic and endometrial cancers. *Dis. Colon Rectum,* 21:165–168.
11. Lynch, H. T., and Frichot, B. C. (1978): Skin, heredity, and cancer. *Semin. Oncol.,* 5:67–84, 1978.

12. Lynch, H. T., Frichot, B. C., Fisher, J., Smith, J. L., and Lynch, J. F. (1978): Spontaneous regression of metastatic malignant melanoma in two siblings with xeroderma pigmentosum. *J. Med. Genet.,* 15:357.
13. Lynch, H. T., Frichot, B. C., III, and Lynch, J. F. (1978): Familial atypical multiple mole melanoma syndrome. *J. Med. Genet.,* 15:352–356.
14. Lynch, H. T., Guirgis, H. A., Harris, R. E., Lynch, P. M., Lynch, J. F., Elston, R. C., Go, R. C. P., and Kaplan, E. (1979): Clinical, genetic, and biostatistical progress in the cancer family syndrome. *Front. Gastrointest. Res.,* 142–150.
15. Lynch, H. T., Harris, R. E., Bardawil, W. A., Lynch, P. M., Guirgis, H. A., Swartz, M. J., and Lynch, J. F. (1977): Management of Hereditary site-specific colon cancer. *Arch. Surg.,* 112:170–174.
16. Lynch, H. T., Harris, R. E., Lynch, P. M., Guirgis, H. A., and Lynch, J. F. (1977): The role of heredity in multiple primary cancer. *Cancer,* 40:1849–1854.
17. Lynch, H. T., Harris, R. E., Organ, C. H., Jr., Guirgis, H. A., Lynch, P. M., Lynch, J. F., and Nelson, E. J. (1977): The surgeon, genetics, and cancer control: The cancer family syndrome. *Ann. Surg.,* 185:435–440.
18. Lynch, H. T., and Krush, A. J. (1971): The cancer family syndrome and cancer control. *Surg. Gynecol. Obstet.,* 132:247–250.
19. Lynch, H. T., Krush, A. J., Thomas, R. J., and Lynch, J. (1976): Cancer family syndrome. In: *Cancer Genetics,* edited by H. T. Lynch, pp. 355–387. Charles C. Thomas, Springfield, Ill.
20. Lynch, H. T., and Lynch, P. M. (1980): Tumor variation in the cancer family syndrome: Ovarian cancer. *Am. J. Surg. (in press).*
21. Lynch, H. T., and Lynch, P. M. (1979): The cancer family syndrome: A pragmatic basis for syndrome identification. *Dis. Colon Rectum,* 22:106–110.
22. Lynch, H. T., Lynch, P. M., Follett, K. L., and Harris, R. E. (1979): Familial polyposis coli: heterogeneous expression in two kindreds. *J. Med. Genet.,* 16:1–7.
23. Lynch, H. T., Lynch, P. M., and Harris, R. E. (1978): Minimal genetic findings and their cancer control implications. *JAMA,* 240:535–538.
23a. Lynch, H. T., et al. (1980): *Arch. Int. Med. (in press).*
24. Lynch, P. M., Lynch, H. T., and Harris, R. E. (1977): Hereditary proximal colonic cancer. *Dis. Colon Rectum,* 20:661–668.
25. Mulvihill, J. J., Miller, R. W., and Fraumeni, J. F., Jr. (eds.) (1977): *Genetics of Human Cancer: Progress in Cancer Research Therapy, Vol. 3.* Raven Press, New York.
26. Pfeffer, L. M., and Kopelovich, L. (1977): Differential genetic susceptibility of cultured human skin fibroblasts to transformation by Kirsten murine sarcoma virus. *Cell,* 10:313–320.
27. Reddy, B. S., Mastromarino, A., Gustafson, C., Lipkin, M., and Wynder, E. L. (1976): Fecal bile acids and neutral sterols in patients with familial polyposis. *Cancer,* 38:1694–1698.
28. Rulon, D. B., and Helwig, E. S. (1973): Multiple sebaceous neoplasms of the skin: An association with multiple visceral carcinomas, especially of the colon. *Am. J. Clin. Pathol.,* 60:745–752.
29. Shiffman, M. A. (1962): Familial multiple polyposis associated with soft tissue and hard tissue tumors. *JAMA,* 179:514.
30. Watne, A. L., Lai, H. Y., Carrier, J., and Coppula, W. (1977): The diagnosis and surgical treatment of patients with Gardner's syndrome. *Surgery,* 82:327–333.

Colorectal Cancer: Prevention, Epidemiology, and Screening, edited by S. Winawer, D. Schottenfeld, and P. Sherlock. Raven Press, New York © 1980.

Cell Proliferation as a Biological Marker in Human Colorectal Neoplasia

Eleanor E. Deschner

Memorial Sloan-Kettering Cancer Center, New York, New York, 10021

The goal of gastrointestinal oncologists and researchers in the United States has been to develop techniques to reduce the high incidence of colorectal cancer and to increase the survival rate for this disease. Mass screening programs such as those operating in Japan for the detection of stomach cancer (14) have not been thought acceptable to the average American adult over 45 years of age, much less cost effective. However, volunteer programs have been initiated at various centers to screen persons over 45 believed to be prone to the formation of polyps and to examine individuals considered high risk for colon cancer, i.e., patients with a previous history of colon cancer or polyps and relatives of familial polyposis patients (17).

One technique found to have great potential in early colon cancer detection is the Hemoccult slide test, which registers the presence of fecal blood in patients on a prescribed meat-free high residue diet. Although hemoglobin is normally present in small amounts of stool, levels detected by this test have been more indicative of gastrointestinal pathology, particularly colonic neoplasia. Thus individuals with one or more Hemoccult-positive (Ho+) slides are scheduled for examination by barium enema with air contrast and by colonoscopy (16).

While biopsies and brush cytology of suspicious areas are obtained during the latter procedure for pathological analysis, other techniques also may be carried out with similar specimens. One procedure involves tritiated thymidine ([3]HTdR) labeling of biopsy material to determine the type of proliferative pattern characterizing the epithelial cells of the mucosa in the area. The nature of the DNA synthesis pattern within a given biopsy may provide a key to the future behavior of the colorectal tissue. Such a marker would be valuable in discriminating cancer-prone patients from those at lower risk.

PROLIFERATION PATTERNS

Normal cell proliferation in colorectal crypts of mammalian species including man has been found to occupy the lower two-thirds of the glands with the major zone of DNA synthesis in the lower third (Fig. 1). However, that is not the only pattern found to occur in normal appearing crypts. The first recog-

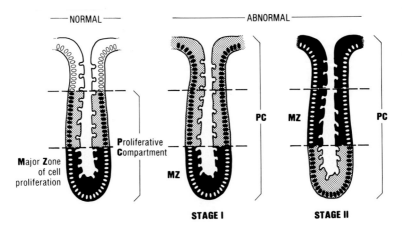

FIG. 1. Diagrammatic representation of the three types of histologically normal-appearing crypts found in colorectal mucosa. At *left,* a crypt with completely normal epithelial cell proliferation. The proliferative compartment (PC) is in the lower two-thirds of the gland with the major zone of cell renewal (MZ) in the low third. In the *middle,* a crypt depicting the stage 1 abnormality which involves extension of the proliferative compartment to the surface, but with the lower third still the major zone of DNA synthesis. Stage 2 abnormality represented by the crypt at *right* shows the proliferative compartment extending from base to surface. However, the major zone of DNA synthesis has shifted to the middle or middle and upper portions of the crypt.

nizable deviation from the normal was an extension of the proliferative compartment to the upper third and along the luminal surface but with the lower third still the major zone of DNA synthesis (Fig. 1). This stage 1 abnormality has been reported in patients with isolated polyps, patients with familial polyposis, symptom-free relatives of familial polyposis patients, patients with a history of cancer, as well as some symptom-free members of the general population (1,3,6,7). More recently, a second abnormality has been described, a pattern demonstrated initially in patients with colorectal cancer (13). Of the 17 biopsies from 13 cancer patients, 6 showed an upward shift of the major proliferative compartments toward the middle and upper portions of the crypts such that the lower zone no longer was the major zone of cell renewal (stage 2 abnormality). DNA synthesizing cells were now located predominantly in the middle or middle and upper third of crypts (Fig. 1).

An example of this can be seen on the analysis of a biopsy from a colon cancer patient when compared with a biopsy from a patient with no gastrointestinal disease (Fig. 2). Expansion of the proliferative compartment to the surface can be recognized as well as an upward shift of the principal site of cell renewal to the middle of the crypts. The altered distribution of labeled cells to the mid and upper crypts in cancer patients is related to an increased labeling index (L.I.) or ratio of labeled to unlabeled cells in these regions of the gland.

This finding has also been observed in mice immediately following 5 weekly injections of the colon carcinogen, 1,2-dimethylhydrazine (DMH) at a dose

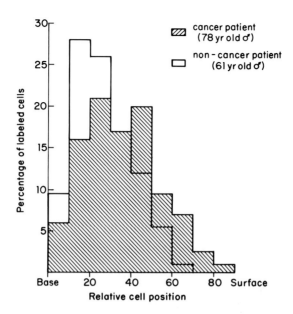

FIG. 2. Labeling distribution and relative position of labeled cells in colorectal crypts of a cancer and control patient. An upward shift of the major zone of DNA synthesis is observed in the cancer patient.

level of 20 mg/kg body weight (5). The repeated delivery of DMH resulted in the expansion of DNA synthesizing cells to the upper third of the glands but with the middle third of the crypt the most active proliferative zone (Fig. 3). Twenty weeks later, mice with this abnormal proliferative pattern had adenomas and carcinomas present primarily in the distal portion of the colon (8,15).

If indeed this parameter (stage 2 abnormality) does forecast the future development of neoplasms, then persons with a previous history of polyps and/or colon cancer could be screened to assess the likelihood of a recurrence. Testing could also be extended to persons in colon cancer-prone families as well as those with a history of long-standing chronic ulcerative colitis.

To acquaint the reader with the procedures followed to obtain information on the nature of the proliferative patterns present in colorectal biopsy or operative material, a brief description of the technique follows.

TECHNIQUES

In each instance biopsy material is fragmented to a size containing approximately five to seven crypts to allow proper diffusion of oxygen to all parts of the specimen; oxygen is required if the radioactive precursor is to be incorporated within the cells. Each biopsy is incubated separately in Eagle's basic medium to which 10% fetal calf serum and approximately 1 μCi of tritiated thymidine

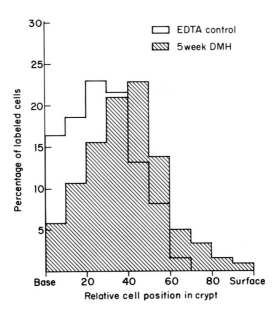

FIG. 3. Distribution of ³HTdR-labeled cells and their relative position in colorectal crypts of a DMH-treated mouse compared with an EDTA-treated control. DMH, a colon carcinogen, was injected subcutaneously for 5 weekly treatments using 20 mg/kg body weight. The major zone of cell proliferation has been shifted in an upward direction in the DMH-treated animal at a time when focal areas of cellular atypism are forming

(³HTdR) or other labeled precursors is added to each milliliter of medium (4). The tissue is incubated for 1 hr to allow incorporation of the isotope, following which the specimen is fixed in 10% neutral buffered formalin. Paraffin sections are prepared, the slides rehydrated and then coated with NTB₂ (Kodak) emulsion. After a suitable exposure time, the slides are developed using standard photographic techniques. After hematoxylin and eosin staining, the slides are cover-slipped in preparation for analysis, using oil immersion. Longitudinal sections through entire colorectal crypts are employed for quantitative studies. The number and positon of ³HTdR-labeled cells is determined for each half of a crypt as well as the total number of epithelial cells per crypt column (half crypt). Cells are scored from the base of the crypt column in an upward direction to the luminal surface. A ³HTdR-labeled cell is one with at least 4 grains appearing over the nucleus.

PATIENT STUDIES

A group of 8 patients ranging in age from 31 to 78 years with no history of gastrointestinal disease was employed as controls for this study. Of the 8 individuals, 2 demonstrated a completely normal incorporation pattern with labeled cells appearing solely in the lower two-thirds of crypts (Fig. 4). However,

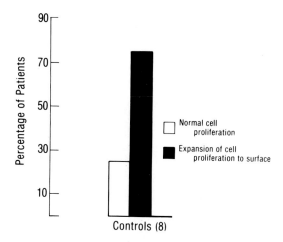

FIG. 4. Distribution of the proliferative patterns among a group of 8 control patients with no history of gastrointestinal disease. Normal cell proliferation exclusively in the lower two-thirds of crypts characterized colorectal biopsies of only 25% of patients tested. The predominant pattern seen was the stage 1 abnormality with extension of the proliferative compartment to the suface. However, in no control patient was the stage 2 abnormality found.

6 of 8 patients (75%) expressed stage 1 alteration in a biopsy, that is, extension of the proliferative compartment to the upper third of the crypt. Between 1.2 and 15.9% of epithelial cells were undergoing DNA synthesis in an abnormal location. However, the major zone of cell proliferation was still the lower third of the crypt. Thus no specimen among the control patients was seen to express the upward shift or stage 2 abnormality.

The distribution of the proliferative patterns among patients belonging to several groups at high risk for colon cancer is presented in Fig. 5. The Ho[+] group will be dealt with separately. The number of patients surveyed in each group ranged from 12 to 18. In each group only a relatively small percentage of the patients had biopsy specimens characterized by totally normal ³HTdR incorporation. Instead, a large percentage showed DNA-synthesizing cells in the upper third of colorectal crypts. This parameter was seen in roughly 60 to 90% of high-risk patients, but a sizeably smaller percentage of these patients with an expanded proliferative zone expressed the second abnormality, this shift in the major zone of cell renewal. This parameter had a reduced frequency in each of the high-risk groups (range 30 to 60%).

Six Ho[+] patients were studied in detail even though barium enema and colonoscopy were essentially negative (Fig. 5). Only one individual had a biopsy with a normal proliferative pattern; 5 patients showed extension of the proliferative compartment to the surface. Three of these patients expressed the stage 2 lesion marked by the shift of the major zone of DNA synthesis.

A review of the results of these various groups would allow us to make some broad generalizations. Certainly, in each group only a relatively small

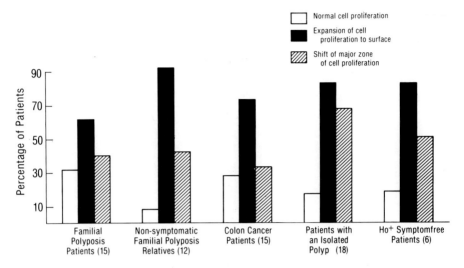

FIG. 5. Colorectal biopsies from patients distributed among five groups at high risk for colon cancer were characterized for their proliferative pattern. The number of patients tested in each group is in parentheses. Note that in all groups, normal cell proliferation occurs less frequently than the other two patterns. Expansion of cell proliferation to the surface (stage 1 abnormality) is seen most frequently. The frequency of the shift of the major zone of cell proliferation (stage 2) is presented as a percentage of stage 1 abnormality and occurs with reduced frequency among all groups, although more markedly in some than in others.

percentage of high-risk patients had biopsy specimens characterized by totally normal ³HTdR incorporation. Even control patients or patients with no gastrointestinal disease were not observed to have this as the predominant proliferative pattern.

Instead, the greater percentage showed DNA synthesizing cells in the upper third of colorectal crypts indicating expansion of the proliferative compartment with loss of regulatory controls which normally suppress DNA synthesis in this region. Since this stage 1 pattern appears to be most characteristic of all patients, this may be an early expression of the aging phenomenon in man. But the marked degree or frequency of labeling in the upper third of crypts may also be a reflection of the presence of the stage 2 abnormality below the surface.

This second abnormality involving a shift in the major zone of cell proliferation is apparently a further stage in the evolution of the mucosa toward neoplasia. Its reduced frequency relative to the surface and upper labeling event would indicate it to be a later stage and a far more discriminatory kinetic parameter in our quest for meaningful tumor markers.

FOLLOW-UP ANALYSES

The observation of the shift of the major zone of the proliferative compartment has been used to analyze biopsies removed from the same patients over a period of years. The results of these follow-up examinations are illustrated by two asymptomatic relatives of familial polyposis patients (Fig. 6). One has been surveyed over a period of 9 years, and the other over 3 years. The male patient was found to have a normal distribution of labeled cells in a biopsy taken at age 15, although some slight enlargement of the proliferative compartment was occurring. This trend continued the following year. The third year demonstrated the displacement of the normal zone of DNA synthesis to the middle and upper zone of the crypts.

The second patient, a female, when first examined showed enlargement of the proliferative compartment in relatively increased levels as well as a borderline response of the lower third of the crypts acting as the major zone of DNA synthesis. A further slight shift toward the more abnormal was seen the next year. Several years later, the biopsy was definitely characterized by a greater frequency of cells in the upper third as well as completely upward shift of the major zone of DNA synthesis.

This shift toward the more abnormal type proliferative pattern was not the predominant trend in most high-risk patients. Instead, values were obtained which revealed little if any change over the time period under surveillance (Fig. 7). Two patients with a history of an isolated adenoma or two have been evaluated and their biopsy shown to have a reasonably stable proliferative character. Biopsies from the patient on the left still have a normal major basal zone of DNA synthesis with some enlargement of the proliferative compartment. Those from the patient on the right, however, appear to be hovering at a transitional stage leading to the more abnormal configuration.

It appears reasonable to state at this point that follow-up analyses of biopsy specimens are of importance and extreme interest in asymptomatic relatives of familial polyposis patients, symptomatic members of colon cancer families, as well as others at high risk for colon cancer. Recognizable focal areas of

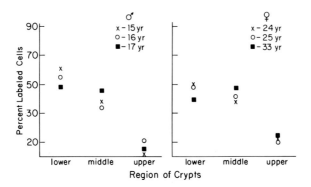

FIG. 6. Percentage of labeled cells distributed in three regions of the colorectal crypts is plotted for 2 asymptomatic familial polyposis patients. At *left,* a male patient followed on 3 successive years, and at *right,* a female followed 3 times over 9 years. The stage 1 abnormality (extension of label to the surface) is seen initially with later appearance of the shift of the major proliferating compartment (stage 2 abnormality).

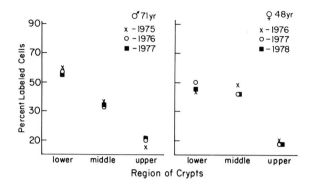

FIG. 7. Percentage of labeled cells distributed in the three regions of the colorectal crypts is plotted for two patients with an isolated polyp surveyed over 3 consecutive years. On the left, a male patient demonstrates only the stage 1 abnormality with relative stability in the proliferative character of the mucosa. The female patient *(right)* demonstrates colorectal mucosa alternating between stage 2 abnormality (shift in the major zone from the lower third to the middle or middle and upper third) and stage 1 abnormality (extension of DNA synthesis to the surface).

cellular atypism or microadenomas have been present in 10 to 15% of biopsies from such patients (10).

Continued study and analysis of human data within these groups may bring to light additional meaningful parameters because significant proliferative alterations may be induced by a combination of genetic, environmental, and temporal factors (2,9,11). It is suggested that the redistribution or shift of the major zone of DNA synthesis within colonic crypts be considered as an early signal of the initiation of a neoplasm at that site.

What is believed to be a microscopic representation of the first visible stage of polyp development appeared in a crypt of a mouse given 3 weekly injections of DMH (Fig. 8). During postnatal growth, the normal course of development of new crypts has been observed from the base of the glands and by a process of bifurcation (12). However, in this instance a bulge or pocket was formed from the middle and upper portion of the crypt. This would coincide with the region found to be most active in cell proliferation during the stage 2 abnormality.

The high incidence of the stage 1 abnormality among all groups tested, including controls, could be related to the aging phenomenon. If the normal regulatory processes break down with increasing age, then the stage 1 abnormality would begin to manifest itself first in one area and then in another, leading to a patchy distribution. The time interval over which this expression of aging occurs might be genetically compressed in certain groups, and thereby a greater likelihood would exist that the stage 2 abnormality manifest itself with subsequent polyp formation. Thus both from the biochemical information and from a theoretical standpoint, this parameter of the upward shift in the major zone of DNA

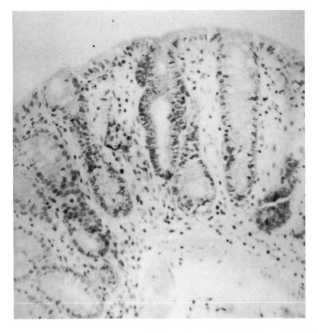

FIG. 8. Distal colonic mucosa from a mouse given 3 weekly injections of DMH at a dose of 20 mg/kg body weight. A bulge is shown arising from the upper region of one crypt (×200).

synthesis appears to have a more selective character and may serve as a more discriminating marker for the early detection of tumor formation in colorectal mucosa.

ACKNOWLEDGMENTS

The author wishes to thank Drs. Sherlock, Winawer, and Lipkin for biopsy material and Florence Long and Mary Hakissian for their dedicated technical assistance. These studies were supported in part by NCI Grants CA-14991 and 08748, and NCI Contract CP 43366.

REFERENCES

1. Bleiberg, H., Mainguet, P., and Galand, P. (1972): Cell renewal in familial polyposis. Comparison between polyps and adjacent healthy mucosa. *Gastroenterology,* 63:240–245.
2. Cohen, B. I., Raicht, R. F., Deschner, E. E., Takahashi, M., Sarwal, A. N., and Fazzini, E. (1980): Biochemical and cell alterations following cholic acid feeding on MNU induced colon tumors in rats. *J. Natl. Cancer Inst.,* 64:573–578.
3. Cole, J. W., and McKalen, A. (1963): Studies on the morphogenesis of adenomatous polyps in the human colon. *Cancer,* 16:998–1002.
4. Deschner, E. E. (1970): Autoradiographic studies of DNA, RNA, and protein synthesis in normal and diseased colonic mucosa. In: *Carcinoma of the Colon and Antecedent Epithelium,* edited by W. Burdette, pp. 222–229. Charles C Thomas, Springfield, Illinois.

5. Deschner, E. E. (1978): Early proliferative defects induced by six weekly injections of 1,2-dimethylhydrazine in epithelial cells of mouse distal colon. *Z. Krebsforsch.,* 91:205–216.
6. Deschner, E. E., and Lipkin, M. (1975): Proliferative patterns in colonic mucosa in familial polyposis. *Cancer,* 35:413–418.
7. Deschner, E. E., Lipkin, M., and Solomon, C. (1966): In vitro study of human epithelial cells. II. H^3-Thymidine incorporation into polyps and adjacent mucosa. *J. Natl. Cancer Inst.,* 36:849–857.
8. Deschner, E. E., and Long, F. C. (1977): Colonic neoplasms in mice produced with six injections of 1,2-dimethylhydrazine. *Oncology,* 34:255–257.
9. Deschner, E. E., and Raicht, R. F. (1979): The influence of bile on the kinetic behavior of colonic epithelial cells of the rat. *Digestion.* 19:322–327.
10. Deschner, E. E., Winawer, S. J., Long, F. C., and Boyle, C. C. (1977): Early detection of colonic neoplasia in patients at high risk. *Cancer,* 40:2625–2631.
11. Lynch, P. M., Lynch, H. T., and Harris, R. E. (1977): Hereditary proximal colonic cancer. *Dis. Colon Rectum,* 20:661–668.
12. Maskens, A. P. (1978): Histogenesis of colon glands during postnatal growth. *Acta Anat.* (Basel), 100:17–26.
13. Maskens, A. P., and Deschner, E. E. (1977): Tritiated thymidine incorporation into epithelial cells of normal-appearing colorectal mucosa of cancer patients. *J. Natl. Cancer Inst.,* 58:1221–1224.
14. Takahashi, K. (1971): Outline of gastric mass survey by x-ray. Early gastric cancer. *Gann,* 11:21–26.
15. Thurnherr, N., Deschner, E. E., Stonehill, E. H., and Lipkin, M. (1973): Induction of adenocarcinomas of the colon in mice by weekly injection of 1,2-dimethylhydrazine. *Cancer Res.,* 33:940–945.
16. Winawer, S. J., Miller, D. G., Schottenfeld, D., Leidner, S. D., Sherlock, P., Befler, B., and Stearns, M. W., Jr. (1977): Feasibility of fecal occult blood testing for detection of colorectal neoplasia. *Cancer,* 40:2616–2619.
17. Winawer, S. J., Sherlock, P., Schottenfeld, D., and Miller, D. G. (1976): Screening for colon cancer. *Gastroenterology,* 70:783–789.

Colorectal Cancer: Prevention, Epidemiology, and Screening, edited by S. Winawer, D. Schottenfeld, and P. Sherlock. Raven Press, New York © 1980.

Measurement of Risk Factors in Identifying Population Groups with Increased Susceptibility to Cancer of the Large Intestine

Martin Lipkin

Memorial Sloan-Kettering Cancer Center, New York, New York 10021

In recent years, newer approaches to the control of large bowel neoplasia have been proposed in several areas. These include attempts to improve the early identification of population groups at increased risk for colorectal cancer, and associated studies of environmental and physiological elements believed to contribute to the pathogenesis of colorectal neoplasms. In parallel studies methods of intervention in population groups at increased risk have been started, and attempts to prevent the origin and progression of colorectal neoplasms have been initiated.

Studies of cell proliferation in the colon of man have contributed to these approaches, because of delineation of the boundaries of the cell proliferation and maturation compartments within the mucosa. In recent years, these findings together with related parameters have been applied to the study of early indices of susceptibility in human population groups at high risk for gastrointestinal cancer. Population groups having increased risk for colorectal cancer are listed in Table 1. The major population groups that have been studied to date are those with hereditary predisposition to colorectal cancer. Phenotypic abnormali-

TABLE 1. *Population groups at increased risk for colorectal cancer*

Familial polyposis syndromes
    Inherited adenomatosis of colon and rectum
    Gardner syndrome
    Turcot syndrome
    Woolf syndrome
    Puetz-Jegher syndrome
    Diffuse gastrointestinal polyposis
Hereditary adenocarcinomatosis
Site-specific colon cancer
Cancer family syndrome
Previous colon, breast, endometrial, or bladder cancer
Single and multiple discrete adenomas
Inflammatory bowel disease
Residence in geographic areas having high frequencies of
    colorectal cancer

TABLE 2. *Phenotypic characteristics recently reported in population groups at increased risk for colorectal cancer*

Phenotypic characteristic	Reference
Colonic epithelial cells	
Adenomatous morphology leading to adenoma-cancer sequence	16,42–44
Abnormal proliferation of cells in individuals with familial polyposis and Gardner's syndrome	1–5,45,46
Extraintestinal neoplasms	16,42,47–52
Immunoparameter	
Inappropriate suppression of normal lymphocyte response to allogeneic stimulus in nonpolyposis familial aggregates and Gardner's syndrome	23
Cutaneous cells	
Heteroploidy of cutaneous epithelial cells in individuals with Gardner's syndrome	19
Growth modifications of cutaneous fibroblasts in familial polyposis and Gardner's syndrome	20–22
Fecal contents	
Decreased fecal degradation of cholesterol in familial polyposis and in some individuals in the general population	24–27
Conversion of bile acids and cholesterol by fecal microflora and modifications of fecal bacterial enzyme activities	53–56
Mutagen activity in feces of human subjects in the general population	28–31
Conversion of nitrogenous compounds to nitrosamines with carcinogenic activity	28–31

ties recently reported in some of these population groups are summarized in Table 2, and are discussed in the following sections.

PROLIFERATIVE ABNORMALITIES IN COLONIC EPITHELIAL CELLS OF INDIVIDUALS WITH FAMILIAL POLYPOSIS

Studies of cell proliferation have aided our understanding of events that develop during neoplastic transformation of colonic cells, in the hereditary diseases leading to large bowel cancer, and in the sporadic large bowel cancers believed to be caused mainly by enviromental or endogenously produced carcinogens. In familial polyposis, colonic epithelial cells predestined to develop neoplasia show characteristic proliferative changes. During progressive stages of abnormal development, cell phenotypes appear in which epithelial cells gain an increased ability to proliferate and to accumulate in the mucosa (1–5).

In the normal colon of man, the major proliferative activity occurs in the lower and mid-regions of the crypts adjacent to the base, occupying about two-thirds of the crypt columns. Approximately 15 to 20% of the proliferating cells are engaged in DNA synthesis, and these rapidly leave the cell cycle as they undergo maturation. The number of cells in the proliferative cycle diminishes as they advance to the lumenal region of the crypts; within hours cells undergo further differentiation, and proliferative activity ceases as they approach the crypt surfaces (6,7).

In individuals with familial polyposis, patches of flat mucosa can be detected having colonic epithelial cells that fail to repress DNA synthesis during migration to the surface of the mucosa (1–5). This finding has been observed in normal appearing colonic epithelial cells of subjects with familial polyposis before as well as after the cells develop adenomatous changes and begin to accumulate as polyps. It has been noted in over 80% of random biopsy specimens (8), and has now been shown to occur with higher frequency than in population groups at low risk of colorectal cancer (9).

Current observations in our laboratory also have now indicated a significantly higher frequency of abnormal proliferative activity of this type in colon cancer-prone families without familial polyposis (9). In our ongoing studies we are continuing to quantitate several proliferative abnormalities as they are observed in colonic mucosa of high and low risk population groups, to further analyze their discriminatory value in pointing to colon cancer risk in subjects in different geographic regions.

A failure of colonic epithelial cells to repress DNA synthesis also occurs in other diseases of man including ulcerative colitis (10). In ways similar to diseases of the colon, in atrophic gastritis, a condition associated with the development of gastric malignancy, epithelial cells also fail to repress DNA synthesis and undergo abnormal maturation as they migrate through the gastric mucosa (11,12). A similar event occurs in precancerous disease of the cervical epithelium in humans (13), and in cervix of rodents after a chemical carcinogen (14). Thus, during the development of neoplasms in other organs as well as in the colon, persistent DNA synthesis occurs in cells that normally would be terminal or end cells. Associated pathological changes accompany this development leading to atypias, dysplasias, and malignancy, as also occurs in familial polyposis.

In familial polyposis, as colonic epithelial cells which do not repress proliferative activity undergo abnormal maturation and accumulate in the mucosa, they develop the morphological changes characteristic of adenomas; these further develop the tubular or villous structures noted above. In terms of cell proliferation kinetics, we have estimated that most epithelial cells in these adenomas are extruded, whereas only a minor fraction are retained to proliferate and induce growth (15). Carcinomas develop with increasing frequency as these adenomatous excrescences enlarge (16).

We believe that a sequence of events leads to malignancy in inherited polyposis (8). Cells having the germinal mutation fail to repress DNA synthesis (phase 1 proliferative lesion) (17). Additional events then occur, giving rise to new clones from the original cell population. An early event leads to the development of the well-known adenomatous cells that proliferate and accumulate near the surface of the mucosa (phase 2 proliferative lesion) (17). In familial polyposis, according to this concept, an additional event then occurs in the cells giving rise to invasive malignancy. This concept allows for a contribution of endogenous or exogenous carcinogenic or promoter elements to interact with the cells having a hereditary predisposition to neoplasia. It also allows for the introduction of preventive measures to block the steps leading to malignant transformation of cells.

CEA IN COLONIC LAVAGE OF INDIVIDUALS AT HIGH RISK FOR LARGE BOWEL CANCER

In addition to abnormal proliferative activity in colonic epithelial cells of familial polyposis, identifiable at an early stage before the development of visible adenomas, increased CEA also has been noted in colonic lavage specimens obtained from members of polyposis family aggregates. Plasma CEA has been disappointing as an indicator of early lesions; however, elevated CEA concentrations have been shown in colonic lavage specimens from individuals with large adenomas and cancer, compared to specimens from individuals without evidence of colonic disease. A recent study was carried out to measure CEA concentrations in colonic lavage of hereditary polyposis families, nonpolyposis colon cancer-prone families, and controls without evidence of colonic disease or familial predisposition to colon cancer. Current findings have indicated a significant elevation of CEA in colonic lavage of many of the individuals in familial polyposis aggregates who do not have visible adenomas (18). The reasons for the CEA elevation are unknown at present, but may be associated with early hyperplasia of the cells or other inflammatory changes that develop within the mucosa in familial polyposis.

STUDIES OF CUTANEOUS CELLS OF INDIVIDUALS WITH FAMILIAL POLYPOSIS

Recent studies also have indicated that phenotypic expressions of the genetic defect leading to familial polyposis can be detected in cutaneous cells. Increased heteroploidy in cutaneous epithelial cells derived from individuals with Gardner's syndrome has been reported (19). It was also noted that cutaneous fibroblasts derived from individuals previously diagnosed as having familial polyposis or Gardner's syndrome have abnormal growth characteristics (20). Two recent studies have shown differences in the distribution of the cytoskeletal protein actin, within cultured cells from individuals with familial polyposis compared to those of normals (21,22). In order to determine the specificity of these observations, additional measurements are presently being carried out on cutaneous cells from larger control groups at low risk for large bowel cancer, and from additional families with various patterns of inherited polyposis and large bowel cancer.

IMMUNOLOGIC STUDIES

Recently, an immunologic abnormality has been reported in individuals from colon cancer-prone families without polyposis (23). When cancer-free individuals from families predisposed to large bowel cancer but without familial polyposis were studied to determine the nature of their cell-mediated immune capacities, 44% demonstrated an apparent perturbation of adherent cell function which manifested itself as an inappropriate suppression of potentially normal lymphocyte ability to respond to an allogeneic stimulus. This *in vitro* defect in recognitive immunity that had developed in these individuals was the same defect demonstrated in individuals with established malignancies. Several patients with Gardner's syndrome also showed the deficit of recognitive immunity (23). These studies also are being extended to asymptomatic individuals in additional familial aggregates having the various disorders leading to large bowel cancer, and offer the possibility of a new immunological approach to the early detection of susceptible population groups.

EXAMINATION OF FECAL CONTENTS

In familial polyposis and related disorders, still other studies are in progress to identify those constituents of fecal contents that may be abnormal, and to examine their potential carcinogenic activity on cells of the colon. The bile acids and their bacterial conversion products are a group of compounds currently under examination. Several recent reports have analyzed and compared the fecal neutral steroids and bile acids in patients with familial polyposis and controls other than relatives (24–26). Individuals with familial polyposis excreted higher amounts of cholesterol and lower levels of the degradation products of cholesterol: coprostanol and coprostanone. Nondegradation of cholesterol also has been found in a minor fraction of individuals in the general population (27), whose background and related characteristics have not been defined.

Current results also have suggested differences in metabolic activity of fecal microflora in members of familial polyposis aggregates, compared to age- and sex-matched controls who consumed similar Western-style diets. Differences in metabolic activity of fecal microflora have previously been shown in population groups at increased risk for large bowel neoplasia. Further studies also are in progress to extend these findings to individuals in the familial colon cancer-prone groups in order to assess the utility of these variations in metabolic activity of fecal microflora and in cholesterol and its metabolites. Findings of this type may contribute to the screening of polyposis family siblings for disease, and could point to mechanisms of initiation or promotion during large bowel carcinogenesis.

Recently, an additional and potentially important lead to the identification of factors involved in colon cancer development was provided by detection of mutagenic activity in the feces of humans (28,29). It was suspected that a nitroso group exchange reaction occurred by transfer from nitrosamine to an amide moiety, resulting in the generation of highly reactive nitrosamide compounds in feces (30), and that endogenous nitrates in humans might lead to formation of carcinogens (31). In current work, patients in the familial polyposis and hereditary large bowel cancer-prone (nonpolyposis) aggregates are under study;

this topic remains an interesting one for further development. We now have a variety of approaches to the analysis of fectal contents of individuals in high and low risk categories underway, including the above parameters.

APPROACHES TO THE PREVENTION OF COLORECTAL CANCER

In view of the numerous observations that have been made on the pathogenesis and early detection of colorectal neoplasia, can reasonable approaches be developed to attempt prevention of onset and progression of these lesions? In support of this possibility are observations, in a variety of experimental model systems and in humans, on modifications of lesion development and growth. Current experimental approaches that have been proposed for the prevention of large bowel neoplasia are summarized in the following references and comprise a new and expanding field of research (32–40). These experimental approaches involve the deletion from or addition to the human diet of naturally occurring substances, or addition of a variety of compounds to experimental model systems.

Thus, in addition to studies on early markers of neoplasm in highly susceptible population groups, a variety of experimental approaches to active intervention and chemoprevention of colorectal neoplasia have been initiated. Experimental programs are in progress in various laboratories to elucidate mechanisms of carcinogenesis and cell transformation in humans, and in cellular and animal model systems that can lead to active intervention by deletion or addition of natural and synthetic substances. As efforts of this type become directed to human populations, the presence of early preclinical phenotypic characteristics can be recorded and quantitated for experimental programs, as described above. Degrees of abnormal cellular change and other related phenotypic abnormalities can be quantitated to characterize current risk, and then to predict the probability of natural evolution of disease in individuals who are at specified ages in well-defined population groups (8,41). Risk profiles for this purpose are being developed and are reported separately (41).

Based on information available on the expected age of development of disease in individuals in these well-defined high risk aggregates, and on the observed evolution of disease when individuals are entered into specified treatment regimens, it will be possible to study the utility of experimental treatment programs on prevention, as well as early detection of phenotypic abnormalities in humans at high risk for colorectal cancer.

REFERENCES

1. Deschner, E. E., Lewis, C. M., and Lipkin, M. (1963): *In vitro* study of human rectal epithelial cells. I. Atypical zone of H3 thymidine incorporation in mucosa of multiple polyposis. *J. Clin. Invest.,* 42:1922–1928.
2. Deschner, E., and Lipkin, M. (1975): Proliferative patterns in colonic mucosa of polyposis families. *Cancer,* 35:413–418.
3. Lipkin, M. (1977): Growth kinetics of normal and premalignant gastrointestinal epithelium. In: *Growth Kinetics and Biochemical Regulation of Normal and Malignant Cells,* pp. 562–589. Williams & Wilkins, Baltimore.

4. Bleiberg, H., Mainguet, P., and Galand, P. (1972): Cell renewal in familial polyposis. Comparison between polyps and adjacent healthy mucosa. *Gastroenterology*, 63:240–245.
5. Iwana, T., Utsunomiya, J., and Sasaki, J. (1977): Epithelial cell kinetics in the crypts of familial polyposis of the colon. *Jpn. J. Surg.*, 7:230–234.
6. Lipkin, M., Sherlock, P., and Bell, B. (1963): Cell proliferation kinetics in the gastrointestinal tract of man. II. Cell renewal in stomach, ileum, colon, and rectum. *Gastroenterology*, 45:721–729.
7. Lipkin, M. (1973): Proliferation and differentiation of gastrointestinal cells. *Physiol. Rev.*, 53:891–915.
8. Lipkin, M. (1978): Susceptibility of human population groups to colon cancer. *Adv. Cancer Res.*, 27:281–304.
9. Lipkin, M., Deschner, E., Blattner, W., Fraumeni, J. F., Jr., and Lynch, H. T. (1980): *(In preparation.)*
10. Eastwood, G. L., and Trier, J. S. (1973): Epithelial cell renewal in cultured rectal biopsies in ulcerative colitis. *Gastroenterology*, 64:383–390.
11. Winawer, S., and Lipkin, M. (1969): Cell proliferation kinetics in the gastrointestinal tract of man. IV. Cell renewal in intestinalized gastric mucosa. *J. Natl. Cancer Inst.*, 42:9–17.
12. Deschner, E. E., Winawer, S., and Lipkin, M. (1972): Patterns of nucleic acid and protein synthesis in normal human gastric mucosa and atrophic gastritis. *J. Natl. Cancer Inst.*, 48:1567–1574.
13. Wilbanks, G. D., Richart, R. M., and Terner, J. Y. (1967): DNA content of cervical intraepithelial neoplasm studied by two wavelength Feulgen cytophotometry. *Am. J. Obstet. Gynecol.*, 98:792–799.
14. Hasegawa, I., Matsumira, Y., and Tojo, S. (1976): Cellular kinetics and histological changes in experimental cancer of the uterine cervix. *Cancer Res.*, 36:359–364.
15. Lightdale, C., and Lipkin, M. (1975): Cell division and tumor growth. *Cancer*, 3:201–215.
16. Morson, B. C., and Bussey, H. J. R. (1970): Predisposing causes of intestinal cancer. In: *Current Problems in Surgery*, pp. 1–50. Year Book Medical Publishers, Chicago, Illinois.
17. Lipkin, M. (1974): Phase 1 and phase 2 proliferative lesions of colonic epithelial cells in diseases leading to colon cancer. *Cancer*, 34:878–888.
18. Poleski, M. H., Blattner, W. A., Chait, M., Winawer, S. W., Fleischer, M., Schwartz, M. D., Fraumeni, J. F., Jr., and Lipkin, M. (1978): CEA in colonic lavage of individuals at high risk for large bowel cancer. *Gastroenterology*, 74:1140.
19. Danes, B. (1977): Brief communication: The Gardner syndrome: A family study in cell culture. *J. Natl. Cancer Inst.*, 58:771.
20. Pfeffer, L., Lipkin, M., Stutman, O., and Kopelovich, L. (1976): Growth abnormalities in cultured human skin fibroblasts. *J. Cell Physiol.*, 89:29–37.
21. Kopelovich, L., Conlon, S., and Pollack, R. (1977): Defective organization of actin in cultured skin fibroblasts from patients with inherited adenocarcinoma. *Proc. Natl. Acad. Sci. U.S.A.*, 74:3019.
22. Kopelovich, L., Lipkin, M., Blattner, W., Fraumeni, J., Lynch, H., and Pollack, R. (1980): *(Submitted for publication.)*
23. Berlinger, N. T., Lopez, C., Vogel, J., Lipkin, M., and Good, R. A. (1977): Defective recognitive immunity in family aggregates of colon carcinoma. *J. Clin. Invest.*, 59:761–769.
24. Reddy, B. S., Mastromarino, A., Gustafson, C., Lipkin, M., and Wynder, E. L. (1976): Fecal bile acids and neutral sterols in patients with familial polyposis. *Cancer*, 38:1694–1698.
25. Drasar, B. S., Bone, E. S., Hill, M. F., and Marks, C. G. (1975): Colon cancer and bacterial metabolism in familial polyposis. *Gut*, 16:824–825.
26. Watne, P. L., Lai, H. L., Mance, T., and Core, S. (1975): Fecal steroids and bacterial flora in polyposis coli patients. Society for surgery of the alimentary tract, May 1975, San Antonio, Texas.
27. Wilkins, T. D., and Hackman, A. S. (1974): Two patterns of neutral steroid conversion in the feces of normal North Americans. *Cancer Res.*, 34:2250–2254.
28. Varghese, A. J., Land, P., Furrer, R., and Bruce, W. R. (1977): Proceedings of the 68th Annual Meeting. *Proc. Am. Assoc. Cancer Res.*, 18:317.
29. Land, P. C., and Bruce, W. R. (1978): Fecal mutagens: A possible relationship with colorectal cancer. *Proc. Am. Assoc. Cancer Res.*, 19:167.
30. Mandel, M., Ichinotsubo, D., and Mower, H. (1977): Nitroso group exchange as a way of activation of nitrosamines by bacteria. *Nature*, [Lond.] 267:248–249.

31. Tannenbaum, S. R., Fett, D., Young, V. R., Land, P. D., and Bruce, W. R. (1978): Nitrite and nitrate are formed by endogenous synthesis in human intestine. *Science,* 200:1487–1489.
32. Wattenberg, L. W. (1972): Inhibition of carcinogenic and toxic effects of polycyclic hydrocarbons by phenolic antioxidants and ethoxygens.*J. Natl. Cancer Inst.,* 48:1425–1430.
33. Wattenberg, L. W., and Fiala, E. S. (1978): Inhibition of 1,2-dimethylhydrazine-induced neoplasm of the large intestine in female CFI mice by carbon disulfide: Brief communication. *J. Natl. Cancer Inst.,* 60:1515–1517.
34. Newberne, P. M., and Suphakarn, V. (1977): Preventive role of vitamin A in colon carcinogenesis in rats. *Cancer,* 40:2553–2556.
35. Ward, J. M., Sporn, M. B., Wenk, M. L., Smith, J. M., Fesser, D., and Dean, R. J. (1978): Dose response to intrarectal administration of N-methyl-N-nitrosourea and histopathologic evaluation of the effect of two retinoids on colon lesions induced in rats. *J. Natl. Cancer Inst.,* 60:1489–1493.
36. Mirvish, S. S., Wallcave, L., Eagen, M., and Shubik, P. (1972): Ascorbate-nitrite reaction: Possible means of blocking the formation of carcinogenic N-nitroso compounds. *Science,* 177:65–68.
37. DeCosse, J. J., Adams, M. B., Kuzma, J. R., LoGerfo, P., and Condon, R. E. (1975): Effect of ascorbic acid on rectal polyps of patients with familial polyposis. *Surgery,* 78:608–612.
38. Lai, H. L., Shields, E. K., and Watne, A. L. (1977): Effect of ascorbic acid on rectal polyps and fecal steroids. *Fed. Proc.,* 36:1061.
39. Troll, W., Meyn, M., and Rossman, G. (1978): Mechanisms of protease action in carcinogenesis. *Carcinogenesis, Vol. 2, Mechanisms of Tumor Promotion and Cocarcinogenesis,* edited by T. J. Slaga, A. Sivak, and R. K. Boutwell. Raven Press, New York.
40. Jacobs, M. M. (1977): Inhibitory effects of selenium on dimethylhydrazine and methylazoxymethanol colon carcinogenesis. *Cancer,* 40:2557–2564.
41. Lipkin, M., Sherlock, P., and DeCosse, J. (1980): Identification of risk factors and preventive measures in the prevention of cancer of the large intestine. *Curr. Probl. Cancer (in press).*
42. Bussey, H. J. R. (1975): *Familial Polyposis Coli.* Johns Hopkins University Press, Baltimore.
43. Lane, N., and Lev, R. (1963): Observations on the origin of adenomatous epithelium of the colon: Serial reaction studies of minute polyps in familial polyposis. *Cancer,* 16:751–764.
44. Spjut, H. (1977): National Large Bowel Cancer Project Workshop, Houston, Texas.
45. Cole, J. W., and McKalen, A. (1963): Studies on the morphogenesis of adenomatous polyps in the human colon. *Cancer,* 16:998–1002.
46. Deschner, E., and Lipkin, M. (1970): Study of human rectal epithelial cells *in vitro.* III. RNA, protein and DNA synthesis in polyps and adjacent mucosa. *J. Natl. Cancer Inst.,* 44:175–185.
47. Gardner, E. J. (1951): A genetic and clinical study of intestinal polyposis, a predisposing factor for carcinoma of the colon and rectum. *Am. J. Hum. Genet.,* 3:167–176.
48. Gardner, E. J., and Richards, R. C. (1953): Multiple cutaneous and subcutaneous lesions occurring simultaneously with hereditary polyposis and osteomatosis. *Am. J. Hum. Genet.,* 5:139–147.
49. Smith, W. G. (1959): Desmoid tumors in familial multiple polyposis. *Mayo Clin. Proc.,* 34:31–38.
50. Turcot, J., Despres, J. P., and Pierre, F. (1959): Malignant tumors of the central nervous system associated with familial polyposis of the colon. *Dis. Colon Rectum,* 2:465–468.
51. Jeghers, H., McKusick, V. A., and Katz, K. H. (1949): Generalized intestinal polyposis and melanin spots of the oral mucosa, lips and digits. *N. Engl. J. Med.,* 241:993–1005.
52. Smilow, P. C., Pryor, C. A., Jr., and Swinton, N. W. (1966): Juvenile polyposis coli: A report of three patients in three generations of one family. *Dis. Colon Rectum,* 9:248–254.
53. Hill, M. J. (1971): The effect of some factors on the faecal concentration of acid steroids, neutral steroids and urobilins. *J. Pathol.,* 104:239–245.
54. Reddy, B. S., and Wynder, E. L. (1973): Large bowel carcinogenesis: Fecal constituents of populations with diverse incidence rates of colon cancer. *J. Natl. Cancer Inst.,* 50:1437–1442.
55. Reddy, B. S., Weisburger, J., and Wynder, E. L. (1975): Effects of high risk and low risk diets for colon carcinogenesis on fecal microflora and steroids in man. *J. Nutr.,* 105:878–884.
56. Hill, M. J. (1975): The role of colon anaerobes in the metabolism of bile acids and steroids, and its relation to colon cancer. *Cancer,* 36:2387–2400.

*Colorectal Cancer: Prevention, Epidemiology,
and Screening,* edited by S. Winawer, D. Schottenfeld,
and P. Sherlock. Raven Press, New York © 1980.

Cancer Risk with Single and Multiple Adenomas: Synchronous and Metachronous Tumors

Göran R. Ekelund

Department of Surgery, Malmö General Hospital, Malmö, Sweden

There has been considerable controversy over the years as to whether colorectal adenomas can transform into carcinoma. This discussion has often been confusing. Generally, there has been no disagreement regarding the cancer risk of villous adenomas, or as they are often called, adenovillous papillomas, papillary adenomas, or villous papillomas. However, the cancer risk for simple tubular adenomatous polyps has been unclear. Most authors agree that all adenomas are qualitatively potential carcinomas (10,17,19). The quantitative magnitude of the risk for malignant transformation of colorectal adenomas into adenocarcinoma is, however, a basis for some disagreement. Morson (18) has suggested one of the major reasons for the confusion, stating that "although the concept of the adenoma-carcinoma sequence has gained increasing acceptance in recent years much of the evidence in its favour remains circumstantial and falls short of direct scientific proof." Table 1 lists the factors increasing cancer risk in patients with adenoma.

NONSTANDARDIZATION OF REPORTING

Another major reason for confusion regarding the polyp-cancer sequence can be found in the variation in nomenclature and classification reported. Many older series include metaplastic (2,15) or hyperplastic (13) polyps among adeno-

TABLE 1. *Factors increasing the synchronous and metachronous cancer risk in patients with adenoma*

Risk factor	Reference
Villous histology	7,10,17
Adenoma atypia	6,17
Size	7,8,10,11,17
Carcinoma and adenoma	9,18
Adenoma adjacent carcinoma	7,10
Multiple adenoma	5,18
Age	10
Male sex	7,12

mas. These are common lesions, often multiple but tiny and easily overlooked at sigmoidoscopy, and overlooked in resected specimens. Since no malignant potential has been attributed to these nonneoplastic polyps, they should be separated from adenomas in the evaluation of cancer risk. In 1976, the World Health Organization proposed a classification of adenomas into tubular adenomas, tubulovillous adenomas, and villous adenomas (16). This is a distinct classification which hopefully will replace all other classifications. It is especially noteworthy that villous lesions are regarded as a category of adenomas and not as a separate entity. The percentages of the various types of adenomas vary slightly among series. Morson (17) reported 75% to be tubular adenomas, 15% tubulovillous, and 10% villous adenomas.

Most available data are from materials consisting of patients highly selected. In an epidemiological, unselected 10-year series of colorectal carcinoma in the city of Malmö, Sweden, coexisting benign polyps were studied. Of the adenomas, 77% were tubular, 21% were tubulovillous, and only 2% were classified as villous adenomas (3,7). In this series there were thus relatively more tubulovillous than villous adenomas as compared to the series reported by Morson, whereas the frequencies of tubular adenomas were similar.

VARYING CRITERIA FOR REPORTING OF CARCINOMA

Another major reason for much of the confusion regarding the polyp-cancer relationship is the use of varying criteria for the diagnosis of carcinoma. There is an established experience that lesions with cytological and histological transformation of the epithelium fulfilling the usual criteria for carcinoma but without invasion through the muscularis mucosae rarely give rise to metastases. Such lesions are thus from a clinical point of view benign and need only local excision for treatment. This fact has led many pathologists to report such clinically benign but histopathologically malignant lesions as benign adenomas in order to prevent unnecessary surgery. This approach, however, results in the underreporting of very early carcinomas in adenomas.

Although there certainly are infinite gradations between the stages, it would be preferable to adopt a standardized classification, such as: (a) adenomas (with or without atypia); (b) adenomas with carcinoma *in situ;* (c) adenomas with foci of intramucosal carcinoma; and (d) invasive carcinoma, i.e., invasion beyond the muscularis mucosae, as described by Enterline (10). The use of such a classification could make comparisons between various series possible.

TYPE OF ADENOMA AND CANCER RISK

Malignant transformation frequently occurs in villous adenomas. Morson (17) has reported the risk to be 40%, as compared to a risk of 5% for tubular adenomas, and 22% for tubulovillous adenomas. The potential for malignant transformation has been reported to be greater when the adenoma has more villous features (1). This is also apparent from the Malmö series in which 11% of tubular adenomas were well differentiated, as compared to only 1% of those which were tubulovillous or villous adenomas. The percentage of adenomas that were poorly differentiated or with advanced dysplasia was 24% for the nonvillous and 40% for the villous types (7). Morson (17) has also reported a definite correlation of increasing epithelial atypia with increasing malignant potential.

SIZE AND CANCER RISK

With increasing size there is an increasing percentage of adenomas with severe atypia, *in situ,* and invasive carcinoma. In the Malmö series, 44% of those adenomas smaller than 5 mm were well or moderately differentiated, in contrast to 27% of those above 10 mm in size (7). In a series of adenomas removed at colonoscopy (11), intramucosal carcinoma occurred in 13% and carcinoma with invasion through the muscularis mucosae in 5.5%. Invasive cancer occurred more frequently in adenomas greater than 10 mm. Morson (17) reported that nearly 50% of adenomas more than 20 mm in size were malignant (i.e., with invasion beyond the muscularis mucosae). Size of adenoma is thus one of the most important parameters when considering the risk of malignancy. An increase in size on repeated radiograms indicates an increased risk that a polyp diagnosed with X-ray is malignant (8).

SITE AND CANCER RISK

The risk of malignant transformation is greater for adenomas located near a coexisting carcinoma and for those located distally in the large bowel. Adenomas having this distribution were more poorly differentiated than those localized elsewhere (7).

SEX AND CANCER RISK

Single and multiple adenomas, as well as multiple carcinomas, are more common in men. In addition, the average grade of differentiation of adenomas tends to be poorer in men than in women. Thus the risk for malignant transformation seems to be slightly more pronounced in men (7). This is also of interest from an epidemiological point of view since carcinoma is relatively more common in females in low risk populations than in populations with a high incidence of colorectal carcinoma (12).

MULTIPLE TUMORS

The risk for malignant transformation is greater for patients with multiple adenomas. In untreated cases of familial adenomatosis, carcinoma arises in almost all cases. However, even the occurrence of one single adenoma indicates a somewhat increased risk that the patient already has or will later develop another adenoma or carcinoma (4). The occurrence of adenoma is at least twice as common in cases with coexisting colorectal carcinoma as in those without and occurs in about two-thirds of those with multiple carcinomas (9). Examined another way, it has been shown that there is a general trend for the incidence of multiple cancers to rise as the number of adenomas increases (5). Multiple colorectal carcinomas are fairly common. In most reports, the frequencies range between 2% and 6%. In the Malmö series, there were 4.6% of cases with multiple synchronous carcinomas, and 2.3% with subsequent metachronous carcinoma (9). There is often a considerable time interval between the initial cancer and the metachronous carcinoma. Lockhart-Mummery and Heald (14) reported it to be on the average 11 years.

RECOMMENDATIONS

Considering the above observations, it is strongly recommended that every patient with a colorectal adenoma or carcinoma have a complete examination of the entire large bowel, i.e., sigmoidoscopy and double-contrast barium enema, as a minimum, and colonoscopy where available and not medically contraindicated, in order to clear the bowel of all synchronous lesions.

After curative removal of colorectal tumors, there is a risk of subsequent metachronous adenomas and carcinomas. A surveillance program for these patients is also critical. When planning such a program, it is necessary to consider the various risk factors mentioned and the methods available for follow-up, i.e., occult blood tests, sigmoidoscopy, barium enema, and colonoscopy.

REFERENCES

1. Appel, M. F., Spjut, H. J., and Estrada, R. G. (1977): The significance of villous components in colonic polyps. *Am. J. Surg.*, 134:770–771.
2. Arthur, J. F. (1962): The significance of small mucosal polyps of the rectum. *Proc. R. Soc. Med.*, 55:703–704.
3. Berge, T., Ekelund, G., Mellner, C., Pihl, B., and Wenckert, A. (1973): Carcinoma of the colon and rectum in a defined population. *Acta Chir. Scand.* [*Suppl. 438*].
4. Brahme, F., Ekelund, G., Nordén, J. G., and Wenckert, A. (1974): Metachronous colorectal polyps; Comparison of development of colorectal polyps and carcinomas in persons with and without histories of polyps. *Dis. Colon Rectum*, 17:166–171.
5. Bussey, H. J. R. (1978): Multiple adenomas and carcinomas. *Major Probl. Pathol.*, 10:72–80.
6. Ekelund, G. (1974): On colorectal polyps and carcinoma with special reference to their interrelationship. Thesis, Studentlitteratur, Lund, Sweden.
7. Ekelund, G., and Lindström, C. (1974): Histopathological analysis of benign polyps in patients with carcinoma of the colon and rectum. *Gut*, 15:654–663.
8. Ekelund, G., Lindström, C., and Rosengren, J. E. (1974): Appearance and growth of early carcinomas of the colon-rectum. *Acta Radiol.* [*Diagn.*] (*Stockh.*), 15:670–679.
9. Ekelund, G., and Pihl, B. (1974): Multiple carcinomas of the colon and rectum. *Cancer*, 33:1630–1634.
10. Enterline, H. T. (1976): Polyps and cancer of the large bowel. *Curr. Top. Pathol.*, 63:95–141.

11. Gabrielsson, N., Granqvist, H., Ohlsén, H., and Sundelin, P. (1978): Malignancy of colonic polyps. Diagnosis and treatment: *Acta Radiol.* [*Diagn.*] *(Stockh.),* 19:479–495.
12. Haenzel, W., and Correa, P. (1971): Cancer of the colon and rectum and adenomatous polyps. A review of epidemiological findings. *Cancer,* 28:14–24.
13. Lane, N., and Lev, R. (1963): Observations on the origin of adenomatous epithelium of the colon. Serial section studies of minute polyps in familiar polyposis. *Cancer,* 16:751–764.
14. Lockhart-Mummery, H. E., and Heald, R. J. (1972): Metachronous cancer of the large intestine. *Dis. Colon Rectum,* 15:261–264.
15. Morson, B. C. (1962): Some peculiarities in the histology of intestinal polyps. *Dis. Colon Rectum,* 5:337–344.
16. Morson, B. C. (ed.) (1976): *International Histological Classification of Tumours, No. 15.* WHO, Geneva.
17. Morson, B. C. (1977): Polyps and cancer of the large bowel. In: *International Academy of Pathology Monograph. The Gastrointestinal Tract,* edited by John H. Yardley, Basil C. Morson, and Murray R. Abell. pp. 101–108. Williams & Wilkins Co., Baltimore.
18. Morson, B. C. (1978): The pathogenesis of colorectal cancer. *Major Probl. Pathol.,* 10:ix.
19. Turell, R. (1978): Colorectal polyps—Revisited. *Am. J. Surg.,* 136:539–540.

Colorectal Cancer: Prevention, Epidemiology, and Screening, edited by S. Winawer, D. Schottenfeld, and P. Sherlock. Raven Press, New York © 1980.

Commentary: Mixed Leukocyte Culture Abnormalities in Inherited Colon Cancer

Norman T. Berlinger

Department of Otolaryngology, National Naval Medical Center, Bethesda, Maryland 20014

Subclinical immunologic deficits have been detected in healthy relatives of family aggregates of lymphoproliferative diseases and gastric cancer suggesting some heritable component of immunopathology in families with a seeming diathesis for malignancy.

We have had the opportunity to study five family aggregates of colon carcinoma who seemed to fulfill the criteria of the heritable cancer family syndrome. These families demonstrated at least two of the following characteristics: (a) carcinoma of the colon apparent in at least three successive generations; (b) carcinoma of the colon appearing with a higher than expected frequency in the family as a whole or in an individual sibship; (c) the occurrence of multiple primary carcinomas of the colon; (d) the occurrence of multiple primary cancers of diverse histological types; (e) the appearance of carcinoma of the colon in the third or fourth decades of life. None of these families demonstrated any evidence of colonic or extracolonic pathology indicating a colonic polyposis syndrome.

Our test of cellular immunocompetence was the mixed leukocyte culture (MLC) reaction. This assay measures the blastogenic response of patient lymphocytes to subtle foreign histocompatibility antigens. It thus represents the *in vitro* counterpart of the allograft response and therefore becomes a model relevant for the tumor situation.

Of the 18 unaffected offspring of individuals with documented colon cancer, 8 (44%) showed significantly decreased lymphocyte responses in MLC as calculated by the relative response method. Interestingly, when patient macrophages were removed from the responding cell population by Sephadex G-10 column filtration, the lymphocytes of the majority of these offspring could manifest significantly improved, and often normal, blastogenesis in MLC.

These results indicate that cancer-free individuals from families with hereditary colon cancer possess a significant cellular immunologic deficit in that their lymphocytes do not optimally respond to an *in vitro* challenge of foreign histocompatibility antigens. Moreover, this deficit appears to be secondary to an inappropriate suppression of lymphocyte responses by autologous macrophages. This was precisely the immunopathologic profile seen in the probands of these families who manifested colon cancer at the time of study. Also, patients with sporadic cancer of the lung, colon, or breast demonstrate exactly the same paradoxical suppression by macrophages of lymphocyte responses to an *in vitro* alloantigenic challenge.

We have also studied affected and unaffected individuals from families with polyposis coli and have found no such immunologic abnormalities. However, two individuals with typical Gardner's syndrome demonstrated decreased MLC responses. These results tend to support the notion of the genetic distinctness of these two clinical entities.

Colorectal Cancer: Prevention, Epidemiology,
and Screening, edited by S. Winawer, D. Schottenfeld,
and P. Sherlock. Raven Press, New York © 1980.

Introduction: Screening Approaches Based on Risk

S. J. Winawer and D. G. Miller

Memorial Sloan-Kettering Cancer Center, New York, New York 10021

The importance of our focus on colorectal cancer in countries at high risk for cancer at this anatomic site is not only because of the high incidence of this disease but also because of the potential for improved survival. This potential for improved survival is based on technological advances over the past few years, accompanied by new insight into concepts of the natural history of colorectal cancer, especially as it relates to associated factors of increased susceptibility. Technologic advances during the past decade have included fiberoptic colonoscopy, colonoscopic polypectomy, flexible sigmoidoscopy, and evolution of the usefulness of select biological markers including fecal occult blood, abnormalities in fibroblast growth patterns and increased chromosomal tetraploidy in tissue culture, mucosal proliferative abnormalities, and mucosal dysplasia (4) (Table 1). Concepts of importance that have evolved fairly recently include identification of high-risk groups including the inherited polyposis and nonpolyposis colon cancer syndromes, the importance of the premalignant adenoma, ulcerative colitis, and the importance of synchronous and metachronous adenomas and cancers. Among the pool of persons at risk for colorectal cancer, the more that can be shifted into the high-risk group for selective screening, the easier the task of identifying those who will be affected by the disease. The greater the number of persons that have to be subjected to general screening, the greater the effort and the greater the cost per case found. Once individuals have been identified as being at high risk, immediate screening and long-term surveillance can reduce the risk of devastating invasive cancer. Most of the information available on

TABLE 1. *Risk and screening*

	Occult blood	Flexible sigmoidoscopy	Barium enema	Colon-oscopy
Standard risk	*	*		
Family history of familial polyposis		*		
Familial polyposis, chronic ulceration colitis		*	*	*
Familial cancer syndromes	*	*	*	*
Personal history of adenoma/cancer	*	*	*	*

the application of screening techniques is based on preliminary results of ongoing trials or small select uncontrolled series. However, based on current understanding of concepts and techniques, rational positions can be assumed for protection of standard and high-risk patients. These positions, of course, will be tempered as data are generated in the future (5).

SUSCEPTIBILITY

Risk for colorectal cancer can be viewed in different subgroups of a population in terms of average risk and high risk: the average-risk patients having no specific predisposing personal or familial factors except for age, and the high-risk groups having identifiable risk factors either personal or familial in nature (Table 2). It is now well-established that risk for colorectal cancer is related to age with the risk beginning at age 40 to 45 in the absence of any underlying genetic factors and increasing approximately twofold in each succeeding decade, reaching a peak at age 75. The risk for men and women is roughly the same.

High-risk subgroups that have been identified in the population include those patients with adenomas of the colon or previous colon cancer, a history of female genital cancer, inflammatory bowel disease, especially ulcerative colitis, and genetic predispositions. The genetic predispositions can be generally divided into nonpolyposis and polyposis types. The polyposis types include the traditional familial polyposis and Gardner's syndrome and their variants; the nonpolyposis genetic syndromes include families with a predilection only for colorectal cancer as well as cancer at other anatomic sites in the gastrointestinal tract, as well as extragastrointestinal cancers especially at female genital sites including breast and uterus. Peutz-Jeghers syndrome has been associated with cancer of the colon, as well as upper gastrointestinal tract cancer, although the majority of polyps are hamartomas located in the small intestine. Juvenile polyposis really consists of sporadic polyps, often only one, and has now been documented to be associated with cancer and adenomas in those families in which these juvenile polyps occur, even though the actual juvenile polyps are benign at the time of discovery in childhood.

Many of these high-risk groups have been further characterized in other parts of this volume in considerable detail. In terms of an approach to screening, it must be emphasized that the usual age-related risk for colorectal cancer changes

---

TABLE 2. *Risks for colorectal cancer*

Average risk:	Age 40 and older, men and women
High risk:	Ulcerative colitis
	Prior colon cancer or adenoma
	Female genital cancer
	Inherited colon cancer
	Polyposis types
	Nonpolyposis types

dramatically as a function of other high-risk factors indicated above. Patients who have had a prior colon adenoma or colorectal cancer are at risk for a subsequent metachronous neoplastic lesion as well as additional synchronous neoplastic lesions at the time the index lesion is discovered, and this is unrelated to age. The age at which members of families with familial polyposis are at risk is at adolescence, and the age at which the nonpolyposis inherited colon cancer family members are at risk begins at age 20. The risk for cancer in ulcerative colitis is related to duration of disease rather than to age. The previous concept of childhood onset of ulcerative colitis providing higher risk is no longer tenable.

TECHNIQUES AVAILABLE FOR SCREENING

Test for Occult Blood

There has been a resurgence of interest in the utilization of occult blood testing in stool for the detection of early colorectal cancer. This test will most likely have its greatest application in patients at average risk who have had no identifiable underlying additional risk factors. It is possible that this test can also be used as an interval examination in other high-risk groups between more aggressive examination by other means including X-ray and endoscopy. The fecal occult blood test, of course, will have no value in patients in whom there is already a predisposition to bleeding, such as patients with ulcerative colitis. It will also be of no value in patients who have known underlying premalignant lesions that may also bleed, such as patients who are already affected with familial polyposis, Gardner's syndrome, or Peutz-Jeghers syndrome. In these patients the search for malignancy by occult blood testing will be of no value since the premalignant polyps may also result in a positive test for occult blood. This test is discussed in detail on other chapters in this volume.

Rigid and Flexible Proctosigmoidoscopy

Proctosigmoidoscopy with the rigid sigmoidoscope has been utilized in many screening programs around the country for many years. It has been of little value on a general population basis because of poor acceptance by patients as a result of discomfort and poor physician application of the test because of lack of interest provided to the physician in training. Where sigmoidoscopy has been utilized it has been demonstrated to be effective. A reasonable estimate of the yield of invasive cancer in asymptomatic patients over the age of 40 is 1.5 in 1,000. In over 26,000 examinations in asymptomatic patients at the Strang Clinic/Preventive Medicine Institute, 58 cancers of the colon were detected. Of the 50 patients followed for 15 or more years, the survival was close to 90% (1). The value of proctosigmoidoscopy cannot be related to rate of detection of invasive cancer alone. Adenomatous polyps are more common than cancer.

The prevalence of polyps on proctosigmoidoscopy in patients over 40 years of age has varied from approximately 4 to 10% in several studies. In addition, it has been shown that periodic proctosigmoidoscopy in an asymptomatic population over a period of 25 years can result in control of cancer of the rectum by identification and removal of premalignant polyps during this examination. It has been shown by later studies with flexible sigmoidoscopy and colonoscopy that rigid sigmoidoscopy is really effective only in the distal 16 cm of rectosigmoid, and that the false negativity is high from 16 to 25 cm.

Flexible sigmoidoscopy with a 60-cm sigmoidoscope has been shown to be of low risk and much higher yield than rigid sigmoidoscopy in the hands of experienced endoscopists (3). Several studies have now indicated this. There now has been a considerable experience with flexible sigmoidoscopy utilizing 60 cm sigmoidoscopes. However, the use of these instruments has been by the experienced colonoscopist, and it remains to be determined what value this scope will have in the hands of the general primary examining physician. It has been previously suggested by our group that a more reasonable approach to examination of the distal 25 cm of bowel may be with a shorter flexible sigmoidoscope of 25 or 30 cm in length which could provide a low-risk, high-yield examination consistently to 30 cm by the primary examining physician who has no prior endoscopic experience. We have been testing this thesis in a feasibility project utilizing a 30 cm prototype instrument in the hands of a family practice physician with low-risk good patient compliance, comfort, and consistent insertion to 30 cm. The problem with this instrument remains its high cost, but it is possible that further technological developments may allow reduction of this cost to provide for its general applicability. This would enable the general medical community for the first time to reconsider its approach to examination of that portion of the bowel that has about 50% of cancers and adenomas located within it. This may provide effective screening of the colon and rectum by coupling with the fecal occult blood test for evaluation of neoplastic lesions above the rectosigmoid. The combination of the two may be especially effective for the average-risk patient since there is a significant false negativity of the fecal occult blood test in the area that can be examined directly by this flexible sigmoidoscope.

Double-Contrast Barium Enema and Colonoscopy in Screening and Diagnosis

For the first time we now have an effective means for surveying the entire colon, either as a screening approach in high-risk patients or as a diagnostic approach in asymptomatic average-risk patients. It has been well demonstrated that the double-contrast barium enema is more productive in the detection of small lesions, especially small polyps, than is the single-column barium enema. The false negativity for the barium enema for polyps is especially high in the upper sigmoid and distal descending colon, where one would normally expect these lesions to occur with greater frequency. It has been shown that colonoscopy complements the air-contrast barium enema exceptionally well in clearing the colon of neoplastic lesions and especially in the detection of additional synchronous lesions in patients who have a single index lesion detected. With current colonoscopes and experience, the physician can reach the cecum in well over 90% of patients in the absence of any serious underlying problems preventing passage of the instrument, such as diverticulitis, severe adhesions, and radiation or tumor fixation of the bowel. The overall complication rate of colonoscopy has been reported to be less than 0.4%. Various tissue sampling techniques can be utilized through colonoscopy, including direct brush cytology, multiple biopsies, and lavage cytology. Lavage cytology was formerly utilized more widely than it is presently, and direct visualization has to a large extent replaced lavage cytology for the detection of colonic neoplasms. Lavage cytology may still be useful in select situations, such as in patients with familial polyposis who have as yet not been operated on and in patients with long-standing ulcerative colitis who are at risk for cancer. In addition to biopsy for the detection of malignancy, biopsy can also be used to evaluate the colon for premalignant changes in ulcerative colitis. This will be discussed in another section in this volume.

In patients who have had a positive screening test for fecal occult blood, both barium enema and colonoscopy are useful in the diagnostic approach for the detection of neoplastic lesions. Colonoscopy and air-contrast barium enema are generally not used for screening purposes in the general population at average risk, but may be useful in high-risk populations. This has not been properly evaluated, but it is generally felt that in certain high-risk populations more aggressive screening by radiologic and endoscopic means is necessary to clear the colon of any neoplastic lesions, and that interval examinations can be done by the less invasive technique of fecal occult blood testing.

Patients with a family history of familial polyposis or Gardner's syndrome can be suitably screened by sigmoidoscopy, especially the more comfortable flexible sigmoidoscopy examination since if they become affected the polyps will be easily identified in the rectum and one need not go on to more extensive examinations. Once it is known that an individual is affected, of course until surgery is performed, surveillance with X-ray and colonoscopy will be necessary on a periodic basis.

In patients with the nonpolyposis types of inherited colon cancer syndromes, no such identifiable biological markers occur in the rectum, and the entire colon has to be surveyed periodically and directly by colonoscopy as well as double-contrast barium enema. This is especially important since it has been shown that there is a reversal of the usual distribution of neoplastic lesions in the colon in such patients, with a higher proportion of these lesions being found on the right side of the colon proximal to the splenic flexure. It is not clear as to the extent of premalignant adenomas that occur in this group of patients prior to the development of colorectal cancer. It is felt that these patients do indeed have a premalignant adenoma that evolves prior to the development of colorectal cancer. Therefore, periodic surveillance would be important in identifying such premalignant lesions and interrupting the polyp cancer sequence in these patients as in the standard-risk patients for colorectal cancer.

Patients who have had an adenoma identified or removed or a colorectal cancer identified and cured need to have aggressive surveillance performed. There appears to be a synchronous rate of approximately 1.5 to 5% for additional cancers in patients with an index cancer, and a synchronous rate of 40 to 50% for additional adenomas in patients with a single adenoma or single cancer of the colon identified (2). In view of this, it is exceedingly important to clear the colon of all additional lesions at some time shortly after identification of the index lesion. It seems that the vast majority of patients who have colorectal cancer identified and operated on do not have colonoscopy performed for routine surveillance of their colon. This is indeed unfortunate since additional premalignant lesions could be uncovered and removed preventing the second metachronous lesion from occurring in these patients. Once the colon has been cleared of all neoplastic lesions, perhaps on two occasions, the colon needs to be put under long-term surveillance at infrequent intervals. This latter concept is based on the very slow evolution of small adenomas *de novo* and their growth to large significant size and transformation to cancers. It has been estimated that this may take 5 or more years, and therefore surveillance intervals need be perhaps every 3 to 5 years in these patients, but should be also done aggressively with at least colonoscopy and perhaps also X-ray. The relative value of colonoscopy and X-ray in all of these groups has not been well established, and in many studies one of the examinations was poor and the other done more expertly, so the comparison demonstrating the benefit of one examination over the other has been biased.

Markers

There has been interest in circulating markers of early cancer and markers obtained by biopsy from mucosa as well as by lavage through endoscopy in patients at risk. At the present time, the only marker that seems to be of potential value in patients at average risk for colorectal cancer is the finding of occult blood in the stool. For various high-risk groups—including the genetic high-risk groups and patients with inflammatory bowel disease—markers are under evaluation and are discussed in much greater detail in other sections of this volume. The current status of the usefulness of markers in average-risk patients is also discussed in another section.

Approach

It is clear that in our approach to screening we must distinguish between average-risk patients and high-risk patients. The screening approaches will be quite different depending on the targeted groups: the general screening approach for average-risk patients and the selective screening approach for high-risk patients, with tailoring of the techniques to the various subgroups. Obviously, the more patients that can be identified as being in a high-risk group, the more productive will be the selective screening of these groups. The interesting question that has been raised is the relationship of sporadic colorectal cancer and colorectal adenomas to the nonpolyposis types of inherited colon cancer, and the relationship to the polyposis types of inherited colon cancer of patients that we see with multiple adenomas. These questions cannot be answered at the present time, and considerably more work will be necessary, but it appears that a much higher percentage of patients than previously considered have genetic factors operating. It is likely that in the future we will be moving towards more aggressive screening of those patients in whom the familial patterns are not truly autosomal dominant but just suggestive of genetic factors operating. Prospective studies in these population groups will need to address these questions and provide data as a basis for guidelines to the medical community in the approach to these various high-risk groups.

REFERENCES

1. Hertz, R. E., Deddish, M. R., and Day, E. (1960): Value of periodic examination in detecting cancer of the rectum and colon. *Postgrad. Med.,* 27:290.
2. Morson, B. C. (1976): Genesis of colorectal cancer. *Clin. Gastroenterol.,* 5:505.
3. Winawer, S. J., Leidner, S. D., Boyle, C., and Kurtz, R. C. (1979): Comparison of flexible sigmoidoscopy with other diagnostic techniques in the diagnosis of rectocolon neoplasia. *Dig. Dis. Sci.,* 24:4:277–281.
4. Winawer, S. J., Poleski, M. H., and Sherlock, P. (1979): Susceptibility for colorectal cancer. Current concepts of screening, diagnosis, and risk. In: *Developments in Digestive Diseases. Clinical Relevance,* edited by J. E. Berk, pp. 73–87. Lea and Febiger, Philadelphia.
5. Winawer, S. J., Sherlock, P., Schottenfeld, D., and Miller, D. G. (1976): Screening for colon cancer. *Gastroenterology,* 70:783–789.

Colorectal Cancer: Prevention, Epidemiology, and Screening, edited by S. Winawer, D. Schottenfeld, and P. Sherlock. Raven Press, New York © 1980.

Fundamental Issues in Cancer Screening

David Schottenfeld

Memorial Sloan-Kettering Cancer Center, and Cornell University Medical College, New York, New York 10021

The process of screening is the efficient application of a relatively simple and inexpensive test to a large number of persons in order to classify asymptomatic individuals as likely, or unlikely, to have colorectal cancer. A program of early cancer detection may also focus on precursor lesions, such as the adenomatous (tubular) and villous polyps of the large intestine. The assumption is that early case finding and therapeutic intervention will restore health and diminish potential morbidity and mortality.

Wilson and Jungner (13) have reviewed the fundamental principles which should guide the planning and development of a program of screening and early detection within any given population. These principles are summarized as follows:

1. Select a disease that is an important public health problem.
2. Have facilities available for diagnosis and treatment, an accepted treatment, and a clearly defined policy about the indications for treatment.
3. Be sure the natural history of the disease is understood. A suitable screening test would identify preclinical or early symptomatic disease.
4. Keep the cost of case finding and treatment reasonable in relation to total health expenditures.
5. Make the screening program a continuing and health maintaining process, acceptable to the target population.

An important objective of epidemiology is to establish the natural history of a disease process. An assumption inherent in a program of early cancer detection is the concept of at least one "critical point" during the latent or preclinical phase of the disease. The application of treatment before any major critical point, rather than after, should result in a substantially better outcome. Indeed, the justification of periodic screening of patients at risk would be the availability of a valid screening procedure to be introduced before the critical point, and where the critical point generally preceded the time of usual diagnosis in symptomatic patients (6).

EVALUATING THE SCREENING PROCESS

The short-term "process" criteria for evaluating the effectiveness of a screening procedure include:

1. Prevalence, incidence, frequency of interval cases
2. Validity
3. Predictiveness
4. Yield in relation to cost
5. Compliance

Validity may be defined as the frequency with which the result of the screening test was later confirmed by an acceptable diagnostic procedure, or in terms of the ability of the test to separate those who have the disease from those who do not. Validity may be determined by measuring sensitivity and specificity. Sensitivity is whether the test can give a positive finding when the person tested truly has the disease under study. Specificity is whether the test can give a negative finding when the person tested is free of the disease under study (Fig. 1).

The sensitivity of a screening program may be increased by (a) allowing the criterion of positivity to be less restrictive; (b) using two or more screening tests in parallel and labeling as positive any subject with a positive response to any test.

In principle, the sensitivity of a screening test may be estimated by administering the diagnostic test to subjects who have screened negatively. However, the use of roentgenographic or endoscopic examinations for determining false negatives in an experimental screening program is impractical and unethical. The usual approach to estimating sensitivity is through the follow-up and rescreening of persons who screen negatively. The number of "interval" cases observed during follow-up in relation to the number detected by the screening test will enable a determination of sensitivity.

The level of specificity may be raised, although usually at the cost of diminishing sensitivity, by (a) allowing the criterion of positivity to be more restrictive; (b) rescreening with the same screening method all subjects found positive on initial screening and considering only those who were positive on two occasions; (c) using two or more screening tests in series and labeling as positive any subject with a positive response to all tests.

Specificity may be estimated after determining the number of false positives or (B) in Fig. 1. The denominator for the determination of specificity is (B + D), which equals the total number of normal persons and approximates the total number of subjects who are tested because of the relative rarity of any single type of cancer. Specificity may be estimated initially from the relationship, $1 - (B/A + B + C + D)$ (3).

With what frequency should the target population be rescreened? Mainly,

		Disease of interest		
		Present	Absent	
Screening test under consideration	Positive	True positives	False positives	A + B
		A	B	
	Negative	False negatives	True negatives	C + D
		C	D	
		A + C	B + D	A + B + C + D

Sensitivity   = A/A + C

Specificity   = D/B + D

Predictive Value   = A/ A + B

FIG. 1. Derivation of measures of validity and the predictive value of a positive test in a screening program.

this should be a function of the rate of progression through the latent period to early clinical disease and the validity of the screening procedure. A practical limitation is imposed by economic, social, and administrative considerations. Annual examination schedules have evolved empirically, and proposed alternative models for optimizing the frequency of screening will require experimental trial or initial evaluation by means of mathematical simulation. An optimal schedule should have high yield and achieve early detection, or minimal detection delay, but not have an excessive number of examinations per person. Obviously, the limits of "early," "minimal," and "excessive" must be specified in relation to the expected outcome of the screening process.

The predictive value of a positive test in a screening program is a measure of program efficiency, rather than of test validity. It may be defined as the proportion of positive individuals who have disease as determined by subsequent diagnostic evaluation (Fig. 1). The predictive value of a positive test is dependent on the validity of the testing procedure and the prevalence of the target disease in the screened population. The rationale for screening high-risk groups is to enhance the predictive probability of a positive test. This would tend to diminish the program cost in relation to the neoplastic yield of a positive test (Table 1).

By identifying groups or individuals at increased risk of incurring cancer at a specific site, the epidemiologist facilitates the selective application of optimal screening methods. For cost-benefit considerations, the principle would be to

TABLE 1. *Risk factors guiding screening for colorectal cancer*

Characteristic	High-risk features
Age	Over 40 in asymptomatic men and women
Associated disease	Ulcerative colitis, granulomatous colitis, familial polyposis syndromes
Past history	Colon cancer with or without polyps
Family history	Colon cancer, isolated or multiple polyps, familial polyposis syndromes.
	In first-degree relatives of patients with large bowel cancer, the risk is increased about 3×. In the studies by Anderson and Romsdahl (1) and Lynch et al. (9), familial colorectal cancer, occurring independently of polyposis, is characterized by early age at diagnosis, vertical transmission, and distribution of lesions as commonly in the right and transverse colon as in the left colon and rectum. Specific families have been characterized by having multiple primary adenocarcinomas of the large bowel and endometrium.

concentrate the greatest proportion of potentially new cases into the smallest proportion of the total population at risk.

However, even with effective and efficient screening procedures and our ability to define risk factors and target populations, there are formidable behavioral barriers in asymptomatic patients. Past studies have attempted to characterize the reluctant participant in a cancer screening program in relation to age, education, social class, current health attitudes, and past illness behavior (5). The Health Belief Model has become a pivotal concept in studies which attempt to distinguish compliers from noncompliers in voluntary preventive programs. The major components of the Health Belief Model are:

1. General health motivation—concern about one's health and about one's capacity to improve it.
2. Perceived susceptibility to a specific disease and its life-threatening consequences.
3. Perceived benefits from recommended health action and potential barriers to compliance.

Kasl and Cobb (7) concluded that the likelihood of a patient engaging in a particular kind of health behavior will be a function of how that individual perceives personal susceptibility to a disease and its life-threatening consequences in relationship to the potential benefits of preventive action.

EVALUATING THE EARLY OUTCOMES OF SCREENING

By assessing the stage distribution of cancers detected, and by analyzing the case fatality rates during the initial 2 or 3 years of the study, the clinical investigators should be able to discern whether the screening program is advancing the time of diagnosis. A concurrent experimental control group, or a historical comparison group, will enable such a judgment to be made. If the cases detected by the screening program do not have a lower early case fatality rate or favorable stage distribution of early lesions, it is unlikely that there will be significant reduction in long-term mortality observed in the experimental group.

Evaluation of both early outcomes is subject to lead time bias and length bias. Lead time may be defined as the interval between the time of detection by screening and the time at which the disease would have been diagnosed in the absence of screening. It is the average duration by which screening advances the diagnosis of cancer. If a valid assessment is to be made of survival in patients detected through a screening program, when compared with that in other patients diagnosed in the absence of screening, then some adjustment must be made for the estimated lead time. If the lead time is 1 year, then the survival rate at 3 years in the experimental group should be compared with the survival rate at 2 years in the nonscreened group. The validity of the screening test, the interval between screening exams, and possibly the age at which screening is conducted will influence the frequency distribution of lead times achieved for screened individuals.

Length biased sampling occurs because of the overrepresentation of persons with slow-growing lesions among the cases detected by a screening examination. This bias is most likely to be expressed at the initiation of a screening program, and diminishes in importance with repeated screening exams at relatively short intervals of time. Length bias may be difficult to estimate, and may influence the prognosis of cancers detected by screening independently of lead time (4,14).

EVALUATING THE LONG-TERM OUTCOMES OF SCREENING

It is the array of unfavorable sequelae of a disease that we hope to prevent or alter through the screening and diagnostic process, subsequent therapeutic intervention, continuing care, and future surveillance. Note that screening is viewed as an extension of the medical care process. The long-term objective of screening must be assessed in terms of reduced cancer-specific mortality and significant alteration of the natural history. In the evaluation of any voluntary screening program, particularly one which includes repeated screening, there are interpretive pitfalls of self selection and motivation in the screened population that bear on the measured outcome or prognosis. Individuals with a major disability (co-morbidity) are unlikely to participate voluntarily in a screening program (12).

The preferred research design for assessing the effectiveness of screening in reducing mortality is a randomized, controlled trial in which the population is randomly divided into a study group offered the screening program and a control group that receives the currently accepted program of routine diagnosis and medical care. Selection of patients through a randomized procedure provides at least three advantages (2): (a) elimination of bias in the assignment of patients to the study or control group; (b) balance in the distribution of risk factors and prognostic factors in the study and control groups, so as to ensure comparability with respect to factors that may influence outcome independently of the effect of screening; and (c) a tendency to enhance the validity of the statistical tests of significance that are used to compare the study and control groups. (A significant experiment is one in which more favorable outcomes occur in the study group than would be expected by random assignment of equally effective case ascertainment methods to study and control groups.)

Various quasi-experimental methods of evaluation have been attempted in the past. For example, mortality may be compared in a defined population before and after the introduction of a screening program, or between two different geographic areas, one with and the other without a screening program, during the same period of time. Quasi-experimental studies may be quite difficult to interpret because of the inability to identify the factors of self selection and the actual screening intensity for individuals within the population.

With respect to the planning and evaluation of preventive and therapeutic services, it is important to estimate the burden of direct and indirect costs. Direct costs (i.e., manpower, supporting services, equipment, and supplies) incurred from case finding in an apparently healthy population include the costs of the screening procedures plus the costs required to provide diagnostic, therapeutic, and follow-up services. Indirect costs include those due to lost earnings and diminished productivity. Indirect costs within an indigent population are less and of a different nature than in the general population because of lower wage rates, greater unemployment, and dependency on income support through public programs. In a screening program, the cost of treatment of patients whose cancers were detected by screening would be compared with the usual cost of treatment of symptomatic patients. The benefits of early diagnosis and treatment include (a) savings in the use of health resources, (b) gains in economic productivity, and (c) enhancement of the quality of life. Indices of economic productivity, rather than social values, would tend to minimize the benefits of averting disability or premature death in the poor and in unemployed women. In program planning, humanitarian considerations and sound economic analysis enter into the formulation of policy decisions (8,11).

ETHICAL CONSIDERATIONS

It has been argued that an experimental trial with random allocation is more ethical than instituting a previously untested preventive program in an unscientific manner. A sound judgment about efficacy requires *a priori* decisions about criteria of eligibility, adequacy of sample size, and measured endpoints.

An important issue is the determination of risks in relation to benefits. The identification of true positives who benefit from successful intervention and of true negatives who experience a sense of well being constitutes a benefit of a preventive program. Treatment of precancers, identified through the screening program, which might not have progressed during a lifetime, represents an indeterminate source of morbidity incurred by the program. In these instances the balance of risks and benefits is facilitated by more precise knowledge of natural history and participation by individual patients in decisions about management. All false positives are disadvantaged by needless exposure to the diagnostic procedures. False negatives are disadvantaged if they fail to take early action after the subsequent occurrence of symptoms, because of a false sense of security aroused by the screening procedure (10).

CONCLUSION

There are important principles in the planning, development, and evaluation of a screening program for cancer. The introduction of screening requires an understanding of natural history, the availability of facilities for diagnosis and optimal treatment, a defined policy about the indications for treatment, and the application of a screening test that is acceptable, effective, and efficient. The short-term "process" criteria for evaluating efficacy include validity, predictiveness, yield in relation to cost, and patient compliance. Distribution of detected cases by stage and their clinical course during the early years of follow-up should compare favorably with the cases diagnosed in the absence of screening. However, evaluation of these early outcomes is subject to lead time bias and length bias. Therefore, the long-term objective of screening must be viewed as the significant reduction in cancer-specific mortality. Other issues range from ethics to economics. The benefits derived from the program must be shown to exceed the risks, and some estimate made of the costs incurred for each year of life saved.

REFERENCES

1. Anderson, D. E., and Romsdahl, M. M. (1977): Family history: A criterion for selective screening. In: *Genetics of Human Cancer,* edited by J. J. Mulvihill, R. W. Miller, and J. F. Fraumeni, Jr. pp. 257–262. Raven Press, New York.
2. Byar, D. P., Simon, R. M., Friedewald, W. T., et al. (1976): Randomized clinical trials: Perspectives on some recent ideas. *N. Engl. J. Med.,* 295:74–80.
3. Cole, P., and Morrison, A. S. (1978): Basic issues in cancer screening. In: *Screening in Cancer,* edited by A. B. Miller, *UICC Technical Report Series Vol. 40,* pp. 7–39. IARC, Geneva.
4. Feinleib, M., and Zelen, M. (1969): Some pitfalls in the evaluation of screening programs. *Arch. Environ. Health,* 19:412–415.
5. Hochbaum, G. M. (1958): *Public Participation in Medical Screening Programs. A Sociopsychological Study.* Public Health Service Publication No. 572, U.S. Government Printing Office, Washington, D.C.
6. Hutchison, G. B. (1960): Evaluation of preventive services. *J. Chronic Dis.,* 11:497–508.
7. Kasl, S. V., and Cobb, S. (1966): Health behavior, illness behavior and sick role behavior. *Arch. Environ. Health,* 12:246–266, 531–541.
8. Klarman, H. E. (1967): Present status of cost-benefit analysis in the health field. *Am. J. Public Health,* 57:1948–1953.
9. Lynch, H. T., Krush, A. J., Thomas, R. J., and Lynch, J. (1976): Cancer family syndrome.

In: *Cancer Genetics,* edited by H. T. Lynch, pp. 355–388. Charles C Thomas, Springfield, Ill.

10. Miller, A. B. (1980): Cancer control by screening: Fundamental issues. In: *Cancer Epidemiology and Prevention,* edited by D. Schottenfeld and J. F. Fraumeni, Jr. W. B. Saunders Co., Philadelphia *(in press).*

11. Pole, J. D. (1968): Economic aspects of screening for disease. In: *Screening in Medical Care,* edited by L. Cohen, E. T. Williams, and G. McLachlan, pp. 141–158. Oxford University Press, London.

12. Sackett, D. (1975): Periodic examination of patients at risk. In: *Cancer Epidemiology and Prevention: Current Concepts,* edited by D. Schottenfeld, pp. 437–454. Charles C Thomas, Springfield, Ill.

13. Wilson, J. M. G., and Jungner, G. (1968): Principles and practice of screening for disease. *Public Health Pap.,* 34:26–39.

14. Zelen, M., and Feinleib, M. (1969): On the theory of screening for chronic diseases. *Biometrika,* 56:601–614.

Colorectal Cancer: Prevention, Epidemiology, and Screening, edited by S. Winawer, D. Schottenfeld, and P. Sherlock. Raven Press, New York © 1980.

World Health Organization Criteria for Screening

Reinhard Gnauck

Department of Gastroenterology, Deutsche Klinik für Diagnostik, Wiesbaden, Federal Republic of Germany

Screening has been defined as "the presumptive identification of unrecognized disease or defect by the application of tests, examinations, or other procedures which can be applied rapidly. Screening tests sort out apparently well persons who probably have a disease from those who probably do not. A screening test is not intended to be diagnostic. Persons with positive or suspicious findings must be referred to their physicians for diagnosis and necessary treatment." This definition was proposed by the United States Commission on Chronic Illness already in 1951 and is accepted by the WHO Regional Committee for Europe (1,2). It should be noted that, by this definition, unrecognized symptomatic as well as presymptomatic disease is included, and that a screening test is or is not intended to be a diagnostic test. Mass screening is a term used to indicate the large-scale screening of whole population groups without selection. Selective screening is screening of high-risk groups in the population; it may still be large scale and can be considered as one form of population screening. Whereas "screening" tends to be thought of as a one-time effort, "surveillance" has been used to convey the idea of continuous observation where screening examinations are repeated periodically. The main object of such screening is "early disease detection" and to bring these patients to treatment (3).

For the evaluation of screening programs the following points need to be considered: validity, reliability, yield, cost, acceptance, and follow-up services (2). The validity of a screening test is its ability to separate those who have the disease sought from those who do not. Applying a screening test to a population will produce the four categories of results shown in Table 1. There will be true and false positives, and true and false negatives. The ideal test would detect only those persons in a population suffering from the disease looked for and would not fail to detect any of them. The ability of a test to classify as positive those persons with the disease is termed "sensitivity," and the ability to class as negative those without the disease, "specificity." Sensitivity is a measure of the false negative rate and specificity of the false positive rate (3,4). The reliability of a screening test involves the variation of the method and its accuracy as well as the error of the observer. The yield may be regarded as the measure of previously unrecognized disease diagnosed as the result of screen-

TABLE 1. *Validity of a screening test*

Screening result	Screened population	
	Persons with disease	Persons without disease
Positive	True positive	False positive
Negative	False negative	True negative

$$\text{Sensitivity} = \frac{\text{Diseased persons with positive test}}{\text{All persons in population with disease}}$$

$$\text{Specificity} = \frac{\text{Nondiseased persons with negative test}}{\text{All persons in population without disease}}$$

From ref. 3.

ing and brought to treatment. The yield is primarily related to the prevalence of the disease in the population, but also to the quality of follow-up examinations.

Before any mass screening is instituted, certain criteria should be met. These criteria are a modification of those proposed by a Canadian-British-U.S.A. group and adopted by the Epidemiology Section of the American Public Health Association (4):

1. Screening must lead to an improvement in end results (defined in terms of mortality, physical, social, and emotional function, pain, and satisfaction) among those in whom early diagnosis is achieved, or in the other members of the community, or both.

   a. The therapy for the condition must alter its natural history favorably by improving survival, function, or both. This improvement should not be confused with the apparent prolongation of survival due to earlier diagnosis. Neither the modification of risk factors nor the fact that the proposed therapy is commonly accepted is sufficient evidence of effectiveness. Claims for therapeutic effectiveness must withstand rigorous methodological scrutiny, and experimental evidence, such as a controlled clinical trial, is essential. The measurement of survival and other end results must be able to withstand epidemiological and biostatistical scrutiny.

   b. Available health services must be sufficient both to afford diagnostic confirmation for those who are found positive and to provide long-term care.

   c. Compliance among asymptomatic patients in whom an early diagnosis has been achieved must be at a level demonstrated to be effective in altering the natural history of the disease in question.

   d. The long-term beneficial effects, in terms of end results, must outweigh the long-term detrimental effects of the therapeutic regimen utilized and the labeling of an individual as diseased or at high risk.

   e. If the benefits of the program accrue to the community at large rather than, or in addition to, the individual identified (e.g., disease carriers, specific occupations), the benefit to the community claimed must be able to withstand scientific scrutiny.

2. The cost/benefit and cost/effectiveness characteristics of the program of screening and long-term therapy must be known. This information is essential in developing an appropriate combination of diagnostic and therapeutic services when manpower and financial resources are limited. A mechanism for the formal periodic weighing of program costs against benefits or effectiveness should therefore constitute a basic component of the initial screening program plan.

   a. The disability resulting from the condition in question must be a sufficient burden (in terms of the frequency, distribution, and severity of the disease, and alternative approaches to its detection and control) to warrant action.

   b. The cost, sensitivity, specificity, and acceptability of the screening test must be known, and it should lend itself to the utilization patterns of the target population.

   c. Ideally, an estimate of the social benefit of preventing, arresting, or curing the condition in question should have been made.

To fulfill all these criteria before starting mass application of a screening test appears somewhat utopian, just as "complete health," as defined by the WHO, resembles heaven on earth. Based on experience in our clinic since 1972 and all other available data, primarily from the United States, it was decided in Germany that starting mass screening for colorectal cancer with Hemoccult is reasonable and justifiable. Therefore, in January 1977, stool testing was added to the scope of the national health check-up program in the Federal Republic of Germany. This program has been in operation since 1972. To approximately 91% of the population—the highest income groups are excluded—a medical examination free of charge is offered annually. Hemoccult testing starts at age 45. In various age groups 6 million people (4.5 million women and 1.5 million men), participate in this check-up every year. This national health program is therefore the largest potential source of information about the effect of Hemoccult screening on colorectal cancer.

Unfortunately, up to now no exact evaluation of this mass screening is possible for technical reasons. In 1980 a new reporting sheet for this check-up will be utilized. At present, no complete registration and statistical analysis of all positive Hemoccult tests, follow-up examinations and cases diagnosed in the screened population can be done. Also, there is no Central Cancer Registry in Germany—except in two states, representing about 5% of the population. For these reasons, to date there have been scanty data from random sampling of the national health program. In 1977, during the first 8 months of Hemoccult usage in this program, a survey was done by Otto and Bunnemann (5); the experience of 100 physicians was recorded. In 30,800 persons tested, a positive test occurred

TABLE 2. *Experience of 100 physicians in 1977*

	No.	%
Persons tested	30,858	
Hemoccult-positive	472	1.5
Colorectal cancers traced	55	0.18
Precancerous polyps traced	53	0.17

From ref. 5.

in 472 (1.5%); 55 colorectal cancers and 53 large polyps were diagnosed in this group, for a total of 3.5 such lesions per 1,000 persons tested (Table 2). Of the 55 cancers, 32 were called "radically resectable."

In another study, done in August 1978, the second year of Hemoccult in this national health check-up, 200 physicians registered their results (MaFo-Institut, Schwalbach/Taunus, *unpublished*). They gave the total number of test persons 52,000, of which 1,050 (2%) had a positive test; 166 "operable" and 48 "advanced" cancers, as well as 109 precancerous polyps were diagnosed in this group (Table 3). The return rate for slides in these surveys was between 80 and 90% respectively, indicating good acceptance of the test.

The State of Hamburg maintains a Cancer Registry for its 1.7 million inhabitants. The annual rate of newly registered colorectal cancers has averaged 111 per 100,000 for the 3 years before introduction of Hemoccult. In 1977 this figure rose to 120 per 100,000. One may speculate that this reflects not a sudden increase in incidence of colorectal cancer, but possibly a more frequent diagnosis due to the mass application of Hemoccult that year. The 1978 figures are not yet available. An update of the continuous monitoring of Hemoccult testing in our clinic is provided in Table 4 (6). Since the State-of-the-Art Conference on Screening for Colorectal Cancer in Washington, D.C., another 3,100 patients coming to our clinic for various reasons have been tested. The records of all patients with a positive test have been reviewed, as well as those with a proven diagnosis of colorectal cancer or adenoma who had negative tests. The slide positivity rate has been 3.6%. It reflects the high percentage of symptomatic patients who come to our clinic with colitis or other gastrointestinal disease causing gastrointestinal blood loss. The false negative and false positive rates

TABLE 3. *Experience of 200 physicians in 1978*

	No.	%
Persons tested	52,000	
Hemoccult-positive	1,050	2.0
Colorectal cancers traced	214	0.41
Precancerous polyps traced	109	0.21

Data from MaFo-Institut, Schwalbach/Taunus *(unpublished)*.

TABLE 4. *Results of Hemoccult testing in the German Diagnostic Clinic 1972-1979*

		1972–78	1978–79	Total
Persons tested		13,000	3,100	16,100
Hemoccult positive	%	3.2	3.6	3.3
	N	411	120	531
Positive patients examined (rectoscopy + BE or coloscopy)		305	80	385
Colorectal cancers		61	14	75
Above rigid rectoscope		43	12	55
Entirely asymptomatic		13	3	16
Younger than 50 years		11	4	15
Large polyps (> 1.0 cm ϕ)		85	21	106
Above rigid rectoscope		63	17	80
Entirely asymptomatic		44	10	54
Younger than 50 years		19	7	26

From ref. 6.

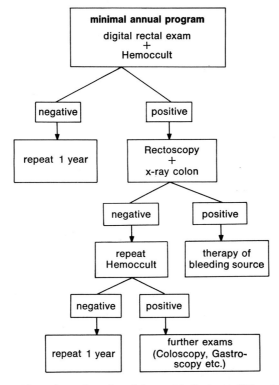

FIG. 1. Minimal screening scheme for colorectal cancer in Germany. This scheme underemphasizes use of colonoscopy because of generally poor availability at present in Germany. If available, colonoscopy of all patients with positive slide tests would be desirable.

have not been determined as yet. About 75% of all cancers and polyps were beyond the reach of the rigid rectosigmoidoscope.

The average age of all cancer patients traced is 61 years; 1 out of 5 is younger than 50 years. For polyps, the average age is 57 years, with 1 out of 4 under age 50. These results, as well as the admittedly scarce data from the national health program, encourage us to continue with Hemoccult screening for colorectal cancer. Considering the limited availability of colonoscopy in Germany, we have recommended for general use in our country the schema shown in Fig. 1 as the *minimal* annual effort.

Starting with 1980, better data should become available from our national study for the evaluation of the effect of this screening approach on individuals and population groups.

REFERENCES

1. Commission on Chronic Illness (1957): *Chronic Illness in the United States: Vol. I. Prevention of Chronic Illness,* p. 45. Harvard University Press, Cambridge, Mass.
2. WHO Regional Committee for Europe (1964): The presymptomatic diagnosis of diseases by organized screening procedures (14th Session, Prague). EUR/RC 14/Tech. Disc./6 (mimeographed).
3. Wilson, J. M. G., and Jungner, G. (1968): Principles and practice of screening for disease. *Public Health Paper* #34. WHO, Geneva.
4. (1971): Mass health examinations. *Public Health Paper* #45, p. 50. WHO, Geneva.
5. Otto, O., and Bunnemann, H. (1978): First experiences in the clinical clarification of positive haemoccult tests within the scope of colorectal cancer screening in the first half of 1977. In: *Kolorektale Krebsvorsorge,* p. 102. Verlag D. E. Wachholz, Nurenberg.
6. Gnauck, R. (1979): Screening and early detection of colorectal cancer. NIH publication No. 80–2075.

Colorectal Cancer: Prevention, Epidemiology, and Screening, edited by S. Winawer, D. Schottenfeld, and P. Sherlock. Raven Press, New York © 1980.

Laboratory Studies on the Hemoccult Slide for Fecal Occult Blood Testing

*Martin Fleisher, *Morton K. Schwartz, and **Sidney J. Winawer

*Departments of *Biochemistry and **Medicine, Memorial Sloan-Kettering Cancer Center, New York, New York 10021*

The high incidence of colon cancer in this country, more than 112,000 new cases annually, should be the catalyst for the improvement and application of screening procedures for the early detection of colon cancer and adenomas. In 1971, Greegor (5) proposed testing the stools of asymptomatic patients for occult blood with the Hemoccult slide as a screening procedure for colon cancer. Numerous investigations followed which were designed to study, evaluate, and confirm the effectiveness of the Hemoccult slide as a screening procedure for cancer of the colon (1,3,4,6,10). It became apparent that in many instances, interpretation, comparison, and corroboration of reports were difficult because conditions were variable. In many cases, investigators made subtle but significant changes in test conditions or experimental design which may have produced dramatically differing results. Inconsistency among the various studies which may have profound effects on the final results of an investigation included such variables as patient selection, frequency of testing, specimen collection, diet, test conditions, and variations in test slide sensitivity and stability. The fact that the Hemoccult slide detection rate varied among studies from 1 to approximately 6% may well reflect variations in screening program design and test protocols (6,9,10). It has also become increasingly clear that this "simple" approach to testing for fecal occult blood is far more complex than formerly perceived. From the points of view of the test itself and acceptable laboratory practice, there are many unknowns that require attention and further investigation. The technical aspects of this test procedure need the same kind of meticulous attention that has been given to all other laboratory test procedures.

A REFERENCE LABORATORY FOR FECAL OCCULT BLOOD TESTING

In order to more effectively address certain aspects of fecal occult blood testing, we have established at the Memorial Sloan-Kettering Cancer Center a special laboratory referred to as a reference laboratory for fecal occult blood testing. It has been proposed that this laboratory serve as an international reference center for fecal occult blood testing and coordinate investigations into:

1. Standardized test procedures for the detection of fecal occult blood;
2. Standard methods for reporting results of tests on patients examined in screening programs for the detection of colorectal cancer;
3. Test sensitivity for the purpose of long-term comparisons of screening programs;
4. Environmental, metabolic, and drug effects on test sensitivity and stability;
5. The development of a reliable, simple, and inexpensive quality assurance program that can serve as the basis for comparative evaluation of screening programs on an international level.

At the time that this chapter was written, medical centers from seven countries including the United States, Australia, Brazil, Germany, Italy, Japan, and Yugoslavia were participating in the activities of the Reference Laboratory. A questionnaire has been developed and distributed to individuals interested in cooperating with our reference laboratory programs. These investigators may form the nucleus for an international workgroup for colorectal cancer. The clinical and technical aspects of each screening program will be surveyed and evaluated. Information such as that listed below will be compiled:

1. Characteristics of patients screened
2. Risk factors of patients screened
3. Symptom status
4. Screening techniques
5. Type of occult blood test used in program
6. Number of smears requested
7. Medication and diet restrictions
8. Interval between slide preparation and laboratory test
9. Test conditions
10. Quality assurance of test procedure
11. Sensitivity of a test procedure used

Following review of this information and based on the findings of the reference laboratory, specific recommendations will be made to standardize the clinical and technical use of test for fecal occult blood.

STABILITY

Our data as well as those reported by others demonstrated the effects of prolonged storage and desiccation on specimen stability on Hemoccult slides

(2,7,8). These studies show a time-dependent conversion of positive to negative Hemoccult slide results which appear to be hemoglobin concentration dependent.

SENSITIVITY

One of the goals of the reference laboratory is to develop a standardized procedure for testing Hemoccult slide sensitivity. The test protocol implemented by the reference laboratory is designed to answer the following questions pertaining to the sensitivity of the Hemoccult slide test:

1. How much blood (hemoglobin) is needed to produce a positive reaction?
2. How does the integrity of the blood cells present at the time of sampling affect the test conditions?

To answer the first question, we use crystalline human hemoglobin dissolved in water as a primary standardization material to establish a criterion of sensitivity. This technique is reliable and can be reproduced in any testing laboratory. The data shown in Table 1 indicate the degree of sensitivity exhibited by the Hemoccult slide. These data clearly indicate that the Hemoccult slide is sensitive to less than 1 μg of human hemoglobin in aqueous solution.

In cooperation with Reinhard Gnauck of the Deutsche Klinik fur Diagnostik in Wiestaden, Germany, and Dieter Kramer, Rohn Pharma GmbH, Darmstadt, Germany, we evaluated a simulated stool material (referred to here as "matrix") as a possible matrix for a quality control program. Crystalline human hemoglobin and human whole blood are homogeneously mixed with the matrix in order to evaluate Hemoccult slide sensitivity in a reproducible and reliable fashion. Table 2 indicates the degree of sensitivity produced by crystalline hemoglobin in the matrix.

This study also indicates the difference in Hemoccult sensitivity between aqueous hemoglobin and the matrix containing hemoglobin. Aqueous hemoglobin at a concentration of 0.12 mg/g is strongly positive (+4) at day 1 while matrix-

TABLE 1. *Hemoccult slide sensitivity*

Days following application of Hb	Amount (μg) hemoglobin applied to slide		
	0.75	1.5	3.2
1	+2	+3	+4
4	+1	+2	+3
7	+1	+2	+3

Color intensity score: +1 (slightly positive); +2 (mildly positive); +3 (moderately positive); +4 (strongly positive).

TABLE 2. *Hemoccult slide sensitivity: human hemoglobin in test matrix*

Days following application	Hb concentration (mg/g matrix)	
	0.12	0.36
1	Trace	+1
3	Trace	+1
5	Neg.	Trace
7	Neg.	Neg.

Sensitivity limit: 36 mg Hb/100 g at day 3.
Color intensity score: neg. (no color); trace (trace color); +1 (mildly positive).

containing hemoglobin produces only a trace color under the same conditions. Although this experiment is at best a simulation of the physiological situation of blood in stool, it does point out the need for a more standardized technique of specimen collection and application.

In answer to the second question regarding the effects of red blood cell integrity on Hemoccult, sensitivity is approached by "spiking" the matrix with human whole blood in which the cells are either intact or hemolyzed.

Table 3 shows the results of human whole blood (intact cells) mixed with the matrix.

Lysing the red blood cells prior to mixing with the matrix thereby making the hemoglobin readily available for reaction results in a greater test sensitivity as compared to intact cells. These data are shown in Table 4.

It can be concluded from these findings that the sensitivity of the occult blood test is a function of the number and physical integrity of the red blood cells present in the stool.

TABLE 3. *Hemoccult slide sensitivity: whole blood (intact cells) in test matrix*

Days following application	Hb concentration (mg/g matrix)		
	0.12	0.24	0.36
1	Neg.	Trace	+1
3	Neg.	Trace	Trace
5	Neg.	Neg.	Trace
7	Neg.	Neg.	Trace

Sensitivity limit: 0.36 mg Hb/g matrix at day 1.
Color intensity score: +1 (slightly positive); neg. (no color); trace (trace color).

TABLE 4. *Hemoccult slide sensitivity: lysed blood in test matrix*

Days following application	Hb concentration (mg/g matrix)		
	0.12	0.24	0.36
1	Neg.	Trace	+3
3	Neg.	Trace	+2
5	Neg.	Neg.	+1
7	Neg.	Neg.	Trace

Sensitivity limit: 0.36 mg/g matrix at day 5.
Color intensity score: +1 (slightly positive); +2 (mildly positive); +3 (moderately positive); neg. (no color); trace (trace color).

REHYDRATION OF HEMOCCULT SLIDE

Rehydration alters the apparent sensitivity of Hemoccult slides to hemoglobin. One of the reasons for this effect involves the dissolution of desiccated hemoglobin before the addition of the alcoholic developing reagent. However, hemoglobin is not the only component "reactivated" following rehydration. Other interfering compounds such as peroxidases, ubiquitous in bacteria and certain foods, are also rehydrated and hence interact to possibly increase false positive results. The nonspecificity possibly resulting from this effect could reduce the effectiveness of the Hemoccult test. Furthermore, this one modification in test procedure may be responsible for some of the variation in positive detection rates reported by different investigators. Our studies on the effects of rehydration indicate a significant increase in sensitivity of the Hemoccult slide following rehydration with water and buffer over a pH range of 4 to 7.5. Figure 1 demonstrates the effect of rehydration on test sensitivity as a function of hemoglobin concentration and storage of Hemoccult slides. It is clear from these data that a strongly positive Hemoccult test remains positive for at least 10 days whether the slides are rehydrated with water or buffer or not hydrated at all. Initial weakly positive results (trace color production) may yield equivocal results on nonhydrated slides after 2 to 4 days of storage. It should be noted that under physiological conditions trace color production may actually be due to components in stool other than hemoglobin. Hence, the test for hemoglobin with the Hemoccult slide may appear more sensitive following rehydration but actually results in a less specific test for hemoglobin in stool.

FECAL OCCULT BLOOD TESTING: THE STATE OF THE ART

Currently there are six products commercially available to the international medical community capable of detecting blood in stool. In the United States, Australia, and Europe, the Hemoccult slide test is the product which has received the greatest attention from the point of view of clinical and technical evaluations. Table 5 summarizes the state of the art of the Hemoccult slide test. There are

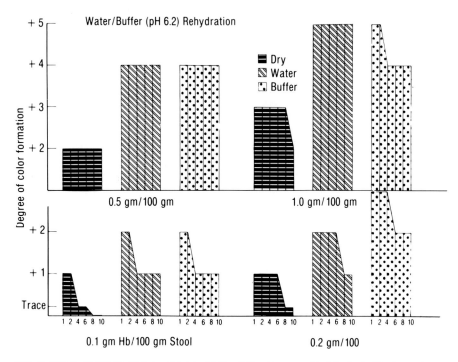

FIG. 1. Effect of rehydration on the sensitivity of the Hemoccult slide test. Stool specimens containing varying concentrations of Hb prepared by *in vitro* addition of hemolyzed whole human blood were applied to Hemoccult slides. After the initial test on day 1, the test slides were developed at 2-day intervals following: (A) no rehydration, (B) rehydration with distilled water, and (C) rehydration with 0.1M potassium phosphate buffer adjusted to pH 6.2. The degree of color formation (intensity) was scored from trace to +5; a trace indication refers to the slightest degree of color formation; a +5 score refers to an extremely dark blue coloration.

TABLE 5. *State of the art: Hemoccult slide test characteristics*

Test reagents	Filter paper impregnated guaiac; hydrogen peroxide and denatured alcohol
Analyte	Hemoglobin
Test rationale	Phenolic oxidation of guaiac in the presence of Hb
Known chemical interference	Compounds with peroxidase activity
Minimum sensitivity	1 μg crystalline human Hb in aqueous solution 0.2 g Hb/100 g stool under simulated conditions[a]
Stability following specimen application	30 days if test is strongly positive (+4) on day 1; 4–5 days if test is weakly positive (+1) on day 1
Stability related to Hb concentration	Yes
Effect of rehydration on sensitivity	Increased sensitivity with increased rate of false positive reactions
Effect of diet on sensitivity	Foods containing peroxidase activity should be avoided (particularly uncooked vegetables). Question of importance of meat is unresolved.
Quality control procedures	Not available at the present time

[a] Blood added to stool *in vitro*.

several other important considerations that impact on the effectiveness of the Hemoccult slide test to detect blood in stool. Such factors include the degree of specimen heterogeneity (i.e., diffuse or small concentrations of blood in stool), type and location of neoplastic lesion, degree of hemolysis of blood in the stool specimen, and assurance that the test conditions are appropriate, including a quality control program for the Hemoccult slide test to assure test validity.

CONCLUSION

The Hemoccult slide test is a potentially effective screening procedure for the detection of early colorectal cancer. In order to better understand the problems related to the Hemoccult screening test and to develop better lines of communication between investigators, a reference laboratory for fecal occult blood testing has been proposed and its establishment at the Memorial Sloan-Kettering Cancer Center has been initiated. The reference laboratory will monitor and assess the effectiveness of the Hemoccult slide test as a screening procedure. The goals of the reference laboratory are as follows:

1. Monitor and investigate sensitivity and stability factors involved in fecal occult blood testing
2. Develop standardized procedures for screening and testing for fecal occult blood
3. Develop a reliable quality control program for fecal occult blood testing
4. Disseminate the findings of the Reference Laboratory to any investigator interested in fecal occult blood screening procedures for early detection of colorectal cancer.

REFERENCES

1. Fleisher, M., Schwartz, M. K., and Winawer, S. J. (1977): The use of fecal occult blood testing in detecting colorectal cancer. *Clin. Chem.,* 23:1157.
2. Fleisher, M., Schwartz, M. K., and Winawer, S. J. (1977): The false-negative Hemoccult Test. *Gastroenterology,* 72:782–784.
3. Glober, G. A., and Peskoe, S. M. (1974): Outpatient screening for gastrointestinal lesions using guaiac-impregnated slides. *Am. J. Dig. Dis.,* 19:399–403.
4. Gnauck, R. (1974): Okkultes Blut im Stuhl als Sushtest nach Kolo-rektalem Krebs und Prakanzerosen Polypen. *Z. Gastroenterol.,* 12:239–250.
5. Greegor, D. H. (1971): Occult blood testing for detection of asymptomatic colon cancer. *Cancer,* 28:131–134.
6. Hastings, J. B. (1974): Mass screening for colorectal cancer. *Am. J. Surg.,* 127:228–233.
7. Ostrow, J. D., Mulvaney, C. A., Hansell, J. R., and Rhodes, R. S. (1973): Sensitivity and reproducibility of chemical tests for fecal occult blood with an emphasis on false-positive reactions. *Am. J. Dig. Dis.,* 18:930–940.
8. Stroehlein, J. R., Fairbanks, V. F., Go, V. L. W., Taylor, W. F., and Thompson, J. H. (1976): Hemoccult stool tests. False-negative results due to storage of specimens. *Mayo Clin. Proc.,* 51:548–552.
9. Winawer, S., Ginther, M., Weston, E., Reichlin, B., Fleisher, M., Cirone, C., Schottenfeld, D., and Miller, D. (1978): Impact of modifications in fecal occult blood test on screening program for colorectal neoplasia. Part 2. *Gastroenterology,* 74:1140 (abst.).
10. Winawer, S. J., Sherlock, P., Schottenfeld, D., and Miller, D. G. (1976): Screening for colon cancer. *Gastroenterology,* 70:783–789.

Colorectal Cancer: Prevention, Epidemiology, and Screening, edited by S. Winawer, D. Schottenfeld, and P. Sherlock. Raven Press, New York © 1980.

Criteria for Validation of Fecal Occult Blood Tests

J. Donald Ostrow

Gastroenterology Section, Northwestern University Medical Schoool, and V.A. Lakeside Medical Center, Chicago, Illinois 60611

As a result of extensive testing over the past 15 years, Hemoccult (Smith-Kline Diagnostics) has become the accepted method for detection of fecal occult blood as a means to screen for colorectal neoplasia (17,20). However, this test is neither specific for blood, nor sensitive in the range of 2 to 10 mg hemoglobin per gram stool (8,13) (up to five-fold increase above the normal limit of 2 mg/g). Consequently, three new tests are under development. HemoFec (Boehringer-Mannheim) (16), and Fecatest (Finnpipette Ky) (1), are variants of Hemoccult that are supposedly more sensitive and specific because of the use of purified guaiac reagent. The third method is a radial immunodiffusion assay of Barrows et al. (2), which is highly sensitive and specific for human hemoglobin. It seems worthwhile to record the criteria that need to be met in order to validate these new tests with the same rigor that has been applied to Hemoccult.

STANDARDIZATION

Guaiac is a natural product of varied composition and purity. Thus each batch of test kits must be standardized for its reactivity. Since guaiac is merely a redox indicator, and the hemoglobin in stool is assayed by its enzymatic peroxidase activity, it is essential that the substrate peroxide be present in saturating concentration, and that pure hemoglobin be used as the enzyme standard. These practices have been ignored previously, and the use of hemoglobin added to stools is to be deplored, since feces contain both inhibitors of the reaction and other substances with peroxidase activity. Also desirable, but not yet practiced, is a means to achieve uniformity in the quantity of stool applied to the assay paper. Optimal times for reading the reaction should be determined, based on the rate of appearance and persistence of the color after the peroxide developer is added. Lots must also be checked for the stability of reagents for 3 years under different storage conditions. In similar fashion, pure hemoglobin should be used as the antigen to standardize the immunodiffusion assay.

SENSITIVITY

These tests are designed to detect blood in the stool, and cannot detect lesions unless they are bleeding (9,18). Thus sensitivity should be defined not in terms of cancers detected, but as milligrams hemoglobin detected per gram stool in patients who are bleeding. To use milliliters of blood lost per day is inappropriate, since the enzymatic reaction is dependent on concentration, not amount of enzyme. Such *in vivo* validation is necessary because an average of 80% of hemoglobin is degraded during passage through the gastrointestinal tract (3,14), rendering it undetectable by either its enzymatic or antigenic properties, and there are inhibitors of the peroxidase reaction in stool. The tests should be assessed against the ^{51}Cr-erythrocyte method (4), which has been extensively validated and has an upper normal limit of 2 mg hemoglobin per gram stool, possibly representing ^{51}Cr excreted in bile after elution from the red cells (11). It is important to avoid contamination of stool by urine because eluted ^{51}Cr is excreted by the kidneys (13). Good reagents will uniformly detect hemoglobin in the range of 2 to 10 mg/g stool, a range in which many lesions bleed occultly (9), but will be negative in the normal range of blood loss. The Hematest (Ames) and old guaiac methods suffered from excessive sensitivity, giving as many false positive reactions in the normal range of blood loss as they did true positive reactions in the minimal bleeding range (8,10). Hemoccult gives few false positive tests, but is negative on over half the stools in the minimal bleeding range (8,13).

SPECIFICITY

The tests ideally should be specific for human hemoglobin. This is not possible with the guaiac-based methods, since fecal peroxidases of vegetable or bacterial origin (14), and hemoglobins or myoglobins in animal meat products, will also react. The immunodiffusion assay is likely to be superior in this regard.

REPRODUCIBILITY

Inhomogeneity of blood in the stool is one reason why multiple samples should be taken from each stool to avoid missing blood loss (17,20). However, the test reagents themselves must be shown, as with Hemoccult (10), to give the same reading more than 95% of the time when the same small portion of stool is tested in duplicate, and read simultaneously by two different observers. The lack of reproducibility was shown to be due to variations in the quality of the tablets with Hematest, but to interobserver differences in interpretation of the color reaction with the old guaiac method (10).

Since stool samples are collected and smeared over a period of several days, and then mailed in for reading, the reaction obtained must not vary with the interval between smearing the stool specimen and addition of the developing reagent (5,8,10,12). This must be assessed with natural sanguineous stools from bleeding subjects, because stools enriched with blood *in vitro* (5) give misleading results. It must also be determined whether the delayed or initial reactions give the most valid readings in relationship to blood loss assessed with ^{51}Cr-erythrocytes (9), and whether prewetting the smear with water before adding peroxide developer (15) enhances or impairs the sensitivity and specificity of the test. These questions have not yet been completely answered (18).

OTHER FACTORS

The effects of different ingesta, including meat, vegetables, roughage, citrus fruits (ascorbic acid inhibits the guaiac reaction) (7), salicylates, laxatives, barium, and oral iron, should be assessed in human subjects. In such studies, a lag or crossover period of at least 3 days is essential if the stools are to reflect the effects of materials taken orally after passage through the intestine (8,10). In this regard, the high-roughage diet proposed by Greegor (6), and widely adopted (20) because it is believed to increase blood loss by abrading the lesions, has never been validated. Theoretically, it might have two unfavorable effects on screening programs. First, it might increase the frequency of false positive tests because of a higher dietary content of vegetable peroxidases. Second, the increased fecal bulk from the high fiber content could dilute fecal hemoglobin concentration below the sensitivity of the occult blood tests.

SUMMARY

The rigorous standardization and validation of tests for fecal occult blood was ignored until recently, resulting in many years of use of the old guaiac and Hematest reactions, which were poorly standardized, nonspecific, excessively sensitive, and poorly reproducible (8,10). Most of these criticisms have been met with Hemoccult, which is currently the only good method among those that have been critically tested. The criteria defined now have to be applied with equal rigor to the three new methods that are under development if they are not to be utilized prematurely in clinical practice and in screening programs.

ACKNOWLEDGEMENT

This work was supported by a Medical Investigator Award from the U.S. Veterans Administration (MRIS #6680).

REFERENCES

1. Adlercreutz, H., Liewendahl, K., and Virkola, P. (1978): Evaluation of fecatest, a new guaiac test for occult blood in feces. *Clin. Chem.*, 24:756–761.
2. Barrows, G. H., Burton, R. M., Jarrett, D. D., et al. (1978): Immunochemical detection of human blood in feces. *Am. J. Clin. Pathol.*, 69:342–346.
3. Burton, R. M., Landreth, K. S., Barrows, G. H., et al. (1976): Appearance, properties and origins of altered human hemoglobin in feces. *Lab. Invest.*, 35:111–115.
4. Ebaugh, F. G., Clemens, T., Rodman, G., et al. (1958): Use of radioactive Cr[51] in patients with gastrointestinal hemorrhage. *Am. J. Med.*, 25:169–181.

5. Fleisher, M., Schwartz, M. K., and Winawer, S. J. (1977): The false negative Hemoccult test. *Gastroenterology,* 72:4:782–784.
6. Greegor, D. (1971): Occult blood testing for detection of asymptomatic colon cancer. *Cancer,* 28:131–134.
7. Jaffe, R. M., Kasten, B., Young, D. S., et al. (1975): False-negative stool occult blood tests caused by ingestion of ascorbic acid (vitamin C). *Ann. Intern. Med.,* 83:824–826.
8. Morris, D. W., Hansel, J. R., Ostrow, J. D., et al. (1976): Reliability of chemical tests for fecal occult blood in hospitalized patients. (Editorial). *Am. J. Dig. Dis.,* 21:845–852.
9. Ostrow, J. D., Hansell, J. R., and Morris, D. W. (1977): Limiting factors in screening for gastrointestinal tumors with Hemoccult. *Digestion,* 16:267 (abst.).
10. Ostrow, J. D., Mulvaney, C. A., Hansel, J. R., et al. (1973): Sensitivity and reproducibility of chemical tests for fecal occult blood with an emphasis on false-positive reactions. *Am. J. Dig. Dis.,* 18:930–940.
11. Stephens, F. O., and Lawrensen K. B. (1969): ^{51}Cr excretion in bile. *Lancet,* 1:158–159.
12. Stroehlein, J. R., Fairbanks, J. R., Go, V. L. W., et al. (1976): Hemoccult stool tests. False-negative results due to storage of specimens. *Mayo Clin. Proc.,* 51:548–552.
13. Stroehlein, J. R., Fairbanks, V. F., McGill, D. B., et al. (1976): Hemoccult detection of fecal blood quantitated by radioassay. *Am. J. Dig. Dis.,* 21:841–844.
14. Thornton, G. H. M., and Illingworth, D. G. (1955): An evaluation of the benzidine test for occult blood in the feces. *Gastroenterology,* 28:593–605.
15. Wells, H. G., and Pagano, J. E. (1977): Hemoccult™ test—Reversal of false-negative results due to storage. *Gastroenterology,* A-125/1148 (abst.).
16. Wielinger, H., and Carstensen, C. A. (1978): *Munch. Med. Wochenschr.,* 120:1095–1096.
17. Winawer, S. J. (1976): Fecal occult blood testing (Editorial). *Am. J. Dig. Dis.,* 21:885–888.
18. Winawer, S. J., Ginther, M., Weston, E., et al. (1978): Impact of modifications in fecal occult blood test on screening program for colorectal neoplasia. *Gastroenterology,* 74:1140 (abst.).
19. Winawer, S. J., Leidner, S. D., Miller, D. G., et al. (1977): Results of a screening program for the detection of early colon cancer and polyps using fecal occult blood testing. *Gastroenterology,* 72:5:2:A-127/1150 (abst.).
20. Winawer, S. J., Sherlock, P., Schottenfeld, D., and Miller, D. (1976): Screening for colon cancer. *Gastroenterology,* 70:783–789.

Colorectal Cancer: Prevention, Epidemiology, and Screening, edited by S. Winawer, D. Schottenfeld, and P. Sherlock. Raven Press, New York © 1980.

Immunochemical Detection of Human Fecal Occult Blood

*Curtis L. Songster, **George H. Barrows, and **Diane D. Jarrett

*Department of Pathology, Bayfront Medical Center, St. Petersburg, Florida 33701; and **Department of Pathology, School of Medicine, University of Louisville Health Sciences Center, Louisville, Kentucky 40232

Early detection and diagnosis of colorectal cancer presents a challenge as well as a formidable problem. Colon and rectal cancer has an estimated annual frequency of greater than 100,000 new cases and causes more than 50,000 annual deaths, surpassing lung cancer and now ranking as the number one cancer killer (18,19). Colorectal cancer discovered early results in very high cure rates: patients with colon cancer detected while clinically asymptomatic have distant metastases less than 5% of the time, and the 5-year survival rates approach 90% (24). No treatment until symptomatology occurs generally voids this optimistic prognosis and there is a dramatic reduction in cure (17). Most workers believe intracolonic bleeding to be the most frequent and persistent consequence of tumor presence (6–9, 24) and such bleeding is generally occult.

Occult blood, and therefore occult hemoglobin, appears to be the most abundant constituent associated with colorectal lesions. Expectedly, positive fecal occult blood tests often lead to the discovery of early colorectal cancers. For this reason, fecal occult blood has been proposed as a satisfactory method to screen for colon and rectal cancer (1,6–9). Traditional chemical tests for occult blood would appear suited to identify those at high risk for colorectal cancer; however, such is less than the case since many dietary ingredients have sufficient peroxidase activity to give a false positive test (11,15,22). Various chemicals have been proven to also interfere, resulting in a false negative test (12,14).

The clinician has not infrequently experienced the frustration and expense of diagnostic work-up in patients with falsely positive occult blood tests. The necessity of a special diet for 3 days to increase reliability (10,13,21) and multiple stool examinations of up to six specimens (23) makes screening programs more cumbersome.

Chemical occult blood tests do not always reliably detect microscopic intraluminal bleeding. A more innovative approach to such a problem appears warranted. Specificity added to the test for fecal occult hemoglobin would reduce special preparatory maneuvers and dietary requirements, thereby greatly improving the method. Most investigators acknowledge the need for an inexpensive and reliable colorectal cancer screening test. This article serves to describe the immunologic approach for the identification of human fecal occult blood and the potential use of such a test in colorectal cancer screening.

Rosenfield et al. (16) were one of the first to devise an immunologic test for human occult blood by using anti-Rh 29 against red blood cell stroma in feces. The sensitivity of that Rh antibody neutralization test has been shown to be 10^8 erythrocytes/gram feces, essentially identical to the Hemoccult test. The rationale for use of Rh antigens was their universal presence on human erythrocytes, and except for a few higher primates, absence on other animal species. Thus employment of this erythrocyte surface antigen test was equal to Hemoccult in sensitivity and additionally offered the distinct advantage of human specificity.

Certain technical factors, however, limited the practical application of this procedure. Some examples include 1 g of stool specimen needed for fractionation, debris separated from red cell stroma through high-speed centrifugation, and special serologic techniques to read the inhibition test results. Additionally, Rh 29 antigen reactivity may deteriorate with prolonged exposure (greater than 24 hr) to fecal stream enzymes resulting in a false negative test. A simpler and more general technique appeared wanting.

Simultaneously, and independent of Rosenfield et al. (16), the present authors devised an immunologic test for occult blood utilizing human hemoglobin as the antigen. It was reasoned that probably the most abundant identifiable compound released by neoplasms within the colonic lumen was blood. Red cell hemoglobin occurs in concentration several magnitudes greater than red cell membrane Rh antigen. A technique to detect soluble hemoglobin as well as intact or hemolyzed erythrocytes was further attractive. Even the anemic patient with a microcytic hypochromic anemia of chronic blood loss generally continues to produce occult blood positive stools. Certainly early lesions associated with substantially higher hematocrits should yield abundant quantities of occult hemoglobin provided a suitably sensitive and specific test was employed.

This communique serves to describe such a test. A specific, accurate, sensitive, simple, inexpensive, noninvasive screening procedure has been developed (20). No special preparation is needed, no foods or drugs have been found to interfere, specimen acquisition is uncomplicated, and the fecal smear is quite stable. This procedure incorporated high titer antibody to human hemoglobin with the radial immunodiffusion (RID) technique. Further, a fecal smear method analogous to the Hemoccult slide test has been perfected, called the fecal smear punch-disc test. In fact, the actual patient unit consisted of guaiac-impregnated paper and a second specially treated paper so that simultaneous companion smears could be prepared from the same stool specimen. These simultaneous companion smears served as the basis for much of this study.

Occasional disagreement between simultaneous companion smears became evident early in the study. Of particular interest was the Hemoccult-positive, punch-disc negative disparity. The authors (4) have previously reported on alteration of hemoglobin antigen during transit through the intestinal tract. This alteration was attributed to small bowel carboxypeptidases and the effect could be demonstrated by hemoglobin electrophoretic mobility. Thus native unaltered hemoglobin could be separated from enzyme-altered hemoglobin. Further application of this observation proved valid when studied by RID application of the punch-disc test.

When transit time was relatively normal so that sufficient contact with small bowel enzymes occurred, small or occult bleeds indeed proved to have enough alteration of the hemoglobin antigen to test negative on the monospecific RID plate. Fortunately, enough peroxidase activity persisted in each case to test positive by the impregnated guaiac paper. This discovery served as a basis for potential separation of occult bleeding into two categories when simultaneous companion smears were made: upper GI tract and lower GI tract. A small pilot study was evaluated to ascertain what clinical impact, if any, such a simultaneous companion test might offer in diagnostic or screening situations.

METHODS AND MATERIALS

Antihemoglobin antibody was incorporated into radial immunodiffusion plates of the Mancini type. When hemolysate was used, minimum hemoglobin concentration detection was 1 mg/dl and standard curves were linear. Cross-reactivity with hemoglobin and myoglobin from usual dietary domestic animals was absent. Human hemoglobinopathies SS, SC, SA, CC, and fetal had no loss of sensitivity. Each batch of antisera was evaluated for cross-reactivity and sensitivity before use. The tests employed in this study used the IgG fraction on one bleed. This work has been described in detail elsewhere (2,4).

For clinical application, the immunochemical hemoglobin test was adapted to filter paper strips. Filter paper was soaked in a pH-adjusted mixture of dextran, streptomycin, penicillin, amphotericin B, and sodium azide. When dry, the treated filter paper was fabricated into patient units similar to Hemoccult.[1] Feces were then tested for occult blood by smearing them on the filter paper analogous to the Hemoccult slide methodology. Subsequently, a uniform dry area of fecal-smeared filter paper was selected and a 1/8 inch disc removed by a commercial conductor's-type punch (McGill Utility). The disc was placed on the surface of an RID plate, rehydrated with 10 μl 0.05 M phosphate-buffered saline (pH 8.5), and incubated at room temperature for 16 to 24 hr. Perpendicular diameters of precipitin rings were measured at equivalence using indirect illumination. Filter paper punch-discs soaked in standard hemoglobin hemolysate were used to validate constant sensitivity of each RID plate and to serve as a known standard for quantitation. To simulate *in vivo* occult bleeding, 1 g aliquots of immunochemical/Hemoccult negative normal stools were mixed with known amounts of hemoglobin hemolysate. With fecal/hemoglobin mixtures, maximum

---

[1] Guaiac paper, Smith Kline Diagnostics, Sunnyvale, CA.

immunochemical hemoglobin sensitivity was 0.3 mg/g stool. A 5- to 10-fold increase in hemoglobin concentration was necessary to achieve similar maximum sensitivity with Hemoccult. The results were essentially identical when intact red cells were mixed with normal stools.

Since commercial guaiac-impregnated paper preparations (Hemoccult) may give false information on storage, storage experiments were conducted. Fecal smears made of fabricated stool and hemoglobin mixtures had unchanged punch-disc sensitivity when stored for periods up to 30 days at room temperature (3).

Filter paper segments were smeared with occult blood positive feces (analogous to Hemoccult smear), allowed to air dry, sandwiched between mylar sheets with an overprinted grid, and then xeroxed. Next, 1/8 inch discs were punched from the smear according to unique coordinates until the entire smear area was exhausted. Each disc was assayed qualitatively and quantitatively for hemoglobin by the RID punch-disc method. Then a smear profile was constructed to reveal the exact amount of hemoglobin and its location according to the geometry of the particular fecal smear.

In order to compare the punch-disc immunochemical method with the standard guaiac-impregnated paper (Hemoccult) method, simultaneous companion smears were prepared for the same location in each acquired stool specimen. The patient units for these simultaneous companion smears consisted of a Hemoccult slide and a prepared segment of punch-disc filter paper for use in the immunochemical test. Explicit printed directions were furnished and the nursing staff of participating institutions were given in-service instruction by the investigators concerning the proper utilization of the units.

From three community hospitals 150 consecutive cases of histologically proven colorectal cancer were prospectively accessioned. These patients, ages 40 to 88 years, were admitted for definitive surgical treatment, although in some instances resection was technically impossible. Since the majority of admissions were elective, no specific time interval existed between admission date and surgical treatment. The range was 12 hr to 10 days with an average time of 3 days. In every case, at least one stool specimen was obtained by nursing personnel or the patient himself and simultaneous companion smears made. The same portion of stool was smeared on both testing papers and the same personnel conducted the interpretation of the tests in a blind fashion. Trace reactions of Hemoccult were considered positive. In order to avoid false negatives as reported by Stroehlein and co-workers (21) and Fleisher et al. (5), Hemoccult specimens were tested within 48 hr of acquisition. Since tests were performed within 48 hr, rehydration was not used.

Prior to or following surgery, every individual in this study was histologically documented to have carcinoma of the colon or rectum. All other types of lower GI tract lesions were excluded. Likewise, all upper GI tract lesions and sources of bleeding were excluded. All surgical pathology material was examined and reviewed by a single investigator (CLS), and the lesions were categorized according to Dukes' staging system. Stage A tumors involved bowel wall only, stage B tumors extended through the bowel wall, and stage C tumors had lymph node metastases. The anatomic categories were divided into cecum, ascending colon, transverse colon, descending colon, sigmoid colon, and rectum. Neoplasm location, Dukes' stage, volume, and area were tabulated.

During the accession of 150 acceptable consecutive colorectal carcinoma cases, many additional patients with simultaneous companion smears for fecal occult blood were accumulated. These 3,686 cases were all unselected hospitalized patients. Companion smears were done each time a Hemoccult test was ordered in the course of the patient's work-up. Patients were known to be bleeding, thought to be bleeding, or simply studied as part of the routine in a complete diagnostic work-up. Discordant results were examined. Preference was given to Hemoccult-positive, punch-disc negative cases. Strict criteria were applied for concluding that occult upper GI bleeding was or was not established. Major criteria included visual documentation of the lesion by fiberoptic endoscopy, conclusive radiographic demonstration, or direct surgical inspection with biopsy. Minor criteria included reliable history with confirmatory laboratory data (ethanol abuse with altered liver function studies, anticoagulant therapy exceeding the therapeutic range, aspirin ingestion with abnormal platelet aggregation studies, and chemotherapy with evidence of toxicity and/or thrombocytopenia). Any case where equivocation existed was excluded. The upper GI tract was divided into esophagus, stomach, duodenum, and jejunoileum, and the bleeding sites localized to these anatomic regions. No patient with established or presumptive lower GI disease was included.

RESULTS

Physician, nurse, and patient prepared fecal smears generally contained enough area to allow punching of 15 to 20 discs. Qualitative presence of hemoglobin varied between 50 and 100% of the discs. Quantitative amounts of hemoglobin also varied among discs. Some loci of the smear were devoid of hemoglobin. Other areas contained expected concentrations and still other areas contained up to a two-fold increase. There was no apparent correlation with specimen, patient, technique of smear, or geometry of smear.

Twenty-nine percent of colorectal cancer cases were found not bleeding by either test. When analyzed by anatomic site, almost 50% of the rectal lesions did not bleed whereas only 25% of the right colon lesions failed to bleed. As summarized in Table 1, occult bleeding was detected by Hemoccult in 40% of the overall cases, whereas the immunochemical test was positive in 65% ($p < 0.001$). By the Hemoccult test 50% of the lesions in the right colon were positive, compared with 63% positive with the immunochemical test. With Hemoccult 34% of lesions in the left colon were positive, and 72% were positive with the immunochemical punch test. Rectal lesions tested 29% positive by Hemoccult and 50% positive by punch-disc. Neoplasm size tended to become

TABLE 1. *Bleeding detected according to anatomic site*

Cancer site	Cancer cases	Positive tests	
		Immunochemical	Hemoccult
Right colon	62	39 (63%)	31 (50%)
Left colon	64	46 (70%)	22 (34%)
Rectum	24	12 (50%)	7 (29%)
Total	150	97 (65%)[a]	60 (40%)[a]

[a] $p < 0.001$ by Chi square.

smaller as the site moved from cecum to rectum (Table 2), but no correlation between size and amount of blood detected immunochemically occurred. Comparison of stage revealed significantly smaller lesions with Dukes' stage A (Table 3). The immunochemical test had a higher frequency of positives in all Dukes' stages.

Adenocarcinoma was found in 146 of the 150 colorectal cancer cases. The exceptions were all rectal cancers. Two cases were Dukes' A squamous cell carcinomas. The remaining two cases were cloacogenic carcinomas, one a Dukes' A and the other a Dukes' B. Preliminary appraisal of each colorectal cancer case fecal smear for mg/dl occult hemoglobin by the immunochemical method revealed great variability. Values ranged from 72 mg/dl in the cecum up to 229 mg/dl in the rectum. No correlation was apparent.

Of the simultaneous companion smears, 86% were found in agreement (74%

TABLE 2. *Companion smear results according to anatomic site*

Cancer site	Cancer cases	Mean surface area (cm²)	Positive tests	
			Immunochemical	Hemoccult
Cecum	25	55	15 (60%)	14 (56%)
Ascending colon	30	30	21 (70%)	14 (47%)
Transverse colon	7	35	3 (43%)	3 (43%)
Descending colon	10	34	6 (60%)	4 (40%)
Sigmoid colon	56	26	40 (71%)	19 (34%)
Rectum	24	10	12 (50%)	7 (29%)

TABLE 3. *Bleeding detected according to Dukes' stage*

Dukes' stage	Cancer cases	Surface area (cm²)	% Positive tests	
			Immunochemical	Hemoccult
A	33	10.9	55	33
B	54	34.7	67	50
C	63	31.7	68	37

TABLE 4. *Major criteria cases with documented bleeding episode according to anatomic site and diagnosis*

Lesion site	Diverticulum	Hiatal hernia	Inflammation and erosion	Active ulcer	Benign neoplasm	Malignant neoplasm	Varices
Esophagus	1	0	2	0	0	0	5
Stomach	0	5	3	3	1[a]	2[b]	0
Duodenum	0	0	0	4	0	0	0
Jejunoileum	0	0	0	1[c]	1[d]	1[e]	0
Other	0	0	1[f]	0	0	0	0

[a] Multiple gastric polyps.
[b] Adenocarcinoma.
[c] Gastrojejunostomy stoma ulcer.
[d] Multiple hemangiomata.
[e] Metastatic adenocarcinoma with mucosal ulceration.
[f] Epistaxis requiring nares packing.

TABLE 5. *Minor criteria cases with presumptive bleeding episode according to final diagnosis*

Salicylate gastritis	Alcohol gastritis	Anticoagulant excess therapy	Renal failure	Chemo-therapy
5	3	2	3	5

both positive, 12% both negative) and not further evaluated; 14% were found discordant (8% being Hemoccult-positive, punch-disc negative and 6% Hemoccult-negative, punch-disc positive). In the former group, 278 patients were examined in detail to determine the reason for guaiac identification of blood when simultaneous immunochemical confirmation was lacking.

Of the 278 cases only 30 patients met the major criteria and an additional 18 patients the minor criteria. Table 4 demonstrates tabulation of major criteria cases and Table 5 a similar presentation for minor criteria. Major criteria cases localized eight lesions within the esophagus, all non-neoplastic. Fourteen lesions were noted in the stomach, six non-neoplastic, two neoplastic, and five instances of hiatal hernia involving as much as 50% of the stomach. The duodenum localized four inflammatory lesions. The jejunoileum revealed a gastrojejunostomy stoma ulcer, one hemangioma, and a metastatic carcinoma with subsequent mucosal ulceration. Additionally, a solitary case presented with epistaxis requiring anterior and posterior nasal packs. The minor criteria patients included three cases each of renal failure and of alcohol abuse. A total of seven cases involved altered coagulation parameters, two on warfarin (Coumadin)-type drugs and the remaining patients on enough aspirin to alter platelet aggregation. An additional five patients were on chemotherapy and had some type of malignant disease ranging from malignant lymphoma to disseminated carcinoma.

DISCUSSION

Variable physical location of erythrocytes and/or hemoglobin within the stool specimen is further reflected in guaiac impregnated paper smears of such specimens. In order to evaluate this problem, guaiac-impregnated paper and non-guaiac-impregnated paper were simultaneously smeared with stool specimens from individuals known to be bleeding and known not to be bleeding as well as from *in vitro* fabricated hemoglobin-positive and hemoglobin-negative specimens. According to a coordinate scheme, the entire fecal smear was "punched-out" using a conductor's-type hand punch. Following determination of hemoglobin present or absent in each individual disc, a map was constructed to reveal the exact geographic location of the hemoglobin. Further, since a radial immuno-diffusion test was utilized, hemoglobin was determined both qualitatively and quantitatively. Even well-prepared specimen smears revealed the presence of hemoglobin to be quite variable.

Hard and well-formed stools might yield smears with no more than 50% of discs positive for hemoglobin. On the other hand, very soft or watery stools might yield 100% of the discs positive for hemoglobin. The quantitative amount of hemoglobin per disc per location was also quite variable. No correlations were established even when the anatomic location of the bleeding colon lesion was known.

It would appear that the Hemoccult test circumvents this potentially discrete location of occult blood in the prepared smeared Hemoccult slide test through the fortuitous addition of chromagen liquid developer, whose aqueous phase presumably solubilizes the entire smear area so that no foci of hemoglobin remain isolated.

The present authors, as well as Rosenfield's group, were one of the earliest to recognize the complexity of occult blood distribution in feces. Prior to the application of immunologic technique, such significant variation was not fully appreciated. Most data imply that GI tract lesions have episodic bleeding, and when compounded with dietary habitus, motility, and other factors, nonhomogeneity of stool occult blood appears to be the rule. Future workers must remain cognizant of these facts when designing immunologic occult blood tests and ponder optimal stool sampling techniques in order to ensure accurate results.

Testing 150 consecutive colorectal carcinomas by the immunochemical fecal smear punch-disc demonstrated marked improvement over the chemical guaiac-impregnated paper (Hemoccult) fecal smear. The immunochemical method increased sensitivity approximately 10-fold over Hemoccult and gave complete specificity. As reported previously, no foods, drugs, or chemicals interfered with the punch-disc interpretation (2). Additionally, all punch-disc test systems may be validated by inclusion of a positive control punch-disc soaked in human hemolysate. The precipitin rings measured in the punch-disc technique allowed quantitation of the occult hemoglobin by comparison with the control hemoglobin. This added feature made the punch-disc test both qualitative and potentially quantitative. The importance of this quantitation was readily apparent during *in vitro* fabricated occult blood companion smear studies: significant variation in commercial quaiac-impregnated paper was discovered in companion smears when all immunochemical punch-disc smears were interpreted for hemoglobin both qualitatively and quantitatively. Unappreciated decreased sensitivity in various lots of Hemoccult may result in increased false negatives. Without positive control and quantitation techniques for Hemoccult, such problems may not be apparent.

Although no more than 10% of the Hemoccult-positive, punch-disc negative patients could be documented to have known bleeding sites, the results appear quite encouraging. Inspection of Table 4 reveals a rather wide spectrum of clinical lesions ranging from inflammation with ulceration to neoplasms, both benign and malignant. The ability to discriminate such bleeding sites may have limited application in the screening environment as many of these individuals would present as chronically ill screenees. Table 5 suggests that more subtle situations may also give rise to occult bleeding, not necessarily elicited even by history.

Some thoughtful comment appears appropriate concerning the potential effect of aspirin in the colorectal cancer screening candidate. More than 900 different proprietary compounds and medicines contain aspirin or its derivatives. Informal studies have shown that on any given day, perhaps as many as one-tenth of the entire population of the United States has ingested aspirin during the previous 24 hr. Many individuals are chronic users, either by habit or by physician's directive. Inhibited platelet aggregation may persist for days. It would appear these individuals are at increased risk to bleed from the upper GI tract in an occult fashion. Perhaps such altered platelets may also promote bleeding from an early colorectal lesion, whether benign or malignant. This would appear a fruitful area for further investigation.

Current screening programs as well as individual users of Hemoccult recommend a total of six slides for adequate testing. Abstinence from meats for the 4 days adds another restriction on screening programs. Sensitivity and specificity of the immunochemical punch-disc technique may reduce the total number of stool specimens required and negate diet restriction, thereby simplifying screening.

Of great importance is the stability of the fecal smear. The Hemoccult smear, as previously discussed, should be tested within 48 hr, whereas the punch-disc smear appears stable for up to 30 days (3). This is particularly valuable when fecal smears must be accumulated, stored, and then mailed.

The disadvantage with the immunochemical punch-disc technique is that a 24 to 48-hr delay occurs between receiving the test and its interpretation. However, since screening programs are by their nature elective procedures, it should not be difficult to effectively organize a screening program utilizing this test. Certainly, successful screening programs for cervical cancer have employed the Pap smear, which may take 3 to 5 days before results are completely interpreted.

The current study suggests that the immunochemical method to detect colorectal bleeding from carcinoma has better sensitivity than existing methods. Since no interference with normal dietary material occurs, the method should simplify screening programs by removing dietary restrictions. Additionally, since the rate of detection for individual smears is higher, it should be possible to screen patients using fewer samples. Lastly, a combination chemical-immunologic test shows a great promise in terms of discriminating between upper and lower GI tract occult bleeding. The immunologic alteration of occult hemoglobin by small bowel enzymes renders the punch-disc test generally specific for the lower GI tract. This appears a decided advantage over guaiac-impregnated paper tests, which detect occult blood irrespective of upper or lower GI tract origin.

Results of simultaneous companion smears found Hemoccult-negative, punch-disc positive were not reported. Those results will be further studied and later published.

ACKNOWLEDGMENTS

Enthusiastic support from the Administrative and Medical Staffs of the Bayfront Medical Center, the Edward H. White II Memorial Hospital, and the Apollo Medical Center, all of St. Petersburg, Florida, made this project possible. The authors thank M. David Alford for technical assistance and Sharon Slosar and Michelle Sebik for manuscript preparation. This investigation supported in part by NCI contract NO1-CB-43968.

REFERENCES

1. Barnett, R. M. (1952): The guaiac test: Correlation and clinical findings. *Gastroenterology,* 21:540–543.
2. Barrows, G. H., Burton, R. M., Jarrett, D. D., Russell, G. G., Alford, M. D., and Songster, C. L. (1978): Immunochemical detection of human blood in stool. *Am. J. Clin. Pathol.,* 69:342–346.
3. Barrows, G. H., Maikranz, P. A., Burton, R. M., and Songster, C. L. (1977): Improved retention of occult blood activity in neutral dried fecal smears. *Gastroenterology,* 72:1027.
4. Burton, R. M., Landreth, K. S., Barrows, G. H., Jarrett, D. D., and Songster, C. L. (1976): Appearance, properties and origin of altered human hemoglobin in feces. *Lab. Invest.,* 35:111–115.
5. Fleisher, M., Schwartz, M. K., and Winawer, S. J. (1977): The false-negative Hemoccult test. *Gastroenterology,* 72(4):782–784.
6. Greegor, D. H. (1967): Diagnosis of large-bowel cancer in the asymptomatic patient. *JAMA,* 201:943–945.
7. Greegor, D. H. (1969): Detection of silent colon cancer in routine examinations. *CA,* 19:330–337.
8. Greegor, D. H. (1971): Occult blood testing for detection of asymptomatic colon cancer. *Cancer,* 28:131–135.
9. Greegor, D. H. (1972): Detection of colorectal cancer using guaiac slides. *CA,* 22:360–363.
10. Humphrey, T. J., and Goulston, K. (1969): Chemical testing of occult blood in feces: "Hematest", "occult test", and guaiac testing correlated with chromium estimation of fecal blood loss. *Med. J. Aust.,* 1:1291–1293.
11. Illingworth, D. G. (1965): Influence of diet on occult blood tests. *Gut,* 6:595–598.
12. Jaffee, R. M., Kaston, B., Young, M. D., and MacLowry, N. (1974): False negative stool occult blood tests caused by ingestion of ascorbic acid (vitamin C). *Ann. Intern. Med.,* 83:824–826.
13. Lehmann, H., and Kitchin, E. G. (1971): A test for occult blood. *Lancet,* 2:258.
14. Markman, H. D. (1967): Errors in the guaiac test for occult blood. *JAMA,* 202:846–847.
15. Ostrow, J. D., Mulvaney, C. A., Hansell, J. R., and Rhodes, R. (1974): Sensitivity and reproducibility of chemical tests for fecal occult blood with an emphasis on false positive reactions. *Am. J. Dig. Dis.,* 18:930–940.
16. Rosenfield, R. E., Kochwa, S., Kaczera, Z., and Maimon, J. (1979): Nonuniform distribution of occult blood in feces. *Am. J. Clin. Pathol.,* 71:204–209.
17. Schudamore, H. H. (1969): Cancer of colon and rectum—General aspects, diagnosis, treatment and prognosis: a review. *Dis. Colon Rectum,* 12:105–114.
18. Seidman, H., Silverberg, E., and Holleb, A. I. (1976): Cancer statistics, 1976. A comparison of white and black populations. *CA,* 22:2–13.
19. Silverberg, E. (1979): Cancer statistics, 1979. *CA,* 29:6–21.
20. Songster, C. L., Barrows, G. H., and Jarrett, D. D. (1980): Immunochemical detection of fecal occult blood, The fecal smear punch-disc test: a new non-invasive screening test for colorectal cancer. *Cancer,* 45:1099–1102.
21. Stroehlein, J. R., Fairbanks, V., Go, V. L. W., Taylor, W., and Thompson, J. (1976): Hemoccult stool tests false negative results due to storage of specimens. *Mayo Clin. Proc.,* 51:548–552.

22. Trujillo, H. P., and Ticktin, H. E. (1966): Influence of uncooked meat on tests for occult blood in the stool. *South. Med. J.,* 59:352–353.
23. Winawer, S. J., Miller, D. G., Schottenfeld, D., Sherlock, P., Befler, B., and Stearns, M. W., Jr. (1977): Feasibility of fecal occult-blood testing for detection of colorectal neoplasia: debits and credits. *Cancer, [Suppl. 5],* 40:2616–2619.
24. Winawer, S. J., Sherlock, P., Schottenfeld, D., and Miller, D. G. (1976): Screening for colon cancer. *Gastroenterology,* 70:783–789.

Colorectal Cancer: Prevention, Epidemiology, and Screening, edited by S. Winawer, D. Schottenfeld, and P. Sherlock. Raven Press, New York © 1980.

Markers in Screening: Overview of Usefulness of Markers

Morton K. Schwartz

Memorial Sloan-Kettering Cancer Center, New York, New York 10021

The search for a constituent useful as an early colon cancer diagnostic test has attracted the attention of physicians and scientists for decades. This search has not yet been completely successful because the sensitivity of described biochemical or immunochemical procedures does not usually permit detection of tumor-specific material until after metastases have occurred; in addition, tests have not been cancer specific and have all produced a significant number of false positives. In recent years, a relationship of the cancer cell to an embryonic state has been widely accepted, and analysis of fetal enzymes and antigens in body fluids has been utilized in an effort to detect tumors and to better understand the relationship of fetal macromolecules to the malignant process. The successful use of blood fetal antigen measurements is, in part, due to the development of immunochemical techniques, particularly the radioimmunoassay, which permit quantitation in the nanogram range.

From the standpoint of general use, the most important tests would be those specific for a single cancer and useful in cancers with the highest population incidence. In the United States, it is projected that there will be 765,000 new cases of cancer in 1980 with 395,000 deaths (1). The new cases include 112,000 patients with colorectal cancer. It is obvious that there is a great need for highly specific and sensitive cancer detection tests. Berlin (2) has pointed out that the successful cancer diagnostic test is one which will detect 75% of all cancers when 90% of these cancers have not undergone metastases. The test should indicate the organ where the cancer resides since this information is essential if curative treatment is to be instituted. Even the oldest and perhaps the most widely known cancer test, serum acid phosphatase, would not meet these criteria. It may be elevated in diseases other than cancer of the prostate, and in cancer of the prostate serum elevations are observed in only 20% of the patients before metastases, but in 80% of patients following metastatic extension of the disease (3).

There are few, if any, diagnostic markers that are useful in primary diagnosis of the major forms of cancer. Most of the well-defined diagnostic biochemical and immunochemical procedures are related to rarer forms of cancer. These include neurogenic amines and their metabolites in neuroblastoma and pheochromocytoma, serotonin metabolites (5-hydroxyindole acetic acid) in carcinoid, chorionic gonadotropin in choriocarcinoma and embryonal testicular tumors, Bence-Jones protein and immunoglobulins in multiple myeloma, α-fetoprotein in hepatocellular carcinoma, and alkaline phosphatase in osteogenic sarcoma and other osteoblastic bone tumors. In these diseases, the assay of biochemical constituents is essential for confirmation of the diagnosis and in following the response to therapy (4).

The problem that exists in the diagnosis of cancer is that as a tumor grows, it reaches a finite size when there is probability for the occurrence of metastasis. However, by the time the tumor is large enough to elaborate sufficient material into the bloodstream or other body fluids in order that a diagnostic test be positive, the chance for metastasis is great; by the time the patient experiences symptoms, there is a significant chance that metastasis has occurred. The probability of metastasis ranges from about 30% in patients with cancer of the body of the uterus to almost 100% in persons with cancer of the pancreas. If improved cure rates are a function of treatment before the cancer is spread, then successful diagnostic testing is essential before clinical symptoms occur. Unfortunately, the state of the art is such at this time that few positive diagnostic tests are observed before the metastatic spread of the cancer. In lung cancer, the probability of metastasis is 20% at a time when the primary tumor is less than 2 cm in diameter, and in breast cancer, 27% when the tumor is only 1 cm in diameter. It has been theorized that metastasis may occur from primary tumors consisting of fewer than 125 cells. It is highly unlikely that a tumor so small would lend itself to clinical detection, or that cancer-specific material detectable in serum or urine would be elaborated by these tumors or the previously described 1 or 2 cm breast or lung cancers. Tests that have been developed, such as chorionic gonadotropin in choriocarcinoma and α-fetoprotein in hepatocellular carcinoma, are in cancers where there is a rapid cell turnover. It has been estimated that the daily turnover is 35% of cells in embryonal tumors, 10 to 15% in squamous cell carcinomas, 4% in sarcomas, and only 1% in adenocarcinomas.

At the present time, screening procedures for the early diagnosis of cancer are essentially limited to the pap smear for cervical cancer and occult blood in colorectal cancer. Many other tests have been proposed but none have had sufficient specificity and sensitivity to meet the criteria for an early screening test. The tests now available are more useful in monitoring disease and following the course of the disease. This is an important and useful role for cancer markers. In order to demonstrate this point, I would like to review the role of several markers other than occult blood in colorectal cancer.

CARCINOEMBRYONIC ANTIGEN

Carcinoembryonic antigen (CEA) is obviously not an organ-specific indicator of cancer, nor can it be as a screening test for early diagnosis. In colorectal cancer, initial values appear to be a good indicator of prognosis. An important use of CEA is serial assays in assessing the status of patients during therapy. Persistent elevations may be indicative of therapeutic failure, whereas following successful surgery or chemotherapy the levels will fall toward normal levels and remain at that level until a recrudescence of the disease occurs. In a prospective study of 102 patients who had no clinically detectable disease following colorectal surgery, CEA levels became elevated in 12 patients. Six of these developed recurrent cancer 0 to 29 months after the elevated CEA was detected. The other 6 patients did not develop a recurrence, and in 2 patients recurrence was observed despite normal CEA (5).

We examined the relation of carcinoembryonic antigen levels to time, site, and extent of recurrence in 358 patients with colorectal cancer (6,7). Recurrence rate was higher in patients with Dukes' B and Dukes' C lesions who had preoperative CEA levels higher than 5 ng/ml. There was a linear inverse correlation between preoperative levels and estimated mean time to recurrence in patients with Dukes' B and C lesions, ranging from 30 months for a level of 2 ng/ml to 9.8 months for a level of 70 ng/ml. In patients with Dukes' C lesions the median time to recurrence was 13 months if preoperative levels were higher than 5 ng/ml, and 28 months if they were lower. Preoperative carcinoembryonic antigen levels in patients with resectable Dukes' B and C cancer provided an additional criterion for assigning these patients to groups at high or low risk for recurrence.

In 16 patients, all of whom had "curative" surgery, prospective studies were conducted. Thirteen of these patients were Dukes' C and three Dukes' B. All were followed clinically and by CEA testing at 3-month intervals and were considered free of disease (NED) at the time of a postoperative CEA elevation. The median disease-free interval was 13 months (range 4 to 57 months), and the median CEA prompting admission for a second-look operation was 21 ng/ml (range 10 to 56 ng/ml). The sites of recurrence were liver in six patients, lung in two and localized disease in six. Two patients had negative exploration for recurrence and were found to have cholelithiasis only (one of these later died of metastases). Resection for cure was done in seven and palliative resection or biopsy only was done in nine patients. Following the second surgery, four patients were NED (12 to 37 months), five were living with disease (10 to 16 months), and seven died of disease 2 to 12 months after treatment. These data indicate that CEA can assist in the early detection of recurrence.

According to Shani and his associates (8), serial CEA measurements are not particularly useful in following the course of patients with metastatic colorectal cancer receiving chemotherapy. In a study of 263 patients, there was a general relation between serial plasma CEA and clinical tumor measurements, but there were discordant correlations in a significant number of patients. Changes in CEA did not correlate with survival although there was a general correlation with disease progression, but this correlation was roughly comparable to that of serum alkaline phosphatase in evaluating the occurrence and progression of liver metastases.

The use of CEA must be weighed against the cost of performing the test. A discouraging report has been published by Meeker (9). He reported that in 299 patients in whom 693 CEA assays were performed, the values altered the clinician's decision making in only four cases. Since the cost per assay was $30, the cost per clinical action was more than $5,000 per patient. When the analysis was confined to patients with colorectal cancer, the effective cost per patient was almost $3,500.

OTHER COLON-RELATED ANTIGENS

Other antigens have been proposed for evaluation of colon cancers. These include CEA-S and the zinc glycinate marker (ZGM) (10,11). This latter antigen does not appear to be related to CEA or antigens known to cross-react with CEA or other well-known antigens such as α-fetoprotein, α_2-microglobulin or blood group substances. ZGM has been detected by immunofluorescence in 90% of adenocarcinomas of the GI tract but in none of non-GI tumors and was present in the deep crypts of the villi, distinguishable from CEA which was stained at the surface epithelium. Further clinical studies are needed to establish the diagnostic role of ZGM.

GLYCOSYLTRANSFERASES

The glycosyltransferases are a family of enzymes which catalyze the sequential addition of monosaccharides (galactose, fucose, sialic acid, etc.) to specific protein and glycoprotein acceptors (most often desialated fetuin).

Sialyltransferase in plasma has been extensively studied. This enzyme catalyzes the transfer of sialic acid from the nucleotide cytidine monophosphate sialic acid to the galactose residue of desialated fetuin. Henderson and Kessel (12) studied the plasma enzyme levels in 134 randomly selected patients with cancer. In normal persons the values were 240 ± 55 units (upper limit, 350 units), but in 18 patients with colon cancer in whom 49 values were obtained the range of activity was from 145 to 1,055 units with a mean value of 492 units. In 46 of the 49 specimens abnormal activity was observed. In 5 patients with cancer of the rectum 7 of 13 specimens were elevated. The range was 247 to 545 units (mean, 376 units). In 10 patients in whom the sialyltransferase activity was related to extent of disease a correct correlation was seen in six patients, but there was a false negative response in two individuals and a false-positive in one. One patient could not be evaluated. In patients with massive metastatic involvement longitudinal sialyltransferase levels were correlated with the clinical course in 90% (18/20) of patients but in only 66% (27/41) of the patients with less extensive tumor involvement. Correlations were observed in 20/26 patients with liver metastases and 11/14 with lung metastases. These data support a conclusion that sialyltransferase may be of some utility in following the patient with metastatic cancer, but is of limited usefulness in early detection.

Podolsky and his associates (13) have studied galactosyltransferase in colon cancer. This enzyme is a uridine diphosphate galactose transferase which catalyzes the transfer of galactose to fetuin. More specifically, these workers have investigated an isoenzyme (galactosyltransferase II) which separates from the other fractions on polyacrylamide gel electrophoresis. The isoenzyme was not detected in any of 58 control serums nor in 12 patients with ulcerative colitis, 8 with Crohn's ileocolitis, 15 with pancreatitis, 9 with viral hepatitis, and 6 with biliary tract disease. It was found, however, in 3 of 15 patients with severe alcoholic hepatitis and 18 to 20 patients with celiac disease.

The isoenzyme was observed in many cancers, but particularly in 85/117 patients with colorectal adenocarcinoma. The enzyme was not detectable in each of 3 patients with Dukes' A disease, 2 of 9 patients with Dukes' B disease, and 9 of 32 patients with Dukes' C disease as well as 5 of 19 patients with distant metastases. In the patients with Dukes' A and B diseases who had presurgical elevated values, the activity became undetectable after curative surgery, and in an additional 14 patients declared free of disease 5 years after surgery there was no detectable enzyme activity. In longitudinal studies, there was a distinct correlation between the clinical status and the enzyme activity.

The isoenzyme was also found in effusions but only in patients whose effusions were cytology positive. No activity was observed in effusions from patients with benign disease or when the cytology was negative. Of particular interest was that total galactosyltransferase activity was present in all effusions, but there was no difference in activity in malignant compared to benign effusions.

OTHER ENZYMES

Other enzymes have also been studied in colorectal cancer. Morgan et al. (14) have found that urinary aryl sulfatase B is elevated in 28% of patients with Dukes' A disease, 55% of those with Dukes' B, and in more than 75% of patients with Dukes' C and D lesions.

In 95 patients who underwent curative resection of colon adenocarcinoma, preoperatively γ-glutamyl transpeptidase (γ-GTP) was elevated in 29% of the patients, lactic dehydrogenase (LDH) in 55%, alkaline phosphatase in 13%, glutathione reductase in 22%, and 5'nucleotidase in 11%. In 31 patients with liver metastases, γ-GTP was elevated in 58%, alkaline phosphatase in 42%, LDH in 44%, glutathione reductase in 50%, and 5'nucleotidase in 42% (15). In another study total serum LDH was elevated in only 24% of patients, but the isoenzyme, LDH5, was abnormal in 52% of these individuals (16).

It is obvious from these data that serum enzymes now available have little to offer in the early detection of colon cancer and may not be of particular use in monitoring metastases to the liver.

CONCLUSION

The introduction of powerful analytical tools, the radioimmunoassay and competitive equilibrium techniques, has made possible quantitation of proteins and other constituents in blood and body fluids at the picogram and femtomole levels. The current interest in CEA, other colon-related antigens, the glycosyl-transferases, and isoenzymes will undoubtedly lead to evaluation of a large series of different antigens and other markers. Success in the search for cancer-specific markers will be a function of the ability to separate and purify individual constituents in sufficient amounts for use in reagent preparation and introducing sophisticated analytical procedures. Well organized clinical trials will then be needed to establish the true role of the marker and both its clinical and economic utility.

REFERENCES

1. Anonymous (1979): Estimated new cancers by sex for all sites—1979. *CA,* 29:14–15.
2. Berlin, N. I. (1975): An overview of research in cancer diagnosis. *Mayo Clin. Proc.,* 50:249.
3. Schwartz, M. K. (1976): Laboratory aids to diagnosis—enzymes. *Cancer,* 37:542–548.
4. Schwartz, M. K. (1975): Biochemical procedures as aids in diagnosis of different forms of cancer. *Ann. Clin. Lab Sci.,* 4:95–103.
5. Herrera, M., Chu, T. M., and Holyoke, E. D. (1976): Carcinoembryonic antigen (CEA) as a prognostic and monitoring test in clinically complete resection of colorectal cancer. *Ann. Surg.,* 183:5–10.
6. Wanebo, H. J., Stearns, M., and Schwartz, M. K. (1978): Use of CEA as an indicator of early recurrence and as a guide to a selected second-look procedure in patients with colorectal cancer. *Ann. Surg.,* 188:481–492.
7. Wanebo, H. J., Rao, B., Pinsky, C. M., Hoffman, R. G., Stearns, M., Schwartz, M. K., and Oettgen, H. F. (1978): Preoperative carcinoembryonic antigen level as a prognostic indicator in colorectal cancer. *N. Engl. J. Med.,* 299:448–451.
8. Shani, A., O'Connell, M. J., Moertel, C. G., Schutt, A. J., Silvers, A., and Go, V. L. W. (1978): Serial plasma carcinoembryonic antigen measurement in the management of metastatic colorectal carcinoma. *Ann. Intern. Med.,* 88:627–630.
9. Meeker, W. R. (1978): The use and abuse of CEA test in clinical practice. *Cancer,* 41:854–858.
10. Eddington, T. S., Astarita, R. W., and Plow, E. F. (1975): Association of an isomeric species of carcinoembryonic antigen (CEA-S) with neoplasia of the gastrointestinal tract. *N. Engl. J. Med.,* 293:103–107.
11. Sanavis, C. A., Oh, S. K., Pusztaszer, G., Doos, W., and Zamcheck, N. (1978): Present status of the zinc glycinate marker (ZGM). *Cancer,* 42:1621–1625.
12. Henderson, M., and Kessel, D. (1977): Alteration in plasma sialyltransferase levels in patients with neoplastic disease. *Cancer,* 39:1129–1134.
13. Podolsky, D. K., Weiser, M. W., Isselbacher, K, J., and Cohen, A. M. (1978): A cancer-associated galactosyl transferase isoenzyme. *N. Engl. J. Med.,* 299:703–705.
14. Morgan, L. R., Samuels, M. S., Thomas, W., Krementz, E. T., and Meeker W. (1975): Arylsulfatase B in colorectal cancer. *Cancer,* 36:2337–2345.
15. Beck, P. R., Belfield, A., Spooner, R. J., Blumgart, L. H., and Wood, C. B. (1979): Serum enzymes in cancer. *Cancer,* 43:1772–1776.
16. Wood, D. C., Varela, V., Palmquist, M., and Weber, F. (1973): Serum lactic dehydrogenase and isoenzyme changes in clinical cancer. *J. Surg. Oncol.,* 5:251–257.

Colorectal Cancer: Prevention, Epidemiology, and Screening, edited by S. Winawer, D. Schottenfeld, and P. Sherlock. Raven Press, New York © 1980.

Multiparametric Approach to Biochemical Surveillance of Large Bowel Cancer

E. H. Cooper and R. Turner

Unit for Cancer Research, University of Leeds, Leeds, LS2 9NL, England

This chapter describes some of the information that can be obtained by various "blood tests" alone and in combination in colorectal cancer. It will be restricted to cases of established disease, as so far there is no evidence that the carcinoembryonic antigen (CEA) test or any other variate in the blood can play any part in the screening or diagnosis of colorectal cancer. Following the diagnosis of a large bowel cancer, its preoperative investigation, and the operative findings, the surgeon has a considerable amount of information on which to base his prognosis. The 5-year survival is correlated with stage so that in Dukes A lesions it ranges from 61 to 81%, in type B lesions 25 to 64%, and in C lesions 6 to 28% as based on five major series with about 4,000 cases in all (10). In those patients in whom tumor is known to be left *in situ* after surgery and there is no attempt at a curative operation, survival can vary considerably from a few weeks to 2 or more years, depending on the tumor load and its rate of growth. Hence although there is general agreement about the survival statistics, prediction of the course of a given individual is far more difficult, and it is now apparent that metastatic disease can have a long asymptomatic period without clinical signs before it produces characteristic indicator lesions.

CARCINOEMBRYONIC ANTIGEN

During the past few years, a major objective in the surveillance of patients after attempted curative surgery has been to detect, as early as possible, those patients in whom disease has not been erradicated in the hope that the institution of further therapy could be beneficial. In patients in whom local recurrence or metastatic disease has been identified, the objective has been to provide the physician with information about the course of the disease and its response to treatment. In common with many other centers, we have used serial CEA determinations to follow our patients (4). The general experience of this test as used as an adjunct to routine surgical follow-up is indicated in Tables 1 and 2.

These measurements were made on average every 6 months and did not involve monthly or bimonthly measurements as has been advocated by some

TABLE 1. *Monitoring of colorectal carcinoma*

Clinical condition	Plasma CEA	No. of patients		
		Colon	Rectum	Total
No evidence of recurrence	Normal	250	275	525
	Rising	23	31	54
Recurrent tumor	Normal	34	32	66
	Antecedent rise	14	23	37
	Synchronous rise[a]	41	48	89
	At operation or first observation[a]	(38)	(43)	
	Other time[a]	(3)	(5)	
Total		362	409	771

[a] The majority of these patients had metastatic tumor confirmed at laparotomy.
From Cooper and Neville (4).

specialist centers. This experience has shown that the rise of CEA can precede the detection of recurrent cancer often by several months, but in the context of routine follow-up on an asymptomatic patient, a rise of CEA was often coincidental with the clinical detection of recurrence. It has been advocated that close monitoring of patients with CEA testing repeated monthly or bimonthly might help in the detection of an "early recurrence" and possibly allow treatment or second look surgery to be undertaken at an opportune moment. So far, the evidence that this ideal is attainable is slight and is often colored with unwarranted optimism at a time when it is still to be proven that such intervention prolongs survival.

Wanebo et al. (18) instituted a program of intensive postoperative monitoring of 55 patients with Dukes' B and 64 patients with Dukes' C lesions and selected 16 for second look operations on the basis of a rising CEA and appropriate ancillary investigations to eliminate distant metastases. Several underwent a

TABLE 2. *Principal metastatic and recurrent sites of colorectal carcinoma*[a]

Tissue	Plasma CEA			
	No change	Synchronous rise	Antecedent rise	Total
Liver	26	61	19	106
Lungs	1	1	2	4
Bone	2	3	1	6
Peritoneum	14	7	4	25
Pelvis	10	8	9	27
Other	13	9	2	24
Total	66	89	37	192

[a] These include patients diagnosed at laparotomy or preoperatively as well as postoperative recurrence.
From Cooper and Neville (4).

second curative resection: 2 were false positive and in 7, only a biopsy or palliative surgery was performed. Optimism is also expressed by Minton and Martin (9) who claim that the shortening of the time between noting a rising CEA and surgery resulted in finding 13 of 18 patients with a resectable tumor; in their previous series based on CEA measurements, they had only 6 of 22 resectable cases. Staab and his colleagues (16) selected 19 colorectal cancers for second look on the basis of CEA levels; 12 were not resectable and of the 8 resectable cases, 4 had evidence of metastatic spread. Again these authors believe that rapid decision making when faced with a rising CEA could result in finding more cases.

On the other hand, Moertel and Schutt (11) considered that the CEA test was fairly insensitive to a small amount of tumor and only 9 of 36 patients with proven local recurrence had an elevated CEA. They point out that generally, the low incidence of positive CEA in Dukes A and B lesions between 28 and 39% reinforces their view. In our own series of residual cancer which included unresectable local disease in the pelvis or apparently small hepatic metastases, only 3 of 42 patients had an elevated CEA when they first presented to chemotherapy clinic 6 weeks after the operation; of the 3 with an elevated CEA, 1 of them was a heavy smoker and the value remained slightly elevated for a year before beginning to rise. Furthermore, this problem of using CEA for the early detection of disease and as the basis for surgical intervention is further confused by the possibility that patients can exhibit transient rises in CEA after curative resection. Rittgers et al. (13) reported that 9 of 25 patients with a raised postoperative CEA exhibited this phenomenon and have even recommended fine-needle biopsy to determine whether there is any evidence of hepatitis prior to exploring patients for a possible recurrence.

The CEA response to chemotherapy in the management of advanced metastatic disease is variable. Although a rise in CEA and tumor progression frequently go together in a patient who is not responding to chemotherapy, the changes in values in those patients who do not respond seem to be less clear-cut. In many publications, there are good examples of a falling CEA on response to chemotherapy followed by a subsequent rise as the patient escapes control. However, once these illustrative cases have been set aside, the broad experience of the clinic may be less clear-cut with either the CEA becoming stable during an apparent clinical response or its course being dissociated from the clinical observation of what is happening to the tumor (15). Moreover, in advanced disease there could well be secondary changes in the metabolism of CEA that alter the level, which must depend on the rate of production and the rate of destruction. Transient rises of CEA have been noted after chemotherapy possibly as the result of release of material from dead cells. It is highly probable that the liver is concerned in CEA metabolism; this may well explain why particularly high values are detected in patients with diffuse hepatic metastases whereas others with relatively large local tumor masses do not produce a similarly high level in the blood (4).

SERUM ENZYMES

As the various shortcomings of the CEA test come to light, several groups have examined whether undertaking parallel measurements of other nonspecific changes in patients with colorectal cancer could give additional information. In the first instance, attention is concentrated on changes in serum enzymes. There have been a large number of enzymes in both serum and urine which have been suggested as tumor markers [see Schwartz (14) for review]. In detecting recurrence of colorectal tumors or monitoring of their treatment by chemotherapy, the level of a single serum enzyme is of limited value in assessing tumor progression before it can be observed clinically. Aronsen et al. (1) in 1970 suggested a multiparametric discriminant analysis approach to the diagnosis of liver involvement in cancer by measuring the serum enzymes γ-glutamyltransferase (γGT), alkaline phosphatase (AP), alanine transferase, and bilirubin. They found a discriminant that could detect 93% of cancer involving the liver in their series. Subsequent studies have not supported the discriminant power of this combination. In the assessment of CEA as a marker for the follow-up of colorectal cancer, we have studied serum enzymes in parallel with CEA. In one study of 109 patients with colorectal cancer and 35 with nonmalignant liver disease, the CEA values alone differentiated hepatic metastases from benign liver disease with a high degree of certainty. It is clear that the CEA may be elevated irrespective of the site of metastases, whereas an elevation of γGT implied hepatic involvement (17).

We will now consider the problem of early detection of metastatic cancer in the liver. Although it was clear that hepatic metastases could be detected by a rising γGT level several months before the liver was large enough to be felt clinically, it subsequently became clear that by the time the γGT begins to rise, the hepatic metastases are well established. This was shown by following the rise of liver enzymes in patients known to have a small hepatic metastasis when the abdomen was closed after resecting the primary tumor. AP, leucine aminopeptidase (LAP), and 5'-nucleotidase (5'-NT) gave results concordant to those with γGT, but their departure from their normal level was later in the evolution of the metastases than that of γGT (4). This experience has recently been repeated in our chemotherapy clinic where the patients are monitored monthly (Table 3).

Munjal et al. (12) confirmed the relationship between CEA and γGT in gastrointestinal cancer. They also showed that serum phosphohexose isomerase was elevated in 57% of their patients compared to elevated values of CEA in 78% and γGT in 58%. In patients in clinical remission, CEA was elevated in 31%, phosphohexose isomerase in 23%, and γGT in 23%. A similar investigation of the usefulness of lactate dehydrogenase showed that overall 45% had a raised value but in clinical remission, only 8% were elevated. Recently, Shani et al. (15) advocated using AP as a substitute for CEA in monitoring colorectal cancer on the grounds that the CEA test is expensive and relatively insensitive.

TABLE 3. *γ-Glutamyltransferase activity 2 months after surgery for colorectal cancer when liver metastases were observed at operation*

< IU/l[a]	30–100 IU/l[a]	> 100 IU/l
38 (38%)	29 (29%)	34 (34%)

[a] Number of months before γ-glutamyltransferase reached 100 IU/l: < 3 months (56%); 3–6 months (8%); 6–12 months (14%); > 12 months (20%).

Our view is that γGT would be a better choice. Although it is acknowledged that occasional bone metastases can cause a rise of AP that would be missed if γGT was used, in our experience, this is rare.

The debate is far from over. Beck et al. (2) have recently described the monitoring of 184 patients with colorectal cancer; once again, γGT emerged as a better indicator of hepatic metastases than AP, 5'-NT, and lactic dehydrogenase. These enzymes were not effective in detecting solitary or local hepatic metastases, and γGT could give false results in preoperative and early postoperative samples. 5'-NT was least liable to give a false elevation, but it was far less sensitive an indicator of metastases.

ACUTE PHASE REACTANTS

In the search for other nonspecific changes in cancer that might be helpful in assessing the biochemical status of the patient, we turned our attention to the behavior of acute phase reactant proteins. An initial survey of the levels of α_1 and α_2 globulin based on a simple electrophoretic technique indicated a strong increase in the α_2 component in active large bowel cancer (6).

In primary tumors and in patients with metastatic cancer, a further analysis showed that in metastatic cancer once the value of α_2 globulin rose above 8 g/liter (normal 5 ± 1.4 g/liter), the level would be sustained or increased in subsequent samples taken over a period of 6 months. Looking at the levels of one of the components of the α_2 globulins, haptoglobin, it became evident that the behavior of this acute phase reactant protein mirrored the general change seen in the mixture of globulins with α_2 electrophoretic mobility. This line of study was then further developed; we used specific immunochemical reactions to examine a series of acute phase reactant proteins (haptoglobin, α_1 antitrypsin, α_1 acid glycoprotein, and ceruloplasmin), as well as prealbumin which tends to behave as a negative reactant (8). The serial measurement of these acute phase reactant proteins tended to follow the clinical evolution of the disease so that they became elevated when there was obvious metastasis and tended to increase with a rising in tumor burden but were relatively insensitive to the smaller amounts of tumor as compared to the change in level of CEA. Nevertheless, when the preoperative levels of the acute phase reactant proteins

TABLE 4. *Serum C-reactive protein in advanced colorectal cancer treated with chemotherapy*

		C-Reactive protein level		
Time	No.	< 10 mg/l (normal)	11–50 mg/l	> 50 mg/l
6–12 months before death	26	18 (69%)	3 (16%)	3 (16%)
3–5 months before death	50	19 (38%)	20 (40%)	11 (22%)
Within 3 months of death	55	6 (10.7%)	14 (25.4%)	35 (63.6%)

were considered in combination with the CEA level, a discriminant index could be derived which appeared to be able to increase the accuracy of prediction of recurrence within 1 to 2 years in patients who had been undergoing curative resections for Dukes B and C lesions.

Recently we have had a similar experience in T3 bladder cancer (Bastable et al., *in preparation*), in which it has been found that the survival of patients with elevated acute phase reactant proteins prior to treatment was worse than that of patients in whom these proteins were at a normal level. This observation of behavior of acute phase reactants in colon cancer has finally led us to adopt the level of C-reactive protein as part of the routine monitoring of colorectal cancer. C-reactive protein differs from the other acute phase reactant proteins as it is normally at about 1,000th the concentration of the other proteins in this series, it responds extremely rapidly to insult, and its level returns to normal soon after the cessation of the stimulus for its elevation (5). In metastatic cancer, an elevation of the C-reactive protein marks a point of biochemical discontinuity in the host reaction to the tumor load.

The majority of patients with advanced metastases show a progressive rise of C-reactive protein (C-RP) during the terminal phases of their illness, but it may have been normal for several months previously (Table 4). This elevation of C-RP reaction can often start when there is no obvious increase of the tumor burden and it clearly helps to stratify patients with indicator lesions who are in moderate balance with their disease from those in whom a cascade of biochemical abnormalities has been initiated.

NUTRITIONAL DISCRIMINANTS

As a further aid to the evaluation of the patient with known metastatic disease, our colleagues (7) have attempted to identify which combination of indices is most helpful in assessing the overall nutrition of the patient. For this purpose, the patients have been divided into 3 groups: first, those with minimal residual disease without indicator lesions; second, a group of patients with indicator lesions but who have survived more than 6 months to make the observation; and third, a group of patients who died within 4 months of making the observation.

A ranking system of analysis was used to show that the progressive fall of hemoglobin is the best discriminant among the groups. Between groups 1 and 2, the decrease of arm fat area, prealbumin, and arm muscle area were the next strongest discriminants. Between groups 2 and 3, it was the fall of albumin, prealbumin, and transferrin that ranked next to the fall of hemoglobin as the most powerful discriminants. Neither calorie intake nor estimated weight loss had much discriminating activity between these groups. Here again, these preliminary studies suggest a series of discontinuities in the biochemical change in the evolution of the cancer-bearing patient. Although some of the processes, such as the fall of hemoglobin, seem to be continuous, others occur early and then move into a fairly stable state such as the loss of body fat. Finally, there is the cascade of the descent of the nutritional proteins with the proteins with the small pool size—prealbumin, transferrin—preceding the fall of albumin, with its much larger pool. In the same fashion, as the C-reactive protein tends to rise quite markedly in the terminal phases, an abrupt fall of prealbumin is often noticed in the last one or two visits to the chemotherapy clinic, prior to death.

In practice, as in malnutrition due to other causes, once the albumin falls below 30 g/liter, the number of biochemical abnormalities rises in parallel with the continuing fall of albumin (19). Because of the immense array of changes that occur as secondary phenomena in cancer, it is possible to devise many different combinations of tests that could be used when following the patients. However, such combinations can increase the warning to the physician that the patient is deteriorating; the lead time of 1 or 2 months they produce (3) is probably too small to be of any practical purpose as there are few alternative treatments available. Indeed, the necessity for accurate biochemical monitoring of patients with advanced cancer seems to be small as the drugs with which they are treated are still fairly ineffective and the markers still too nonspecific and lacking in sensitivity. Clearly, a further impetus for detailed monitoring will be the development of more effective treatment of advanced disease. At present in postoperative patients:

1. A relatively "late," in biological terms, but "early" warning, in clinical terms, of recurrence can be achieved.
2. Such a warning might be useful for testing adjuvant therapy by randomizing patients to treatment or no treatment. It would be less hazardous than second look but difficult to organize logistically.
3. The current methods would enable advanced patients with indicator lesions to be stratified more accurately, which could influence the interpretation of phase 1 and 2 studies.

ACKNOWLEDGMENTS

We wish to thank The Yorkshire Gastroenterology Cancer Research Group for their cooperation in these studies. This research has been funded by the

National Institute of Health, contract No. 1-CM-43727, and the Yorkshire Cancer Research Campaign. The CEA assays were performed by the staff of the Ludwig Institute, London (director: Professor A. M. Neville).

REFERENCES

1. Aronsen, K. F., Noslin, B., and Phil, V. (1970): The value of γ-glutamyl transpeptidase as a screen test for liver tumour. *Acta Clin. Scand.,* 136:17–22.
2. Beck, P. R., Belfield, A., Spooner, R. T., Blumgart, L. H., and Wood, C. B. (1979): Serum enzymes in colorectal cancer. *Cancer,* 43:1772–1776.
3. Bullen, B. R., Cooper, E. H., Turner, R., Neville, A. M., Giles, G. R., and Hall, R. (1977): Cancer markers in patients receiving chemotherapy for colorectal cancer: A preliminary report. *Med. Pediatr. Oncol.,* 3:289–300.
4. Cooper, E. H., and Neville, A. M. (1978): Logic and logistics of monitoring large bowel cancer. In: *Gastrointestinal Tract Cancer,* edited by M. Lipkin and R. A. Good, pp. 437–455. Plenum Press, New York.
5. Cooper, E. H., and Stone, J. (1980): Acute phase reactants in cancer. *Adv. Cancer Res.,* 30:1–44.
6. Cooper, E. H., Turner, R., Geekie, A., Neville, A. M., and Goligher, J. C. (1976): Alpha globulins in the surveillance of colorectal cancer. *Biomedicine,* 24:171–178.
7. Hall, J. C., Lawton, J. O., Appleton, N., Stocks, H., and Giles, G. R. (1980): The assessment of protein-calorie malnutrition in patients with gastrointestinal cancer. *J. Natl. Cancer Inst. (submitted).*
8. Milford Ward, A., Cooper, E. H., Turner, R., Anderson, J. A., and Neville, A. M. (1977): Acute phase reactant protein profiles: An aid to monitoring large bowel cancer by CEA and serum enzymes. *Br. J. Cancer,* 35:170–178.
9. Minton, J. P., and Martin, E. W. (1978): The use of serial CEA determinations to predict recurrence of colorectal cancer and when to do a second look operation. *Cancer,* 42:1422–1427.
10. Moertel, C. G. (1973): Large bowel. In: *Cancer Medicine,* edited by J. F. Hollard and E. Frei, pp. 1597–1627. Lea and Fibiger, Philadelphia.
11. Moertel, C. G., and Schutt, A. J. (1978): Carcinoembryonic antigen test for recurrent colorectal cancer: Inadequacy for early detection. *JAMA,* 239:1065–1066.
12. Munjal, D., Chawla, P. L., Lokich, J. J., and Zamcheck, N. (1976): Carcinoembryonic antigen and phosphohexose isomerase levels in patients with and without liver metastases. *Cancer,* 37:1800–1807.
13. Rittgers, R. A., Steel, G., Zamcheck, N., Lowenstein, M. S., Sugarbaker, P. H., Arayer, R. J., Lokich, J. L., Maltz, J., and Wilson, R. E. (1978): Transient carcinoembryonic antigen (CEA) elevations following resection of colorectal cancer: A limitation in the use of serial CEA levels as an indicator for second look surgery. *J. Natl. Cancer Inst.,* 61:315–318.
14. Schwartz, M. K. (1973): Enzymes in cancer. *Clin. Chem.,* 19:10–22.
15. Shani, A., O'Connell, M. J., Moertel, C. G., Schutt, A. J., Silvers, A., and Go, V. L. W. (1978): Serial plasma carcinoembryonic antigen measurements in the management of metastatic colorectal carcinoma. *Ann. Intern. Med.,* 88:627–630.
16. Staab, H., Anderer, A., Stumpf, E., and Fisher, R. (1978): Carcinoembryonic antigen follow up and selection of patients for second look operation in management of gastrointestinal carcinoma. *J. Surg. Oncol.,* 10:273–282.
17. Steele, L., Cooper, E. H., Mackay, A. M., Losowsky, M. S., and Goligher, J. C. (1974): Combination of carcinoembryonic antigen and gamma glutamyl-transpeptidase in the study of the evolution of colorectal cancer. *Br. J. Cancer,* 30:319–324.
18. Wanebo, J. H., Stearns, M., and Schwartz, M. K. (1978): Use of CEA as an indicator of early recurrence and as a guide to a selected second look procedure in patients with colorectal cancer. *Ann. Surg.,* 188:481–491.
19. Whitehead, R., Coward, W. A., and Lunn, P. G. (1973): Serum albumin concentration at the onset of kwashiorkor. *Lancet,* 1:63–66.

Colorectal Cancer: Prevention, Epidemiology,
and Screening, edited by S. Winawer, D. Schottenfeld,
and P. Sherlock. Raven Press, New York © 1980.

Current Status of CEA

Norman Zamcheck

*Mallory Gastrointestinal Research Laboratory, Mallory Institute of Pathology, Boston City
Hospital, and Harvard Medical School, Boston, Massachusetts 02118*

In the 10 years since Thomson's original report of a serum assay for CEA, the use of the assay has been clarified and may be summarized as follows:

The plasma CEA assay does not make the diagnosis of any cancer; but it does aid in the detection of CEA-producing tumors, including most colorectal cancers. CEA plasma levels tend to correlate with Dukes' staging of colonic malignancy, highest CEA levels occurring in patients with widespread malignancy, especially when the liver is involved. The assay is of little value for screening for early colonic cancer. Thus the CEA assay is a better indicator of widespread disease than it is of early colon cancer. A preoperatively negative assay does not exclude the diagnosis of cancer. Generally, the higher the level of CEA, the poorer is the prognosis, but not invariably.

In order to use the CEA assay intelligently, one should appreciate that the circulating CEA level depends on several factors including (a) the total mass of CEA-producing tumor; (b) the stage and (c) degree of differentiation of the primary tumor; (d) the invasion of lymphatics, blood vessels, or perineural spaces (59); (e) the sites and (f) extent of distant spread of tumor; and (g) liver involvement and its functional status. The key role of the liver in regulating circulating levels is increasingly apparent.

Serial CEA determinations are helpful as an adjunct to the clinical management of patients in assessing prognosis, in detection of recurrence and of metastasis, in decision making for "second-look" surgery, in monitoring the effects of chemotherapy, radiation therapy, or combined therapy, and in altering therapy.

The clinical usefulness of measuring CEA in body fluids—such as pleural and peritoneal effusions, cerebrospinal fluid, cysts and digestive fluids—is being defined. Immunohistochemical localization of CEA in pathological tissues points to additional applications in immunohistopathological diagnosis. The use of radiolabeled anti-CEA antibody in the radioimmunodetection of CEA-producing malignancies is under initial exploration. Its potential for radiation therapy remains unexplored.

NONSPECIFICITY OF THE CARCINOEMBRYONIC ANTIGEN ASSAY

None of the present assays for CEA is specific for colon cancer or for digestive tract cancer. The high rates of positivity initially reported in patients with pancreatic cancer were largely due to the fact that pancreatic cancer is often diagnosed late in its course. Approximately 52% positivity was reported in unselected patients with breast cancer, 40% in prostatic cancer, 33% in bladder cancer, and 72% in cancer of the bronchus (61).

CARCINOEMBRYONIC ANTIGEN IN BENIGN DISORDERS (19)

With the exception of some heavy cigarette smokers, 97% of healthy normal individuals have "normal" blood CEA levels (8). Patients with benign disease have normal CEA levels, and elevations, when observed, are usually modest. Perhaps more than any other common benign clinical condition, liver disease of all types, especially severe alcoholic cirrhosis (1,2,11,30), may give elevated CEA levels. Some patients with benign obstructive jaundice may also have CEA elevations, which are usually reversed on release of the obstruction, provided persistent biliary inflammation or liver abscess does not supervene (21). "Active" inflammatory bowel disease may be associated with transient elevations. Ulcerative colitis of long duration is known to predispose to colonic cancer, but there is no convincing evidence yet available that CEA levels will detect early colon cancer in this disease (19).

SCREENING

Thus, although "malignancy" may be differentiated from "nonmalignancy," in part by the circulating CEA levels, there is no sharp threshold value between the two. A high proportion of patients with "early" colonic cancer have normal or low CEA values. These two facts militate against successful screening for early cancer by use of the CEA assay alone (3).

The higher the threshold level applied, the more reliable is the detection of cancer, however, and the more advanced are the cancers detected. Thus screening for advanced cancer is presently feasible. Quantitation by dilution (without prior perchloric acid extraction) has revealed very high levels of CEA (above 1,000 ng/ml) in some patients with advanced cancer; such levels are not reported in benign diseases.

SERIAL ASSAYS IN THE ASSESSMENT OF COLON CANCER

All workers (5,14,20,22,31,37,58) confirmed the initial report of Thomson et al. (53) that preoperatively elevated assay levels fell to normal levels after complete resection of colonic cancers. A single negative postoperative CEA level, however, did not exclude the presence of residual tumor, as was initially hoped. Rising CEA levels following tumor resection correlated with residual, recurrent, or metastatic tumor.

To determine whether serial CEA assays would help to detect recurrence after resection, Sorokin et al. (44) studied prospectively 102 patients who had undergone potentially curative resection for colorectal cancer. When first studied, none had detectable metastases or evidence of recurrent cancer. Eighteen patients showed CEA levels greater than 2.5 ng/ml. Six of these had progressively rising CEA levels; all six subsequently developed recurrent cancer. Holyoke et al. (9), Mach et al. (22), Dykes et al. (1) and Mackay et al. (23) reported similar series of patients, whose rising CEA levels preceded clinical evidence of tumor recurrence by 2 to 18 months. Despite this general agreement that serial assays help detect recurrent colon cancer in asymptomatic patients, Ravry and co-workers (35) at the Mayo Clinic reported that tumor recurrence was readily detected by "other clinical means" in such patients. Sugarbaker et al. (51) also showed that careful symptom review and clinical examination were indispensable in assessing such patients, especially since some colonic cancers (as well as many other cancers) may produce no plasma elevations of CEA.

Mach et al. (22) at Lausanne, Switzerland, reported eight patients who had recurrent colonic cancer after apparently complete tumor resection. All patients had elevated values (greater than 5 ng/ml) preoperatively and some fell to "normal" levels postoperatively, whereas others did not fall at all or very much. All had rising levels thereafter. Clinical evidence of recurrence was observed 2.5 to 10 months later. In patients after complete tumor resection who had no evidence of recurrence, the serial CEA levels remained flat and normal.

Nine patients with completely resected colorectal cancers studied at the Peter Bent Brigham Hospital had CEAs which remained low for more than 2 years after surgery (Fig. 1): none had evidence of metastasis (51); CEA levels were

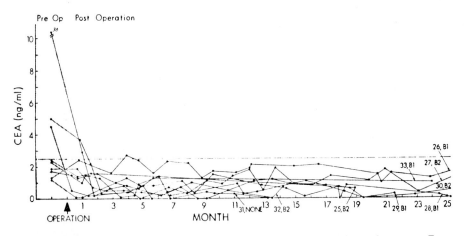

FIG. 1. Serial CEA levels in 9 patients with completely resected colorectal cancers. From Zamcheck (58).

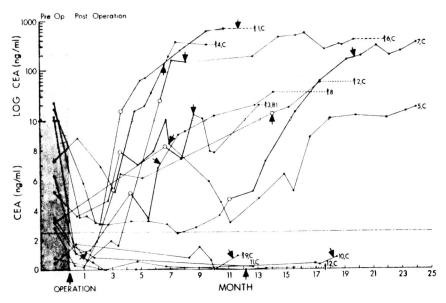

FIG. 2. Serial CEA levels in 12 patients who developed recurrent or metastatic colorectal cancer. From Sugarbaker et al. (51).

drawn monthly and the patients were examined physically at 3-month intervals. Note that all but three of these patients had normal CEA levels preoperatively.

The monthly serial CEA titers in 12 patients who developed recurrent or metastatic colorectal cancer are seen in Fig. 2. The arrows indicate when the first objective clinical evidence of recurrence was detected. The circles indicate when it was determined clinically that a significant rise in the CEA levels had occurred. In 7 patients, the rising CEA trends gave the first objective evidence of recurrence (excluding nonspecific symptoms). In contrast to Mach's cases, four of our patients did not show rising CEA levels preceding objective evidence of recurrence. They had minimal or no elevations of CEA preoperatively and their CEA levels remained low for at least 1 year. Three of these were poorly differentiated cancers. It was initially thought that such colorectal cancers were "non-CEA" producers. Subsequent studies have shown that CEA staining is demonstrable immunochemically in the tissues of virtually all large bowel cancers. Poorly differentiated cancers show lesser amounts and some, very little indeed. The smaller amounts, once in circulation, do not cause elevated plasma levels since they appear to be cleared by the normal liver.

SECOND-LOOK SURGERY

When it became apparent that rising serial CEA levels could provide evidence of recurrence in otherwise asymptomatic patients, it was logical that they be considered for use as an indicator for "second-look" surgery, and several groups have assessed the potential usefulness of this approach.

Martin et al. (24) performed second-look surgery on 32 patients primarily on the basis of rising serial CEA levels. They found resectable localized disease in 13 (41%) of patients, one of whom survived for 5 years after reoperation. None of these lesions had been diagnosed preoperatively. Exploration was negative in only 3 patients (9%). Martin et al. recommended, therefore, that after recognized benign causes of CEA elevations were excluded, re-exploration be performed when two consecutive CEA levels increased "significantly" above the postoperative base-line. They constructed a nomogram depicting graphically the assay reproducibility in their laboratory in order to provide for ready recognition of this increase.

In Tubingen, Dr. Staab and associates (45) combined computerized serial CEA surveillance curves and clinical diagnostic methods to select 30 patients for second-look surgery. They differentiated between local recurrence and generalized metastases by calculating the differing slopes of the rising serial CEA curves. A slowly rising CEA rate, i.e., a 30 to 50% increase of the CEA level compared with the postoperative baseline levels, could usually be correlated with a local tumor recurrence, whereas a rapidly rising CEA rate (with consecutive CEA increases greater than 50% and levels exceeding 10 ng/ml) could generally be correlated with distant tumor spread, predominantly liver metastases. Martin et al. (24), Staab et al. (45–47), Steele et al. (48), and Wanebo et al. (56) have all recommended CEA as a guide to second-look surgery. Steele et al. recommended that studies be done to determine whether initiation of systemic chemotherapy without second-look surgery would be beneficial for patients with CEA rises greater than 2.1 ng/ml per 30 days.

TRANSIENT RISES IN CEA: A LIMITATION IN THE USE OF SERIAL CEA LEVELS AS AN INDICATOR FOR SECOND-LOOK SURGERY

In reviewing our experiences with 69 patients with colorectal cancer, Rittgers et al. (39) found 24 who demonstrated significant rises (greater than the 95% confidence limits (3.0–9.8 ng/ml)). Nine subsequently showed unexplained falls in CEA levels approaching the base-line. These patients had an average of 18 postoperative determinations. Only one, 14 months after surgery, developed a recurrence (anastomotic site). The other 8, followed for a mean of 27 months postoperatively, showed no evidence of recurrence. CEA levels in these 8 increased by a mean of 6.6 ng/ml above the postresection base-line. Four of these had alkaline phosphatase elevations at the peak CEA, suggesting liver dysfunction, and one of these had biopsy-proven hepatitis. Staab et al. also observed transient rises which they were unable to account for. Possible explanations for reversible CEA rises include heavy smoking, liver malfunction, and transfusion of CEA-positive blood (four of our patients had received transfusions).

Thus, even when laboratory variation as a cause of the CEA rises is eliminated, biologic causes other than cancer, especially nonmalignant liver disease, are not ruled out. It must be emphasized that although rising serial CEA levels are undoubtedly helpful in making the decision for re-exploration, they do not substitute for complete clinical assessment. We recommend that complete liver assessment be done as part of the preoperation work-up when a rising CEA is the sole indication of tumor recurrence.

CEA AS A MONITOR OF CHEMOTHERAPY

Numerous collaborative studies underway in many countries are testing the effectiveness of combinations of surgery, chemotherapy, radiation therapy, and immunotherapy on metastatic digestive tract cancer. There is urgent need for objective monitors of the patient's response to treatment to supplement clinical, laboratory, and roentgenographic examinations. Serial CEA determinations appear to provide such objective evidence, and in some clinics changing CEA trends are being used as one indicator for making therapeutic decisions.

We have studied several series of patients at the Sidney Farber Cancer Institute. Most recently Mayer and associates (26) studied 47 patients with documented metastatic colorectal cancer. Thirty patients received chemotherapy and had serial CEAs. Four (13.3%) demonstrated probable tumor regressions, and seven (23.3%) had stable diseases. Of 19 (63.3%) who showed "disease progressions," 11 died; and in 14 (74%) the CEA value doubled.

CEA titers declined in all four responders (Fig. 3), but in only one instance did the level fall to below 4.0 ng/ml and provide evidence of a tumor response

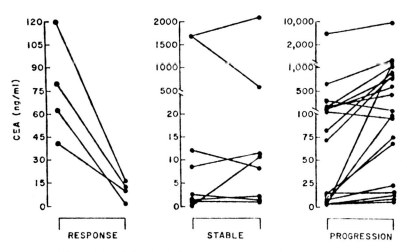

FIG. 3. Changes in serial CEA levels during chemotherapy. (Note difference in the ordinate scales of the three categories.) From Mayer et al. (26).

not appreciated clinically. The only cytotoxic drugs effecting tumor regression in this series were 5-fluorouracil (5-FU) and fluorodeoxy-uridine (5-FUDR). CEA levels usually rose as disease progressed, but once elevated, absolute values did not correlate directly with tumor burden.

Examples from These Series

A 52-year-old man with metastatic rectal cancer had an apparent response to hydroxyurea and 5-FU with disappearance of adenopathy, but this response did not persist as was indicated by the rising CEA trend (Fig. 4).

A 73-year-old woman who underwent sigmoid resection for a Dukes' adeno-carcinoma showed a progressive rise in CEA titer 8 months before any other sign of tumor recurrence could be detected (Fig. 5). Note that the elevated preoperative CEA never fell to normal. This is a poor prognostic finding.

Mayer summarized the role of CEA as a monitor of chemotherapy in meta-static colorectal cancer as follows:

1. If elevated, serial CEA levels provide a measurable index of residual disease otherwise clinically undetectable.

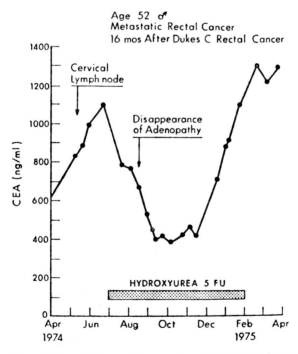

FIG. 4. Rapidly rising CEA in a 52-year-old man with metastatic rectal cancer signaled the need to change chemotherapy. From Sugarbaker et al. (50).

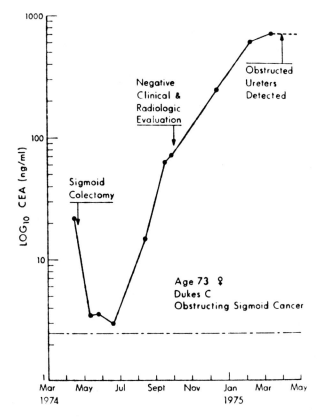

FIG. 5. A progressive rise in CEA was seen 8 months before any other sign of recurrence was detected. From Sugarbaker et al. (50).

2. Rising CEA levels may pre-date clinical evidence of tumor resistance to previously effective chemotherapy, indicating the need for a change in therapy.
3. A rising CEA level is incompatible with disease regression.

Although most workers agree that serial CEA determinations are useful in monitoring the course of patients with digestive tract cancer, some, especially the Mayo Clinic group (35), state that the use of the assay adds relatively little to complete clinical and laboratory assessment of the patient. Moertel and co-workers (41) point out a lack of statistical correlation between falling CEA trends and improved patient survival in their data. It is generally agreed that the ultimate test of the usefulness of CEA assays in monitoring disseminated colorectal cancer must await the development of improved chemotherapeutic agents.

CEA MONITORING OF RADIATION THERAPY

Findings by Sugarbaker and associates (49) at the Peter Bent Brigham Hospital suggested that serial plasma CEA levels are also useful for monitoring radiation therapy for rectal cancer. Serial CEA assays were performed on 16 patients receiving preoperative radiation therapy of rectal cancer or radiation of recurrent or metastatic colorectal cancer. Radiation therapy of localized colorectal cancer reliably reduced previously elevated circulating titers. Significant decrease of elevated CEA titers with accumulating doses of radiation indicated that the bulk of CEA-producing tumor was within the radiation treatment portal. When the amount of disseminated disease was extensive compared to that of the treated lesion, radiation therapy failed to lower CEA values. A rebound in CEA levels strongly suggested that the initial decline did not presage long-term control. Thus the serial trends assisted in management decisions—including the timing, nature, and extent of surgery. Sugarbaker was careful to point out, however, that such decisions must be made cautiously with full understanding of the entire clinical and laboratory status of the patient, as well as of the limitation of the assay.

Patient Example

A 43-year-old man received 4,500 rads of preoperative radiation therapy for a large posteriorly fixed rectal cancer (Fig. 6). The CEA level fell to undetectable levels and abdominal-perineal-sacral resection was then carried out. The patient

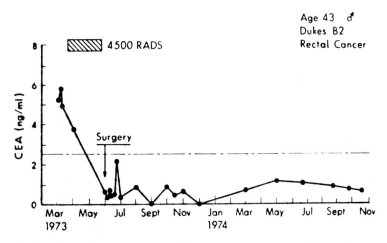

FIG. 6. Serial CEA levels in radiation-treated rectal cancer followed by surgical resection. From Sugarbaker et al. (49).

remained apparently disease-free for 3 years after therapy, confirmed by the serial CEA levels.

ROLE OF THE LIVER

Understanding the liver status of patients with digestive tract cancer is essential for interpreting serial CEA levels (18,19,43). Using the original Thomson radio-immunoassay for CEA, Moore et al. (30) showed that CEA elevations were obtained in 45% of patients with severe alcoholic liver disease, none of whom had evidence of gastrointestinal malignancy. Circulating CEA levels were usually lower in patients with alcoholic liver disease than in patients with colonic or pancreatic cancer.

Khoo and Mackay (10) found elevated serum CEA levels using MacSween's method in primary biliary, cryptogenic, and alcoholic cirrhosis and noted that the levels correlated with degrees of impairment of liver function as indicated by BSP retention and alkaline phosphatase and transaminase levels.

Early clinical evidence suggested a role of the hepatobiliary system in the regulation of circulating CEA levels. In patients with digestive tract cancer, a rapid rise of CEA was often associated with the onset of jaundice (43). Whether this was due to increased production of CEA by tumor, to impaired metabolism due to liver cell failure, or to biliary obstruction was uncertain. Accordingly, Lurie et al. (21) studied 29 jaundiced patients with benign extrahepatic biliary tract obstruction and inflammation. During the obstructive and inflammatory phase, 52% of the patients had CEA levels greater than 2.5 ng/ml. Elevated levels were associated more frequently with common duct stones (and cholangitis) than with gallbladder stones (and cholecystitis) without obstructive disease. Some with common duct stones had levels greater than 5.0 ng/ml, which returned to normal following surgical relief of obstruction in 7 of 10 patients. The levels increased, however, in 3 patients with progressive inflammation. The highest values were seen in 2 patients with liver abscesses.

Highest CEA levels are repeatedly found in metastatic disease of the liver. Terminal failure of the liver to metabolize and/or excrete CEA in the face of an increasing CEA load probably contributes to the rapid rises so often observed. It is unlikely that such elevations are caused solely by a rapid increase in production of CEA by the tumor. Thus concomitant monitoring of the liver function is essential for the correct interpretation of CEA levels. Cooper et al. (4) showed that liver involvement by metastatic colorectal cancer could be reliably predicted many weeks in advance by combined measurement of CEA and gammaglutamyl transpeptidase. Similarly, Munjal et al. (32) found that elevations of phosphohexose isomerase occurred commonly in the presence of liver metastases from colorectal, breast, and lung cancer, whereas nonhepatic metastases less frequently gave rises.

O'Brien et al. (34) have reported the association of intrahepatic cholestasis in postmortem liver tissue with extraordinarily high preterminal plasma levels of CEA (levels of 1,000 ng/ml or higher).

COMBINATIONS OF MARKERS

McIntire et al. (28) showed that the combined measurement of alpha-fetoprotein and CEA detected more patients with gastric cancer than either alone, although alpha-fetoprotein measurement did not help detect more colon cancers.

Several groups (60,61) are actively studying combinations of different markers in the same patient in the effort to improve further the usefulness of the CEA assay. Such tumor markers include enzymes—such as alkaline and acid phosphatase, phosphohexose isomerase, gamma-glutamyl transpeptidase, 5-nucleotidase, and aldolase—and ectopic hormones, including adrenocorticotropic hormone, human chorionic gonadotropic hormone, gastrin, and parathormone among many others. Neville et al. (33) recently reviewed the role of CEA in association with other tumor markers in colorectal and mammary carcinoma.

CEA ACTIVITY IN OTHER BODY FLUIDS

CEA active substances have been measured in all extravascular body fluids including saliva (25), meconium (40), digestive fluids (29), gastric fluid (54), duodenal juice (16), biliary juice (52), pancreatic juice (27,36,42), pleural effusions (38), ascitic fluid (13,17), urine (55), cerebrospinal fluid, cyst fluids (6), and small and large bowel washings (7,57). Winawer stated that assay of CEA concentrations in colonic lavage may have potential application in the further assessment of the mucosa at risk for colon adenomas and for colon cancer. Whether it will prove accurate enough for the detection of cancer in patients at risk requires further study.

These studies have indicated an association between high levels of CEA and the presence of a CEA-producing malignancy, thus supporting their potential clinical usefulness especially when combined with other determinants of malignancy including cytological or immunohistological testing. However, nonmalignant causes of CEA-like elevations must also be taken into account. More study is needed.

METHODOLOGY

Several methods are now widely used for assay of CEA. Effective use of the CEA assay, as with any laboratory test, requires understanding of the limitations of the method used. With the Hansen method (CEA—Roche), widely used in the United States, plasma specimens are first tested by an "indirect" method in which perchloric acid extraction precedes the actual radioimmunoassay; this indirect assay measures CEA concentrations reliably up to approxi-

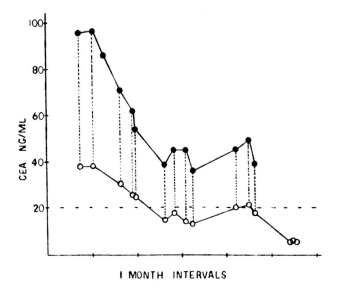

FIG. 7. Disparity between indirect and direct CEA methods. Dotted lines join values obtained on the same plasma specimen. Rising CEA values [from Loewenstein et al. (15)].

mately 20 ng/ml. Specimens shown to have CEA concentrations greater than 20 ng/ml by the initial assay are reassayed by a "direct" method (without perchloric acid extraction), and the latter values are reported. Values obtained by the direct method are higher than those obtained by the indirect method on the same specimen. This is relevant to the use of serial levels.

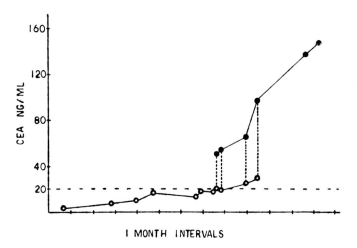

FIG. 8. Falling CEA values. From Zamcheck (58).

An apparent sudden increase in a patient's rising serial values at 20 ng/ml (Fig. 7) may be caused by the shift in method rather than by a worsening in the patient's status due to tumor growth or spread. Similarly, a sudden decline in reported results from, i.e., 52 to 19 ng/ml (Fig. 8) may largely reflect the change in method rather than tumor regression. The existence of the discrepancy need not impair the clinical usefulness of the assay; but clinicians who are unaware of the methodological switch may misinterpret serial levels traversing 20 ng/ml.

ACKNOWLEDGMENTS

This research was supported in part by Grants CA-04486 from the National Cancer Institute and IM-18 from the American Cancer Society.

REFERENCES

1. Booth, S. N., Jamieson, G. C., King, J. P. G., Leonard, J., Oates, G. D. and Dykes, P. W. (1974): Carcinoembryonic antigen in management of colorectal carcinoma. *Br. Med. J.,* 2:183–186.
2. Booth, S. N., King, J. P. G., Leonard, J. C., and Dykes, P. W. (1973): Serum carcinoembryonic antigen in clinical disorders. *Gut,* 14:794–799.
3. Chu, T. M., and Murphy, G. P. (1978): Carcinoembryonic antigen: Evaluation as screening assay in non-cancer clinics. *N.Y. State J. Med.,* 78:879–882.
4. Cooper, E. H., Turner, R., Steele, L., Neville, A. M., and Mackay, A. M. (1975): The contribution of serum enzymes and carcinoembryonic antigen to the early diagnosis of metastatic colorectal cancer. *Br. J. Cancer,* 31:111–117.
5. Dhar, P., Moore, T. L., Zamcheck, N., and Kupchik, H. Z. (1972): Carcinoembryonic antigen (CEA) in colonic cancer: Use in pre- and postoperative diagnosis and prognosis. *JAMA,* 221:31.
6. Fleisher, M., Robbins, G. F., Breed, C. N., Fracchia, A. A., Urban, J. A., and Schwartz, M. K. (1973): Biochemistry of breast cyst fluid. *Clin. Bull.,* 3:94–97.
7. Go, V. L. W., Ammon, H. V., Holtermuller, K. H., Krag, E., and Phillips, S. F. (1975): Quantification of carcinoembryonic antigen-like activities in normal human gastrointestinal secretions. *Cancer,* 36:2346–2350.
8. Hansen, H. J., Snyder, J. J., Miller, E., Vandervoorde, J. P., Miller, O. M., Hines, L. R., and Burns, J. J. (1974): Carcinoembryonic antigen (CEA) assay. A. laboratory adjunct in the diagnosis and management of cancer. *J. Hum. Pathol.,* 5:139–147.
9. Holyoke, E. D., Reynoso, G., and Chu, T. (1972): Carcinoembryonic antigen in patients with carcinoma of the digestive tract. In: *Embryonic and Fetal Antigens in Cancer, Vol. 2,* edited by N. G. Anderson, J. H. Coggin, E. B. Cole, and J. W. Holleman, pp. 215–219. USAEC Report CONF-720208, Department of Commerce, Springfield, Virginia.
10. Khoo, S. K., and Mackay, I. R. (1973): Carcinoembryonic antigen in serum in diseases of the liver and pancreas. *J. Clin. Pathol.,* 26:470–475.
11. Khoo, S. K., Warner, N. L., Lie, J. T., and Mackay, I. R. (1973): Carcinoembryonic antigenic activity of tissue extracts: A quantitative study of malignant and benign neoplasms, cirrhotic liver, normal adult and fetal organs. *Int. J. Cancer,* 11:681–687.
12. Kupchik, H. Z., Loewenstein, M. S., Feil, M., Rittgers, R. A., and Zamcheck, N. (1978): The disparity of indirect and direct zirconyl gel assays for carcinoembryonic antigen. *Cancer,* 42:1589–1594.
13. Kupchik, H. Z., Zamcheck, N., and Saravis, C. A. (1973): Immunochemical studies of carcinoembryonic antigens: Methodologic considerations and some clinical implications. *J. Natl. Cancer Inst.,* 51:1741–1749.
14. Laurence, D. J. R., Stevens, U., Bettelheim, R., Darcy, D., Leese, C., Turberville, C., Alexander, P., Johns, E. W., and Neville, A. M. (1972): Evaluation of the role of plasma carcinoembryonic

antigen (CEA) in the diagnosis of gastrointestinal, mammary and bronchial carcinoma. *Br. Med. J.,* 3:605.

15. Loewenstein, M. S., Kupchik, H. Z., and Zamcheck, N. (1976): Disparity between CEA-Roche "indirect" and "direct" carcinoembryonic antigen values: Clinical relevance. *N. Engl. J. Med.,* 294:1123.

16. Loewenstein, M. S., Rau, P., Rittgers, R. A., Adhinarayanan, B. G., Kupchik, H. Z., and Zamcheck, N. (1980): CEA of duodenal aspirates in patients with benign and malignant disease: Preliminary observations. *J. Natl. Cancer Inst.,* 64:235–239.

17. Loewenstein, M. S., Rittgers, R. A., Feinerman, A. E., Kupchik, H. Z., Marcel, B. R., Koff, R. S., and Zamcheck, N. (1978): Carcinoembryonic antigen assay of ascites and detection of malignancy. *Ann. Intern. Med.,* 88:635–638.

18. Loewenstein, M. S., and Zamcheck, N. (1977): Carcinoembryonic antigen and the liver. *Gastroenterology,* 72, 161–166.

19. Loewenstein, M. S., and Zamcheck, N. (1978): CEA levels in benign gastrointestinal disease states. *Cancer,* 42:1412–1418.

20. LoGerfo, P. J., Krupey, J., and Hansen, H. J. (1971): Demonstration of an antigen common to several varieties of neoplasia. *N. Engl. J. Med.,* 285:138.

21. Lurie, B. B., Loewenstein, M. S., and Zamcheck, N. (1975): Elevated carcinoembryonic antigen levels and biliary tract obstruction. *JAMA,* 233:326–330.

22. Mach, J. P., Jaeger, P. H., Bertholet, M. M., Ruegsegger, C. A., Loosli, R. M., and Pettavel, J. (1974): Detection of recurrence of large bowel carcinoma by radioimmunoassay of circulating carcinoembryonic antigen (CEA). *Lancet,* 2:535–540.

23. Mackay, A. M., Patel, S., Canter, S., Stevens, U., Laurence, D. J. R., Cooper, E. H. and Neville, A. M. (1974): Role of serial plasma CEA assays in detection of recurrent and metastatic colorectal carcinoma. *Br. Med. J.,* 1:383–385.

24. Martin, E. W., James, K. J., Hurtubise, P. E., Catalano, P., Minton, J. P. (1977): The use of CEA as an early indicator for gastrointestinal tumor recurrence and second-look procedures. *Cancer,* 39:440–446.

25. Martin, F., and Devant, J. (1973): Carcinoembryonic antigen in normal human saliva. *J. Natl. Cancer Inst.,* 50:1375–1379.

26. Mayer, R. L., Garnick, M. G., Steele, G. D., and Zamcheck, N. (1978): Carcinoembryonic antigen as a monitor of chemotherapy in disseminated colorectal cancer. *Cancer,* 42:1428–1433.

27. McCabe, R. P., Sharma, M. P., Gregg, J. A., Loewenstein, M. S., and Zamcheck, N. (1976): Carcinoembryonic antigen (CEA) activity in pancreatic juice of patients with pancreatic carcinoma and pancreatitis. *Cancer,* 38:2457–2461.

28. McIntire, K. R., Waldmann, T. A., Go, V. L. W., Moertel, C. G., and Ravry, M. (1974): Simultaneous radioimmunoassay for carcinoembryonic antigen (CEA) and alpha-fetoprotein (alpha-FP) in neoplasms of the gastrointestinal tract. *Ann. Clin. Lab. Sci.,* 4:104–108.

29. Molner, I. G., and Gitnick, G. L. (1976): CEA levels in fluids bathing gastrointestinal tumors. *Gastroenterology,* 70:313.

30. Moore, T. L., Dhar, P., Zamcheck, N., Keeley, A., Gottlieb, L., and Kupchik, H. Z. (1972): Carcinoembryonic antigen(s) in liver disease. I. Clinical and morphological studies. *Gastroenterology,* 63:88–94.

31. Moore, T. L., Dhar, P., Zamcheck, N., and Kupchik, H. Z. (1971): Carcinoembryonic antigen (CEA) in diagnosis of digestive tract cancer, pp. 393–400. *Proc. 1st Conference and Workshop on Embryonic and Fetal Antigens in Cancer.* Oak Ridge National Laboratory. Oak Ridge, Tennessee.

32. Munjal, D., Chawla, P. L., Lokich, J. J., and Zamcheck, N. (1976): Combined measurement of carcinoembryonic antigen, phosphohexose isomerase, gammaglutamyl transpeptidase, and lactate dehydrogenase levels in patients with and without liver metastases. *Cancer,* 37:1800–1807.

33. Neville, A. M., Patel, S., Capp, M., Laurence, D. J. R., Cooper, E. H., Turberville, C., and Coombes, R. C. (1978): The monitoring role of plasma CEA alone and in association with other tumor markers in colorectal and mammary carcinoma. *Cancer,* 42:1448–1451.

34. O'Brien, M. J., Bronstein, B., Zamcheck, N., Saravis, C., Burke, B., and Gottlieb, L. S. (1980): Cholestasis and hepatic metastases: A factor contributing to very high plasma carcinoembryonic antigen (CEA) elevations. *J. Natl. Cancer Inst. (in press).*

35. Ravry, M., Moertel, C. G., Schutt, A. J., Go, V. L. W. (1974): Usefulness of serial serum carcinoembryonic antigen (CEA) determinations during anticancer therapy or long term follow-up of gastrointestinal carcinoma. *Cancer,* 34:1230–1234.

36. Rey, J. R., Krebs, B. P., and Delmont, J. (1978): CEA activity in pure pancreatic juice. In: *Clinical Application of CEA Assay,* edited by B. P. Krebs, C. M. LaLanne, and M. Schneider, pp. 116–120. Excepta Medica, Amsterdam.

37. Reynoso, G., Chu, T. M., Holyoke, D., Cohen, E., Valensuela, L. A., Nemoto, T., Wang, J. J., Chuang, J., Guinan, P., and Murphy, G. P. (1972): Carcinoembryonic antigen in patients with different cancers. *JAMA,* 220:361–365.

38. Rittgers, R. A., Loewenstein, M. S., Feinerman, A. E., Kupchik, H. Z., Marcel, B. R., Koff, R. S., and Zamcheck, N. (1978): Carcinoembryonic antigen levels in benign and malignant pleural effusions. *Ann. Intern. Med.,* 88:631–634.

39. Rittgers, R. A., Steele, G., Zamcheck, N., Loewenstein, M. S., Sugarbaker, P. H., Mayer, R. J., Lokich, J. J., Maltz, J., and Wilson, R. E. (1978): Transient carcinoembryonic antigen (CEA) elevations following resection of colorectal cancer: A limitation in the use of serial CEA levels as an indicator for second-look surgery. *J. Natl. Cancer Inst.,* 61:315–318.

40. Rule, A. M. (1973): Carcinoembryonic antigen (CEA); Activity of meconium and normal colon extracts. *Immunol. Commun.,* 2:15–24.

41. Shani, A., O'Connell, M. J., Moertel, C. G., et al. (1978): Serial plasma carcinoembryonic antigen measurements in the management of metastatic colorectal carcinoma. *Ann. Intern. Med.,* 88:627–630.

42. Sharma, M. P., Gregg, J. A., Loewenstein, M. S., McCabe, R. P., and Zamcheck, N. (1976): Carcinoembryonic antigen (CEA) activity in pancreatic juice of patients with pancreatic carcinoma and pancreatitis. *Cancer,* 38:2457–2461.

43. Skarin, A. T., Delwiche, R., Zamcheck, N., Lokich, J. J., Frei, E., III (1974): Carcinoembryonic antigen clinical correlations with chemotherapy for metastatic gastrointestinal cancer. *Cancer,* 33:1229–1245.

44. Sorokin, J. J., Sugarbaker, P. H., Zamcheck, N., Pisick, M., Kupchik, H. Z., and Moore, F. D. (1974): Serial CEA assays: Use in detection of recurrence following resection of colon cancer. *JAMA,* 228:49–53.

45. Staab, H. J., Anderer, F. A., Stumpf, E., Fischer, R. (1977): Carcinoembryales antigen (CEA): Klinische vertung der rezidiverungs und metastasierungs-prognosen mittels CEA-verlaufsanalyse bei patienten mit adenokarzinomen des gastrointestinaltraktes. *Dtsch. Med. Wochenschr.,* 102:1083–1086.

46. Staab, H. J., Anderer, F. A., Stumpf, E., and Fischer, R. (1978): Slope analysis of the post-operative CEA time course and its possible application as an aid in diagnosis of disease in gastrointestinal cancer. *Am. J. Surg.,* 136:322.

47. Staab, H. J., Anderer, F. A., Stumpf, E., and Fischer, R. (1978): Carcinoembryonic antigen follow-up and selection of patients for second-look operation in management of gastrointestinal carcinoma. *J. Surg. Oncol.,* 10:273–282.

48. Steele, G., Zamcheck, N., Wilson, R. E., Mayer, R., Lokich, J., Rau, P., and Maltz, J. (1980): Results of CEA-initiated "second-look" surgery for recurrent colorectal cancer. *Am. J. Surg.,* 139:544–548.

49. Sugarbaker, P. H., Bloomer, W. D., Corbett, E. D., and Chaffey, J. T. (1976): Carcinoembryonic antigen monitoring of radiation therapy for colo-rectal cancer. *Am. J. Roentgenol.,* 127:641–644.

50. Sugarbaker, P. H., Skarin, A. T., and Zamcheck, N. (1976): Patterns of serial CEA assays and their clinical use in management of colorectal cancer. *J. Surg. Oncol.,* 8:523–537.

51. Sugarbaker, P. H., Zamcheck, N., and Moore, F. D. (1976): Assessment of serial carcinoembryonic antigen (CEA) assays in postoperative detection of recurrent colorectal cancer. *Cancer,* 38:2310–2315.

52. Svenberg, T. (1976): Carcinoembryonic antigen-like substances of human bile. Isolation and partial characterization. *Int. J. Cancer,* 17:588–596.

53. Thomson, D. M. P., Krupey, J., Freedman, S. O., and Gold, P. (1969): The radioimmunoassay of circulating carcinoembryonic antigen of the human digestive system. *Proc. Natl. Acad. Sci. USA,* 61:161.

54. Vuento, M., Engvall, E., Seppala, M., and Ruoslahti, E. (1976): Isolation from human gastric juice of an antigen closely related to the carcinoembryonic antigen. *Int. J. Cancer,* 18:156–160.

55. Wahren, B., Edsmyr, F., and Zimmerman, R. (1975): Measurement of urinary CEA-like substance: An aid in management of patients with bladder carcinoma. *Cancer,* 36:1490–1495.
56. Wanebo, H. J., Sterns, M., and Schwartz, M. K. (1978): Use of CEA as an indicator of early recurrence and as a guide to a selected second-look procedure in patients with colorectal cancer. *Ann. Surg.,* 188:481.
57. Winawer, S. J., Fleisher, M., Green, S., Bhargava, D., Leidner, S. D., Boyle, C., Sherlock, P., and Schwartz, M. K. (1977): Carcinoembryonic antigen in colonic lavage. *Gastroenterology,* 73:719–722.
58. Zamcheck, N. (1978): Serial CEA determinations in management of colo-rectal cancer: Update. In *Cancer Campaign, "Colon Cancer," Vol. 2,* edited by E. Grundmann, pp. 149–161. Fischer Verlag, Stuttgart.
59. Zamcheck, N., Doos, W. G., Prudente, R., Lurie, B. B., and Gottlieb, L. S. (1975). Prognostic factors in colon carcinoma: Correlation of serum carcinoembryonic antigen level and tumor histopathology. *Hum. Pathol.,* 6:31–45.
60. Zamcheck, N., and Kupchik, H. Z. (1974): The interdependence of clinical investigation and methodological development in early evolution of assays for carcinoembryonic antigen. *Cancer Res.,* 34:2131–2136.
61. Zamcheck, N., and Pusztaszeri, G. (1975): CEA, AFP and other potential tumor markers. *Cancer,* 24:204–214.

Colorectal Cancer: Prevention, Epidemiology, and Screening, edited by S. Winawer, D. Schottenfeld, and P. Sherlock. Raven Press, New York © 1980.

Leads from Animal and Human Models for Possible Use as Biological Markers

M. Earl Balis and Josephine S. Salser

Laboratory of Cell Metabolism, Memorial Sloan-Kettering Institute for Cancer Research, New York, New York 10021

Many investigators have shown that a variety of molecules differ in a number of ways between tumors and nonmalignant counterparts. Few of these have turned out to be of significant magnitude or generality to be useful as diagnostic or prognostic tools. In view of the morphologic changes seen as intestinal cells change from dividing to differentiated cells, there was realistic hope that one would be able to distinguish between resting and dividing cells enzymatically. If this could be done, it might also be possible to do the same thing between normal and malignant cells. For wherever there are morphological criteria that distinguish cell types, one can reasonably expect to find biochemical changes.

In early studies, using the small intestine as a model system, we were able to show that a large number of enzymes varied quantitatively as cells migrated toward the lumen (3). Furthermore, it soon became apparent that not only were there changes in amount but there were changes in the nature of the regulation of the production of the enzyme protein (4). Some enzymes were apparently synthesized from stable messenger RNA (mRNA), whereas others depended on rapidly renewed mRNA systems. Later studies revealed that there were differences in the enzymes themselves (or their milieu) in view of the fact that heat stability was greater in crypt variants (2).

With these findings as a background, we decided to pursue similar studies on the mucosa of the normal and malignant colon. Colorectal tumors have been found to differ qualitatively and quantitatively from normal mucosa in several biochemical parameters. In particular, the enzymes thymidine kinase and adenosine deaminase have shown altered physico- and immunochemical properties. A major theoretical and practical consideration in this regard is the relationship of the changes in these properties associated with malignancy to those that occur as a concomitant of normal maturation. As mucosal cells move from mitotically active crypts to differentiated nondividing flat mucosa, one would expect to find enzyme changes that reflect the new roles of the cells. Tumors that are found in the midst of the flat mucosa are mitotically active and might be expected to contain enzymes that resemble those of the dividing crypt. In studies of adenosine deaminase of rats, it had been found that in the jejunum, a villus-specific form of the enzyme was synthesized as cells migrated toward the lumen. This form could be distinguished by its isoelectric point and slightly greater molecular weight (8).

These findings led to similar studies of the colonic mucosa and colonic tumors (9). A tumor-related form of adenosine deaminase could be identified by an altered isoelectric point and changed substrate specificities and inhibitor sensitivities. Extension of these studies to humans led to the demonstration that in normal colonic mucosa, adenosine deaminase exists in a single form with a molecular weight of approximately 100,000. On the other hand, adenocarcinomas of the colon contain adenosine deaminase variants having a range of molecular weights. The primary forms have molecular weights of approximately 35,000 and 72,000. No striking differences in specific activity, substrate specificity, or sensitivity to inhibitors have been observed. Neutralization studies with antisera to various adenosine deaminase preparations have also failed to reveal differences between the 35,000 molecular weight form from adenocarcinomas and the enzyme of adjacent normal mucosa. The 72,000 form did exhibit a diminished capacity to react with antisera directed against normal human adenosine deaminase. Evidence suggests the possibility that identification of these peculiar forms of adenosine deaminase in cellular material obtained by colonic lavage has potential diagnostic value.

A second marker of potential utility is the enzyme thymidine kinase. This enzyme has been found to exist in two forms in normal human colon: (a) a crypt form and (b) a flat mucosal form (7). The most striking differentiation between the two forms is that afforded by immunochemical studies. Antisera against preparations of thymidine kinase prepared from human colon indicate that it is possible to distinguish between thymidine kinase from the crypt and that from the flat mucosa. Tumors contain a form of kinase not distinguishable from that of the flat mucosa by this criterion. A similar form has been purified from human placentae. Antibodies to this placental enzyme show several lines in immunodiffusion studies, suggesting the possibility that we may be able to distinguish between tumor and normal enzymes.

THYMIDINE KINASE STUDIES

We have recently obtained data in a collaborative study with Paul Higgins of Sloan-Kettering Institute that one of these antibody preparations is able to discriminate carcinoma *in situ* from normal cells. The full potential of this specificity awaits further exploration.

The response to effectors and stability studies further distinguish between normal and tumor thymidine kinase. Studies in experimental animals indicate the possible value of the specific forms of this enzyme as indicators of premalignant and malignant states. These studies in rats suggest a use for these altered enzyme variants as biological markers of colon cancer.

ANIMAL STUDIES

Early studies in our laboratory showed that although the activity of thymidine kinase as normally measured was much higher in crypt than in nondividing mucosal cells (4,5), when the assay was carried out in the presence of bacterial phospholipase C, there was enormous activation of the enzyme, especially in the differentiated cells (5). As a result, the activity in surface cells was higher than in those of the crypt (6) (Table 1). This enzyme had heretofore been viewed as one found almost exclusively in mitotically active cells. Thus it was quite surprising to find relatively large amounts of apparent kinase activity in the cells of the flat mucosa and villus tips.

We then investigated changes in thymidine kinase in the colon of rats of various ages from fetal to maturity. We also examined the enzyme in the colons of rats that had been given dimethylhydrazine (DMH), a well established colon carcinogen. These animals had tumors of the colon of varying sizes and histologic patterns. The enzyme was assayed as were the responses to phospholipase C (PC), dithiothreitol (DTT), and glutathione (GSH) (Table 2). The fetal tissue had the highest activity, and the level dropped steadily with increasing age of the rats. There was a somewhat higher activity in the colons of the DMH-treated animals. The tumors had activities ranging from that of the DMH-treated normal appearing colons (31) to values almost as high as those of the fetal intestines, 395 versus 400. Similarly, PC treatment caused the smallest increase (1.3-fold) in the fetal tissue and the highest in the old rat intestines (15-fold), while the tumors showed a range of from 1.5 to 11. The effect of DTT was also age related. This compound caused a slight stimulation in the fetal intestines and a 20% inhibition in the adult colon. The tumors ranged in values from 0.85 to 1.08 times that of control. GSH produced an inhibition in thymidine kinase activity that decreased with age, and here, too, the tumors had values ranging from near adult to near fetal values.

TABLE 1. *Effects of PC on TdRK in colon*

Fraction	Control activity	PC activity
Upper	5.1	32
Mid	10.3	34
Lower	13.8	28

Control activity is that of the total homogenate in μ units/mg protein. This was separated by centrifugation at $127,000 \times g$. The ratio of values in PC to standard assay is reported. The kinase activities of the upper, mid, and lower layers of the colon were 16%, 29%, and 55%, respectively, of the total activity under standard assay conditions. In the presence of PC, the activity is essentially equally distributed among the three layers.

TABLE 2. *Rat colonic TdR kinase*

Tissue source	TdRK activity	Relative PC	TdRK DTT	Activity GSH
Fetus	400	1.3	1.09	0.17
Neonatal	143	2.3	1.01	0.33
Wealing	185	2.9	0.95	0.16
200 g	30	6.9	0.83	0.21
325 g	31	12.0	0.79	0.54
475 g	16	14.0	0.82	0.79
475 g treated with DMH	30	15.0	0.70	0.55
DMH-induced tumors	31–395	1.5–11	0.85–1.08	0.26–0.52

PC (phospholipase C), dithiothreitol, and glutathione values are the ratio of activities in assay containing crude PC to the assay done without it. Assays were done with 0.42 mM dithiothreitol and 0.25 mM glutathione, respectively. DMH-treated animals received 2 mg/kg injections s.c. for 21 weeks.

HUMAN STUDIES

These studies indicated a wide range of values in colonic thymidine kinase and suggested that the tumor enzyme had some properties that resembled that of flat mucosa and placenta in response to rabbit anti-thymidine kinase, as mentioned above. These more recent findings urged us to assay the enzyme in fibroblasts of normal subjects and patients with familial polyposis. Through the cooperation of Dr. Martin Lipkin of this Institute, we have obtained a series of samples of such tissues from five patients with familial polyposis. In this preliminary group, two had Gardner's syndrome (Table 3). We assayed activity of the enzyme per 10^3 cells and the effects of deoxythymidine triphosphate (dTTP), DTT, GSH, and thermal inactivation. The enzyme in fibroblasts from normal subjects had lower values, that in fibroblasts from the polyposis patients higher, and that in tumor fibroblasts the highest activities. dTTP inhibited all preparations, but that from normals the least. DTT stimulated thymidine kinase in all cells: most from tumors, least from normal fibroblasts. GSH inhibited normal cell preparations the least and tumors the most. Normal cell enzymes were the most heat stable; tumor enzymes, the least. Throughout all these studies with fibroblasts, however, one of the three normal subjects was distinctly abnormal. The enzyme level in the fibroblasts from this subject was twice as high as that in the others. The response of this enzyme to DTT, GSH, and thermal inactivation was more like that seen with thymidine kinase in fibroblasts from the polyposis patients. Colonoscopic biopsies revealed large areas of epithelial atypia in this subject. We were thus encouraged to carry these studies further.

Since no difference between Gardner and non-Gardner polyposis subjects was seen, all polyposis fibroblast studies are now reported together in this next study. We restricted our measurements to specific thymidine kinase activity calculated per microgram DNA, and the effects of DTT and heating. Eleven

TABLE 3. *Comparison of TdRK in human cells*

Control fibroblast	TdRK activity cpm/10³ cells	Relative activity			
		dTTP	DTT	GSH	Heating
1	2.9, 3.3, 2.0	0.53	1.8	0.80	0.66
2	3.6	0.60	1.5	0.62	0.59
3	6.9, 7.3	0.48	4.0	0.38	0.35
Gardner fibroblasts					
1	28.1	0.33	3.2	0.32	0.35
2	35.4, 19.0	0.35	4.0	0.26	0.28
Non-Gardner polyposis fibroblasts					
1	20.6, 19.4	0.35	2.7	0.25	0.29
2	15.6, 22.3	0.38	3.9	0.30	0.24
3	13.6, 14.2	0.40	3.8	0.29	0.19
Tumor cells					
HT29	66.6, 78.5	0.30	5.2	0.19	0.15
SKCO-1	53.6, 58.2	0.28	4.6	0.24	0.19

Thymidine kinase (TdRK) was done by standard radioactive assay. Multiple values represent independent cultures grown from the same cell stock at different times.

controls (Table 4) had a range of values from 1.3 to 3.7, values in seven patients with polyposis ranged from 6.8 to 17.7, and those in two tumors from 27 to 40. Mean values with standard deviations are 2.08 ± 0.23, 10.03 ± 1.08, and 32.84 ± 4.93, respectively. DTT increased control activities from 1.4 to 4.0 × in normal (but only 1.4 to 2.6 if we ignored subject 3 who had the atypia), 2.7 to 3.9 × in the skin fibroblasts from polyposis patients, and 4.9 × in the tumors. Means were 1.9 ± 0.03, 3.35 ± 0.14, and 4.85, respectively. Heat lability gave the same general picture. Residual activity was 0.60 ± 0.04 in normal, 0.28 ± 0.02 in polyposis patients, and 0.17 in tumors. The only overlap was in subject 3 who resembled the polyposis group and it was seen in all parameters. Quite clearly, as with the rat system, we can define biochemical parameters that appear to distinguish thymidine kinase from normal, abnormal, and malignant cells.

In an effort to determine something more about the basis for these differences, we have examined the thymidine kinase from colon, placenta, and colon carcinomas as well as fibroblasts by polyacrylamide gel electrophoresis (PAGE). Several peaks of enzyme activity were eluted from the gel. We have concentrated our attention on what we refer to as peaks A and B. As can be seen from the top graph of Fig. 1, a peak is seen in normal colonic mucosa indicated as A, and another is found in placenta with a slightly faster rate of migration which is marked B. The A peak and very little B are found in fibroblasts from normal subjects. A typical normal run is shown in the second plot. Five normals were examined and the ratio of A:B was 5.5. Two polyposis runs are diagrammed;

TABLE 4. *TdRK activity in cultured human cells: individual data of thermal lability and response to DTT*

Group	Subject	TdRK activity cpm $\times$ 10^{-3}/μg DNA	Relative activity DTT	Relative activity Heat lability
I. Cutaneous fibroblasts				
A. Control	1	1.5, 1.7, 1.0	1.7	0.68
	2	1.8	1.5	0.59
	3	3.5, 3.7	4.0	0.35
	4	1.4	1.4	0.68
	5	1.8	1.6	0.65
	6	1.7	1.3	0.68
	7	1.3	1.5	0.65
	8	2.4	1.8	0.78
	9	2.1	1.5	0.62
	10	3.5	2.6	0.46
	11	1.9	2.0	0.50
Mean $\pm$ SE		2.08 $\pm$ 0.23	1.9 $\pm$ 0.03	0.6 $\pm$ 0.04
B. Familial polyposis				
	1	10.3, 9.7	2.7	0.29
	2	7.8, 11.2	3.9	0.24
	3	6.8, 7.1	3.8	0.19
	4	14.3	3.2	0.35
	5	17.7, 9.5	3.8	0.28
	6	8.2	2.9	0.28
	7	7.6	3.2	0.30
Mean $\pm$ SE		10.03 $\pm$ 1.08	3.35 $\pm$ 0.14	0.28 $\pm$ 0.02
II. Colon carcinoma cells	HT29	40.6, 33.3, 3.93	4.9	0.15
	SKCO1	26.8, 29.6	4.8	0.19
Mean $\pm$ SE		32.84 $\pm$ 4.93	4.85	0.17

three were run all together and the mean ratio of A:B was 0.92. Two colon carcinoma lines were run with A:B ratio of 0.60. Thus, by this criterion, also, fibroblasts of polyposis subjects can be distinguished from those of normal subjects. The polyposis enzyme is more placenta-like and more tumor-like than the normal. These are preliminary investigations that were derived from our animal model studies.

CLINICAL RELEVANCE

Similarly striking quantitative changes in other enzymes, e.g., methyltransferases and ornithine decarboxylase, have been seen with the onset of malignancy. Some may be qualitative, others quantitative but so extensive as to be characteristic of abnormal growth. It must be borne in mind that no single marker may be forthcoming, but the interrelationships of many may be highly indicative of malignant changes and may have value as prognosticators of the course of the disease.

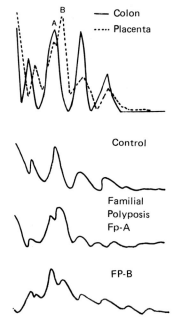

FIG. 1. Electrophoretic patterns of human cytosolic activities. Polyacrylamide gel electrophoretic analyses were carried out in 5% polyacrylamide gel as previously described (1). The horizonal axis represents the migration (relative to bromophenol blue from left to right); the vertical axis represents relative TdRK activity. Normal colon and term placenta are included in the first panel to define peaks A and B. The ensuing panels represent control (normal) fibroblasts, familial polyposis (FP-A and FP-B) fibroblasts, and colon carcinoma cells in culture.

REFERENCES

1. Balis, M. E., Salser, J. S., Trotta, P. P., and Wainfan, E. (1978): Enzymes of purine and pyrimidine metabolism as tumor markers. In: *Biological Markers of Neoplasia: Basic and Applied Aspects,* edited by R. W. Rudden, pp. 517–534. Elsevier North-Holland, Amsterdam.
2. Balis, M. E., Brown, G. F., and Cappucino, J. G. (1971): Heat stability of AMP pyrophosphorylase in differentiating intestinal epithelial cell. *Biochem. Biophys. Res. Comm.,* 42:1007.
3. Imondi, A. R., Balis, M. E., and Lipkin, M. (1969): Changes in enzyme levels accompanying differentiation of intestinal epithelial cells. *Exp. Cell Res.,* 58:323.
4. Imondi, A. R., Lipkin, M., and Balis, M. E. (1970): Enzyme and template stability as regulatory mechanisms in differentiating intestinal epithelial cells. *J. Biol. Chem.,* 245:2194.
5. Salser, J., and Balis, M. E. (1973): Distribution and regulation of deoxythymidine kinase activity in differentiating cells of mammalian intestines. *Cancer Res.,* 33:1889.
6. Salser, J. S., and Balis, M. E. (1974): Enzymatic studies of normal and malignant intestinal epithelium. *Cancer,* 34:889–895.
7. Salser, J. S., and Balis, M. E. (1976): Foetal thymidine kinase in tumors and colonic flat mucosa of man. *Nature,* 260:261–263.
8. Trotta, P. P., and Balis, M. E. (1977): Structural and kinetic alterations in adenosine deaminase associated with the differentiation of rat intestinal cells. *Cancer Res.,* 37:2297–2305.
9. Trotta, P. P., and Balis, M. E. (1978): Characterization of adenosine deaminase from normal colon and colon tumors. Evidence for tumor-specific variants. *Biochemistry,* 17:270–278.

Colorectal Cancer: Prevention, Epidemiology, and Screening, edited by S. Winawer, D. Schottenfeld, and P. Sherlock. Raven Press, New York © 1980.

Introduction: Physician Awareness of Concepts in Colorectal Cancer

Owen Dent

Australian National University, Canberra, Australia

Currently, there is no evidence that assumed methods of prevention of colorectal cancer are effective or that improvements in therapeutic techniques are extending patient survival beyond that attained two decades ago. Hope for the future appears to lie in detection of lesions in the asymptomatic stage through population screening or, more efficiently, by selectively screening high-risk groups. The success of any screening program depends on the willingness of doctors to carry it out, their understanding of recent advances in screening techniques, and their awareness of colorectal cancer incidence and distribution and of high-risk groups in the population.

The degree of physician awareness of these issues is largely unknown, although recent studies in Australia are showing significant gaps in knowledge which need to be redressed through initial and continuing medical education. There is no reason to believe that similar short-comings do not exist in other countries as well.

A major problem for first-contact doctors is that, despite the relatively high incidence of colorectal cancer and its significance as a cause of death, the disease is not commonly encountered and does not loom large in their usual activities. The cases they do see are, on referral, taken out of their hands by specialists and often lost to them thereafter. Lack of follow-up presumably leads to lack of awareness, and a recent British study attributed a significant proportion of delay in colorectal cancer diagnosis to delay by the family doctor as a result of failure to recognize symptoms and failure to perform a rectal examination (2).

The relative incidence of colorectal cancer as compared with other forms of cancer needs to be emphasized to physicians in high-incidence countries. Both public and professional awareness of lung, breast, and cervical cancer is heightened because of the emphasis these are given in the popular press, whereas, in Australia at least, colorectal cancer has had little publicity in either lay or professional media, despite its high rank in incidence. First-contact doctors in particular need to be made more aware of colorectal cancer incidence.

Similarly, both first-contact physicians and specialists in gastroenterology need to be made aware that neither patient delay in presenting symptoms nor doctor delay in diagnosis has decreased in the past 20 years, nor has survival improved. On all three counts, we have found a degree of overconfidence among both specialists and family doctors (1). Notwithstanding, the relatively high survival rate for colorectal cancer as compared with other forms of cancer should be emphasized, as opinions of Australian physicians have shown an unwarranted degree of pessimism.

The delineation of categories at increased risk is an important research task, the results of which need to be carried through quickly to first-contact doctors to encourage them towards an aggressive approach to early detection. Australian studies have shown a distinct lack of awareness of the magnitude of increased risk in first-degree relatives and even of the risk of metachronous cancer after successful resection. We also found a distinct lack of aggressiveness in approaching relatives for screening via the index case. First-contact doctors are particularly well placed to identify high-risk families and should be encouraged to impress upon patients the importance of regular screening of relatives. Further effort is needed to discover effective means of convincing a reluctant patient that relatives should be made aware of their increased risk and of their need for regular screening.

There is a need for training of first-contact doctors in sigmoidoscopy and encouragement of its use in general practice. Nevertheless, overconfidence as to the proportion of cancers that can be detected at sigmoidoscopy should be cautioned against, as should overconfidence about the proportion detectable on digital rectal examination.

Education of new medical graduates in early detection of colorectal cancer should be enhanced, though they need to be given an awareness of the cost-effectiveness of available techniques, and responsible selective application should be encouraged. With fecal occult blood testing in particular, physicians need to be made aware of improvements in specificity and selectivity. Australian studies have shown a sizeable proportion of doctors who flatly reject all fecal occult blood testing on the grounds that the adequacy of earlier methods has been questioned, and a further proportion who still employ these methods.

Pressure for increased awareness of colorectal cancer and an aggressive approach to screening must take account of existing knowledge as well as entrenched opinion among both first-contact doctors and specialists in gastroenterology.

REFERENCES

1. Dent, O., Bassett, M., and Goulston, K. (1978): Knowledge and attitudes of gastroenterologists in colorectal cancer. *Aust. N. Z. J. Surg.,* 48:331.
2. Holliday, H. W., and Hardcastle, J. D. (1979): Delay in diagnosis and treatment of symptomatic colorectal cancer. *Lancet,* 2:309.

Colorectal Cancer: Prevention, Epidemiology, and Screening, edited by S. Winawer, D. Schottenfeld, and P. Sherlock. Raven Press, New York © 1980.

Introduction: Factors Influencing Patients' Attitudes Toward Screening for Colorectal Cancer

LaSalle D. Leffall, Jr.

American Cancer Society, Inc., New York, New York 10017

During the past 5 years, the American Cancer Society (ACS) through its local units reached more than 3 million persons over 40 years of age with educational programs (films, speakers, discussion) on colorectal cancer. Many of these programs provided opportunities for target population groups to take the actions recommended, i.e., offering the guaiac slide test, demonstrating the value of the test(s), as well as encouraging their adoption as good health habits.

To support and give direction to these and other ACS Public Education activities involving the priority cancer sites (lung, colorectal, breast, and uterus), the Society conducts ongoing research to obtain up-to-date information about public attitudes toward cancer and cancer tests and conducts demonstration projects from time to time to measure the relative impact of various educational methods.

This chapter briefly reviews two such studies which have a bearing on efforts to control colorectal cancer in the future.

PUBLIC ATTITUDES

The first study, "A Basic Study of Public Attitudes Toward Cancer and Cancer Tests," was conducted for the Society by Lieberman Research, Inc., in May 1979. Based on a nationwide sample of 1,553 men and women 18 years of age and older, the study examines the two major detection tests for colorectal cancer—digital and proctoscopic examinations. Although 34% of adults report they have regular digital exams, only 4% report that they have regular proctoscopic exams. Only a minority of people know why doctors do digital rectal exams. Less than 1 of 2 (47%) people are aware that this exam is a check for colorectal cancer, and even fewer—only 1 of 7 people (15%)—know that this is a check for prostate cancer.

About 16% of adults have heard of the do-it-yourself guaiac slide test, and 3% have done it. Although relatively few people have heard of the test, over one-third (36%) indicate that they would be interested in doing it. Even more importantly, 72% indicate that, if they did the do-it-yourself test and the results showed possible complications, they would likely go to a doctor for a procto-scopic exam. Thus the guaiac test offers strong potential as a screening device to encourage people at risk to go for further follow-up tests.

MOTIVATIONAL FACTOR

A second study was done to evaluate the public's willingness to perform the guaiac test and to assess the relative effectiveness of alternative means of persuading people to do the test. Volunteers in four different parts of the United States contacted a total of 11,115 members of the American Association of Retired Persons (AARP), using five methods that differed in the extent of personal and impersonal contact involved. Other variables such as the inclusion of postage and dietary restrictions were studied and cost efficiencies were estimated. Findings of this study suggest that the guaiac test does have the potential for reaching a significant proportion of the nation's older population.

The five different methods used to persuade people to do the test were the following:

1. The total mail-out method. This involved mailing members three slides along with literature describing the purpose of the test and how to perform it.
2. The selective mail-out method. This involved mailing literature describing the test to members, asking them to send back a card if they were interested in doing the test. Slides were then sent to those requesting them.
3. The come-in method. This involved mailing literature describing the test to members, asking them to come to a specified location (e.g., hospital, clinic) where the purpose of the test was discussed and slides were distributed to those requesting them.
4. The group meeting method. This involved having volunteers attend regular chapter meetings where they discussed the purpose of the test and distributed slides to those who requested them.
5. The at-home method. This involved having specially trained volunteers visit members in their homes where they described the test and left slides with those who were interested in performing it.

The findings of the study definitely indicate that there is both an interest and a willingness to do the test. Considering all ways of persuading individuals to do the test, about 15% of those contacted accepted the slides, did the test, and returned the slides for processing. It is significant that these results were achieved despite the absence of any prior publicity or promotion of the program. The findings suggest that with added promotional efforts and appropriate selection of method, it would be possible to reach a significant proportion of an elderly population.

The group meeting method was the most effective personal distribution method used. If mail or nonpersonal distribution methods are used, the selective mail-out method (where individuals are informed of the test and slides mailed only to those who request them) is the one recommended for future use.

The rate of return was higher when the envelope in which the slides were placed contained postage than when individuals had to provide their own postage. The increased rate of return overshadowed the extra cost involved.

Incorporating certain dietary restrictions (e.g., a meat-free diet) into the testing did not markedly reduce participation in the program. Since meat products may lead to the occurrence of false positives on the test, it is worth knowing that the inclusion of special diets does not lower participation to any significant degree.

The return rate was no greater when a digital examination was offered in connection with the screening. This finding suggests that a considerable savings of time and effort can be made by not including a digital examination in future undertakings of this sort.

An additional factor which was included in the study was the identification of specific sponsors of the screening program. The results showed that equal return rates were achieved when ACS and AARP were identified on a separate basis as sponsors of the program. The findings reveal that the type of sponsorship had little differential impact on either the return rate or the cost per return achieved.

The importance of colorectal cancer as a disease affecting the elderly of this nation warrants the serious consideration of effective early detection programs such as the guaiac slide test. The findings of this study offer practical information for those who are interested in the effective delivery of such a test program to older age groups.

REFERENCE

1. '76 American Cancer Society (1975): Cancer Facts and Figures. New York, N.Y. 10017.

Colorectal Cancer: Prevention, Epidemiology,
and Screening, edited by S. Winawer, D. Schottenfeld,
and P. Sherlock. Raven Press, New York © 1980.

Review of Screening for Colorectal Cancer Using Fecal Occult Blood Testing

S. J. Winawer, M. Andrews, C. H. Miller, and M. Fleisher

Memorial Sloan-Kettering Cancer Center, New York, New York 10021

Use of the fecal occult blood test as a screen for colorectal cancer must be considered within the framework of critical issues that must be addressed in screening. These issues include the long-range potential benefit of screening at a particular anatomic site in a specific population group or country with the major objective of mortality reduction, the target population to be screened and their associated risk factors, the availability and appropriateness of other screening tests as well as their sensitivity and specificity, the sensitivity and specificity of diagnostic tests, without which the screening tests are of no value, the potential compliance of patients and the awareness of physicians of the concepts involved in screening and diagnosis, and the related cost factors. Screening for colorectal cancer based on occult blood detection in the stool has become a focus of interest because of the development of better materials and methods for this test. The effectiveness of this test in screening, however, must be evaluated within the framework of the above critical issues (12,17).

Prior tests for occult blood in the stool including the Hematest (orthotoludine), Benzidine test, and guaiac solutions utilizing a single stool specimen brought in by the patient on an uncontrolled diet have been discarded because of unreliability and a high percentage of false negativity and false positivity. There was a resurgence of interest in fecal occult blood testing with introduction of the impregnated guaiac slide test with stabilized reagent. In a series of papers from 1967 through 1971, Greegor (7,8) reported on the use of this test in his private practice suggesting its feasibility among asymptomatic patients at risk for colorectal cancer by virtue of age only, when placed on a high-roughage, meat-free diet with six smears obtained. Within his own experience as well as in a cooperative study with a group of other physicians, Greegor observed that the test was useful as an indicator of early colorectal cancer in truly silent cases with a low rate of known false negatives. These initial observations were followed by studies in Hawaii by Glober and Pescoe (5); in the United States by Hastings (9) and Miller (10); and the studies in Germany by Frühmorgen and Demling (4) and Gnauck (6). All of these studies supported the concept that this test may be useful as a screening approach for colorectal cancer. Since then two controlled trials were initiated, one at The Preventive Medicine Institute–Strang Clinic in New York in 1974 (14), followed by initiation of a study at the University of Minnesota (1). In addition to these two controlled trials, several community programs as well as uncontrolled trials were started around the world utilizing a variety of approaches in different types of populations and, in addition, a national program was instituted in West Germany.

In Greegor's initial series, 5% of the patients had positive tests. One of this group had a colon cancer, two had diverticulosis, and one had a polyp, and in only one could no disease be found. In his latter experience the frequency of positive reactions decreased to 2.8% but the pathology remained the same. His later personal experience *(personal communication)* indicated that the frequency of positive reactions further decreased to approximately 1%. In a collaborative study in which 103 physicians reported on use of this approach, 139 cancers were detected (8). Of all the patients who had colon cancer and followed the instructions for the test, only one patient had a false negative test. No other false-negatives were found in Greegor's personal experience over 10 years. In 47 cases that were considered to be silent, 85% were pathologically localized to the bowel wall. Only 20 of the 139 cases of cancers were within reach of the standard sigmoidoscope.

Hastings' study (9) was a community-wide study of mass screening over a short period of time. Among 1,835 individuals, age 40 or above, five colon cancers were discovered in the diagnostic follow-up examination of 41 of 114 persons with a positive test. In the study of 2,323 people by Miller and Knight (10), 7 patients with polyps and 3 with cancer were identified in 39 patients with positive slides undergoing diagnostic examinations. In the Hawaiian study of Glober and Pescoe (5), in 1,539 Japanese Americans four asymptomatic cancers and three polyps were detected in the work-up of 32 positive screenees. The program of Frühmorgen and Demling in 1975 (4) included the participation of 5,016 persons in a newspaper-advertised campaign. In the Hemoccult-positive group of 117 persons, 13 carcinomas and numerous large polyps were found.

Gnauck's program (6), in progress since 1972, included 5,007 patients. The program continued until 1975. The rate of positive tests varied among his groups from 1.5 to 4.8%. In 144 of the 202 positive patients, a complete diagnostic examination was performed yielding 22 carcinomas and 29 polyps larger than 1 cm in diameter. Of the carcinomas, 14 were beyond the reach of the sigmoidoscope.

The frequency of positive slides in these studies ranged from 1 to 3% except for Hastings' study in which 6% of patients were positive. The predictive value for neoplasia (cancer or adenoma) varied from 18 to 50%.

In the reported studies, many variations of technique were used but all have used the impregnated guaiac slide test with stabilized reagent. This test is based on the peroxidase activity of substances in the stool which convert the colorless group of guaiac compounds from their phenolic state by oxidation to the quinone state which is blue in color, utilizing a stabilized hydrogen peroxide reagent.

It must be emphasized that this reaction is a reaction produced not only by the peroxidase-like activity of human hemoglobin, but also by the peroxidase activity of a variety of substances, including nonhuman hemoglobin, bacteria, and vegetable peroxidases. In addition, when human hemoglobin is the substance producing the positive test, it may be hemoglobin from a bleeding neoplastic or non-neoplastic lesion, or from physiologic blood loss, and the hemoglobin producing a positive test could result from blood loss anywhere in the gastrointestinal tract.

CONTROL TRIALS

The first controlled clinical trial to be initiated utilizing fecal occult blood testing was at The Preventive Medicine Institute-Strang Clinic in collaboration with Memorial Sloan-Kettering Cancer Center in 1974 (14) (Tables 1 and 2). In this trial, asymptomatic men and women age 40 and older coming to The Preventive Medicine Institute receive a comprehensive medical examination including a medical questionnaire, rigid sigmoidoscopy; in addition, the study group is sent a fecal occult blood test kit to prepare at home. This initially consisted of single Hemoccult (Smith Kline Diagnostics, Sunnyvale, CA) slides, and later the Hemoccult II slide. Patients are asked to prepare six smears over

TABLE 1. *Control trial of screening: clinical factors*

Men and Women
Mostly asymptomatic
Age 40 and older
Mostly average risk
No past history of colorectal cancer
Medical questionnaire administered
Past medical history ascertained
Family history ascertained
Comprehensive medical examination
Rigid sigmoidoscopy
Fecal occult blood testing with Hemoccult slides (study group)

From Winawer et al. (16).

TABLE 2. *Control trial of screening: technical factors[a]*

Single Hemoccult slides used previously
Hemoccult II slides used currently
No rehydration
Meat-free diet
High-bulk diet (including fiber)
Number of smears: 6
Storage interval: 4 days

[a] See text for details.
From Winawer et al. (16).

3 days on a meat-free, high-fiber diet with restriction of vitamins and medications. They are asked to perform this within 4 days of their examination and to bring the slides in on their examination date at which time slides are tested. Diagnostic tests are performed, including double-contrast barium enema and colonoscopy, if the slides are positive. An upper gastrointestinal series is performed if no colonic neoplasm is found and, when indicated, an upper gastrointestinal endoscopy. Routine blood studies are also obtained. Approximately 22,000 patients have been enrolled in this study completing more than 40,000 examinations, including comprehensive examinations, fecal occult blood testing, and proctosigmoidoscopy (Kobayashi and Samec, *this volume;* 10–16) (Table 3).

The compliance in the different subgroups of the Strang Clinic study for fecal occult blood testing ranged from 70 to 80%, and 95% of all patients completed proctosigmoidoscopy (Table 4). The overall rate of positive slides was 2.5%, but this varied depending on the type of slides used, patient status, and age. The rate of positivity for the single Hemoccult slides was 1%, with a predictive value for neoplastic lesions of 50%, including 12% for cancer and 38% for adenomas. With the Hemoccult II slides the rate of positivity increased to 3.7%, with a predictive value of 44%. When the Hemoccult II slides were rehydrated, the rate of positivity increased to 5.4%, and the predictive value for neoplasia decreased sharply to 19% (Fig. 1). There was an increase of slide positivity with age by decade (Table 5). The majority of patients (85%) with

TABLE 3. *Overall population characteristics*

Total enrolled:			21,961		
Total by patient status:		*Annual*	*Initial*		
	N	9,512	12,449		
	%	43	57		
Total by study status:		*Study*	*Control*		
	N	13,127	8,834		
	%	60	40		
Total by sex:		*Male*	*Female*		
	N	9,757	12,204		
	%	44	56		
Total by age:		*40–49*	*50–59*	*60–69*	*70+*
	N	7,200	7,660	5,386	1,715
	%	33	35	25	8
Total reported symptomatic:		N	1,593		
		%	7		
Total reported family history of cancer:		N	3,547		
		%	16		
Total reported personal history of cancer:		N	1,558		
		%	7		
Total reported personal history of polyps:		N	837		
		%	4		

From Winawer et al. (16).

TABLE 4. *Control trial of screening: results summary*

Patient compliance with proctoscopy	95%
Patient compliance with fecal occult blood test	
Annual patients	69%
Initial patients	80%
First slide	69%
Subsequent slides	80%
Rate of slide positivity	
Single Hemoccult	1%
Hemoccult II	3.7%
Predictive value for neoplasia	
Single Hemoccult	50%
Hemoccult II	44%
Predictive value by age	1.6–6.6%
False positivity	0.5–2.1%
False negativity	
Adenomas in rectosigmoid	76%
Dukes' staging	Favorable in screened group
Diagnostic studies: cancers	Double-contrast barium enema and colonoscopy = complementary
Diagnostic studies: adenomas	Colonoscopy = more sensitive
Rigid proctoscopy	Sensitive only below 16 cm

significant neoplastic lesions had between one and three Hemoccult slide tests positive (Table 6). Analysis of daily smears indicated that only 41% of neoplastic lesions would have been detected if only one smear per day was examined rather than two smears (Table 7). Preliminary data indicate that colorectal cancers detected by Hemoccult slides alone had a more favorable staging than those detected by either proctosigmoidoscopy or symptoms.

The double-contrast barium enema was fairly sensitive for cancers but had a low sensitivity for colorectal adenomas as compared to colonoscopy. In patients

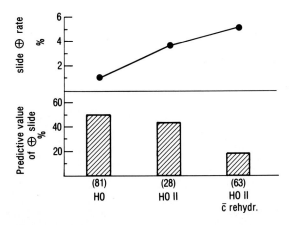

FIG. 1. Rate of positivity and predictive value of Hemoccult (HO) slides in 3 screening periods. Reprinted with permission from ref. 13.

TABLE 5. *Correlation of colorectal neoplasia with age in HO-positive patients*

Age	No. patients HO positive with completed investigation	Colon cancer	Polyps			Predictive value for neoplasia
			≥ 5 mm	≤ 5 mm	Other	
40–49	33	—	9	2	22	27% (9/33)
50–59	56	6	19	2	29	45% (25/56)
60–69	88	10	31	6	41	47% (41/88)
> 69	21	3	8	1	9	52% (11/21)
Totals	198	19	67	11	101	43% (86/198)

Predictive value for neoplasia of HO-positive test correlates with age, the lowest being in 40–49 group. No cancers were observed in 40–49 group.

TABLE 6. *Distribution frequency of Hemoccult-positive slides*

No. of slides positive	No. of patients with positive slides		No. of patients with positive slides and neoplasia	
	No.	(%)	No.	(%)
1	87	(44)	34	(40)
2	65	(33)	30	(35)
3	16	(8)	9	(10)
4	10	(5)	4	(5)
5	6	(3)	3	(3)
6	14	(7)	6	(7)
Total	198	(100)	86	(100)

TABLE 7. *Hemoccult-positive slides (A/B) and neoplastic lesions*

	One or more A/B pairs positive	
Cancer	3/0	(50%)
Adenoma	6/16	(38%)
Total	9/22	(41%)

From Winawer (13).

having a flexible endoscopic examination, it was determined that there was a high false negativity for rigid sigmoidoscopy and that most of the lesions missed were in the 16 to 25 cm range from the anal verge. The false negativity for adenomas within the rectosigmoid was 76%, this being known because all patients had rigid sigmoidoscopy performed. The false negativity for cancers has not yet been determined, nor has the false negativity for adenomas above the rectosigmoid.

A second control trial evaluating the Hemoccult slide in fecal occult blood testing as a screening test for colorectal cancer was initiated at the University of Minnesota by Gilbertsen and Bond (1). In this study, participants were randomized into one of three study groups consisting of those who received Hemoccult slides each year; those who received the slides every other year; and a control group. Persons found to have positive Hemoccult slides were requested to have diagnostic examinations including X-rays and colonoscopy. The X-rays were of the single-column type rather than double contrast. Of the patients who had positive tests and who underwent diagnostic evaluation, approximately 9% had cancer of the colon, the majority of which were Dukes' A or B cancers. It was of interest that only 39% of the lesions of the colon that were detected were found on the barium enema, and 61% were found only on the colonoscopy. The plan of this study is to continue screening for 5 years, followed by a 5-year period for follow-up data among the various groups. The data generated from this program so far suggest that fecal occult blood testing is a useful method for screening for neoplasms of the intestine. In this particular study, screening began at age 50 as compared to age 40 in the Strang Clinic–Memorial Sloan-Kettering Cancer Center study. The highest yield appears to be in patients 63 years of age and over. The sensitivity of the barium enema in this particular study was low, but the type of barium examination performed was a single-column examination rather than a double-contrast examination. A progress report of this program is presented elsewhere in this section.

OTHER STUDIES IN PROGRESS

Additional studies have been performed or are in progress around the world utilizing fecal occult blood testing as a screening test for colorectal cancer. In a county-wide screening program, Bralow and Kopel (2) reported a public response twice as great as anticipated. The compliance ratio in this study was 79%, and approximately 10% of the returned slides had at least one positive specimen. Among the patients who had positive tests and who had diagnostic evaluation, 15% were found to have polyps and 9% were found to have cancers, which were early, localized lesions. This study demonstrated that a community-wide screening program is feasible with a high yield of early cancer at a reasonable cost and with good patient compliance. There was a problem with follow-up evaluation among patients, with only 30% of individuals cooperating.

The American Cancer Society has had a keen interest in this area, and in November 1976 initiated an area-wide screening program using guaiac slide testing (3). Professional and public education was emphasized. The age at which screening was allowed was 21 years or older. Of 49,157 tests distributed, 19,707 (40%) were returned. Patients who had positive tests on an unrestricted diet had the test repeated with a restricted diet and were worked-up only if the second test was positive. This was an approach similar to that used by Gnauck, and also in the Sarasota community program by Bralow. A total of 130 patients completed a diagnostic work-up, resulting in 101 cases with intestinal pathology, including 15 colorectal cancers and 18 polyps. The pathology of the cancers was favorable as compared to the tumor registry data in general for the area.

Another community-wide program initiated in the Chicago area utilized a heavy emphasis on public education and motivation through use of the media, including television (18). This program also had encouraging results but like other community programs had the same problem of a low frequency of follow-up diagnostic examinations in patients who screened positive. In all of the community programs where this problem existed, the underlying difficulty appeared to be lack of sufficient physician awareness of the importance of thorough diagnostic evaluation of patients who have had positive tests on a single screening examination.

Although fecal occult blood testing has been little utilized in Japan because of the low incidence of colorectal cancer, one program by Kobayashi *(this volume)* reported results of a screening program utilizing this approach. His preliminary observations were encouraging for the use of fecal occult blood testing as a screening test for colorectal cancer in Japan. Interest has evolved in other countries for screening large bowel cancer. The incidence of large bowel cancer in Israel is similar to that in Europe but lower than in the United States, and a rising trend has become apparent. It appears now to be the most common malignancy following breast cancer in females and lung cancer in males in the Israeli population. In one study by Rozen and associates *(this volume),* the target population was high-risk groups rather than the average-risk patients, in order to increase yield and lower the cost. Their early results appear to be encouraging. In Austria where the frequency of large bowel cancer has increased in recent years, Samec *(this volume)* reported screening results with fecal occult blood testing. Of 5,323 people given tests, 4% showed a positive reaction, and in this group a variety of gastrointestinal lesions, including cancers, were detected.

A large, rather ambitious study has been initiated in the Federal Republic of West Germany encouraging screening of men and women who are asymptomatic in doctors' offices on a periodic basis utilizing fecal occult blood testing. This program has already entered several million persons who have had fecal occult blood testing, a percentage of which have had positive tests and further diagnostic evaluation. The study now is in the process of developing a data collection system and follow-up program for gathering results. The results of this program will be looked at with keen interest from the standpoint of patient compliance, follow-up diagnostic examination by the community physicians, as well as cost and mortality, and other aspects of their evaluation. With such a wide-scale national study, it may be difficult to provide many of these critical elements of data (see Schwartz, *this volume*).

INTERPRETATION OF RESULTS OF PROGRAM UTILIZING FECAL OCCULT BLOOD TESTING

It has become difficult to interrelate the results of the various screening programs utilizing fecal occult blood testing as a screen for colorectal cancer. The problems are in the reporting of patient characteristics, methodology, and results.

In many of the reports it is not stated whether patients are asymptomatic or symptomatic, and often not even the age at which screening has been initiated is included in the data. Furthermore, the type of slides used is often not stated, that is, whether it is the single Hemoccult slide, Hemoccult II slide, or other type of slide; whether six slides have been used or three slides; and what the time interval is between preparation of smears by the patient and laboratory testing. Usually no comment is made on whether the slides are rehydrated prior to testing with the reagent. In many reports the diet is initially unrestricted and when patients have positive tests, the test is repeated on an restricted diet and only persistent positivity is worked up. In other studies the diet is restricted from the beginning, with work-up of all patients who are positive. These variations in approach may have a strong impact on the degree of false negativity and false positivity. The type of diet used, whether it is meat-free or high bulk and, if high bulk, whether it contains fiber, is often not stated, and this too may have a profound effect on false positivity and false negativity. It has been shown by Goulston and associates *(this volume)* that an unrestricted diet is associated with a high rate of false positives and false negatives. Clearly, more work needs to be done in this area. Few data have been generated from these programs in terms of the yield related to a control group, since most studies are uncontrolled.

The diagnostic work-up has varied greatly in studies: sigmoidoscopy and single-column barium enema were performed in some studies, double-contrast barium enema in other studies, and in some studies, both double-contrast barium enema and colonoscopy. Conclusions about the sensitivity and specificity of colonoscopy as compared to the barium enema are often made even when the barium enema is suboptimal and a single-column examination rather than a double-contrast type is used.

The reasons for false negativity are not yet known, nor is the degree of false negativity known, except perhaps in the rectosigmoid, from the Strang Clinic–Memorial Sloan-Kettering Cancer Center study. False negativity may relate to methodology but undoubtedly also relates to the intermittent quality of bleeding from neoplastic lesions. False positivity, of course, can result from a variety of sources. False positivity can be defined as false positivity for blood or false positivity for neoplastic lesions or, even more specifically, false positivity for cancer; and this can be further categorized on an anatomic basis, in terms of colon, rectum, and upper gastrointestinal tract. Vegetable peroxidases can certainly produce a positivity in the absence of any bleeding. False positivity can also occur from physiologic blood loss, and perhaps to a lesser extent from meat in the diet, and from non-neoplastic bleeding lesions such as angiodysplasia, diverticulosis, hemorrhoids, and inflammatory bowel disease. The immunochemical method discussed elsewhere in this volume could eliminate the false positivity from vegetable peroxidases and non-human hemoglobin but will not eliminate the false positivity from human hemoglobin arising from non-neoplastic bleeding sources and physiologic blood loss. However, there is clearly a need for a more specific slide that would reduce the nonhemoglobin false positivity (11).

In all of the above studies reported to date, short-term objectives have been described, including feasibility of the approach, yield, compliance, false positivity, sensitivity and specificity of the diagnostic tests, and staging of detected cancers. Patient compliance and physician awareness have had special emphasis in few studies. The long-term objectives that need to be achieved for acceptance of this approach as a valid screening test are related not only to survival of those patients with a positive screening test who have demonstrated a favorable pathological stage of cancer at surgery but also to the mortality benefit to the screened group as compared to the control group. Hopefully, this will be forthcoming from the ongoing clinical trials, but will take considerably more time.

NEED FOR STANDARDIZATION OF REPORTING

It is quite clear that for any order to occur in the data being reported around the world, a standardization of reporting must be developed. We must know clearly the specific details of the patient characteristics, clinical methodology, and results from each program that is reported. In addition, laboratory quality control must also be added to all programs. The sensitivity and reproducibility of the slide tests being utilized in the screening programs must be evaluated in the laboratory and monitored during the progress of studies. It is possible that variations in data being obtained in different studies not only are related to the clinical methodology of the screening approach, the demographics of the patients, and the type of diagnostic investigation being performed on those patients who are positive, but also are related to the sensitivity of the slides being used. At the present time, a Reference Laboratory (at Memorial Sloan-Kettering Cancer Center) has been established and has the capability of determining the sensitivity of slides being used, providing a quality control program. A number of laboratories working with screening programs throughout the world have indicated a willingness to cooperate with this Reference Laboratory. This is further discussed elsewhere in this volume. In order to enhance collection of meaningful data in this area and to provide greater cooperation of those groups who are interested in screening for colorectal cancer, an International Workgroup is being organized. One of the goals of this International Workgroup will be to heighten awareness of the needs for standardization of reporting and quality control among investigators interested in this area. Hopefully, this will aid achievement of the common goal of many workers in the field, the secondary prevention of colorectal cancer through detection of early cancers and premalignant lesions and prevention of the devastating consequences of invasive colorectal cancer.

REFERENCES

1. Bond, J. H., and Gilbertsen, V. A. (1977): Early detection of colonic carcinoma by mass screening for occult stool blood: Preliminary report. *Gastroenterology,* 72:5:A-8/1031.

2. Bralow, S. P., and Kopel, J. (1979): Hemoccult screening for colorectal cancer. Impact study on Sarasota, Florida. *J. Fla. Med. Assoc.,* 66:915–919.
3. Elwood, T. W., Erickson, A., and Lieberman, S. (1978): Comparative educational approaches to screening for colorectal cancer. *Am. J. Public Health,* 68:2:135–138.
4. Fruhmorgen, P., and Demling, L. (1978): First results of a prospective field study with a modified guaiac test for evidence of occult blood it the stool. In: *Early Detection of Colorectal Cancer,* edited by K. Goerttler. Verlag DE, Wachholz KG, Nurnberg.
5. Glober, G. A., and Peskoe, S. M. (1974): Outpatient screening for gastrointestinal lesions using guaiac-impregnated slides. *Am. J. Dig. Dis.,* 19:399–403.
6. Gnauck, R. (1977): Screening for colorectal cancer with the Hemoccult test. *Leber Magen Darm,* 7:32–35.
7. Greegor, D. H. (1967): Diagnosis of large bowel cancer in the asymptomatic patient. *J.A.M.A.,* 201:943–945.
8. Greegor, D. H. (1971): Occult blood testing for detection of asymptomatic colon cancer. *Cancer,* 28:131–134.
9. Hastings, J. B. (1974): Mass screening for colorectal cancer. *Am. J. Surg.,* 127:228–233.
10. Miller, S. F., and Knight, R. A. (1977): The early detection of colorectal cancer. *Cancer,* 40:945–949.
11. Winawer, S. J. (1976): Fecal occult blood testing (Editorial). *Am. J. Dig. Dis.,* 21:885–888.
12. Winawer, S. J. (1978): Colorectal neoplasia: Current techniques for early diagnosis. *N. Y. State J. Med.,* 78:12:1892–1894.
13. Winawer, S. J. (1979): Colorectal cancer screening and early diagnosis. In: *Screening and Early Detection of Colorectal Cancer,* edited by Dorothy R. Brodie, Consensus Development Conference Proc., pp. 193–210. June 26–28, 1978. NIH Publication No. 80-2075, Washington, D.C.
14. Winawer, S. J., Leidner, S. D., Miller, D. G., et al. (1977): Results of a screening program for the detection of early colon cancer and polyps using fecal occult blood testing. *Gastroenterology,* 72:5:2:A-127/1150 (abst.).
15. Winawer, S. J., Miller, D. G., Schottenfeld, D., et al. (1977): Feasibility of fecal occult blood testing for detection of colorectal neoplasia: Debits and credits. *Cancer,* 40:5:2616–2619.
16. Winawer, S. J., Miller, D. G., Schottenfeld, D., and Sherlock, P. (1980): Progress report on controlled trial of fecal occult blood testing for the detection of colorectal neoplasia. *Cancer (in press).*
17. Winawer, S. J., Sherlock, P., Schottenfeld, D., and Miller, D. G. (1976): Screening for colon cancer. *Gastroenterology,* 70:783–789.
18. Winchester, D. P., Shull, J. H., and Scanlon, E. F. (1979): A mass screening program for colorectal cancer using chemical testing for occult blood in the stool. Presentation at The Society of Surgical Oncology 32nd Annual Meeting Scientific Program, April, Atlanta, Ga.

Colorectal Cancer: Prevention, Epidemiology, and Screening, edited by S. Winawer, D. Schottenfeld, and P. Sherlock. Raven Press, New York © 1980.

Colon Cancer Control Study: An Interim Report

*Victor A. Gilbertsen, **Richard B. McHugh, **Leonard M. Schuman, and *Stanley E. Williams

*Department of Surgery, University of Minnesota, Minneapolis, Minnesota 55414; and **School of Public Health, University of Minnesota Health Sciences Center, Minneapolis, Minnesota 55455*

Many questions remain concerning the early detection of cancer of the colon and rectum through the finding and investigation of occult blood in the stool in a population which is ostensibly asymptomatic and at high risk for colorectal disease (7). The Colon Cancer Control Study at the University of Minnesota is a randomized, controlled clinical trial of the Hemoccult form of the guaiac test for stool blood as an aid in the detection of early carcinoma of the colon and rectum. The detection of lesions proceeds from the indication of occult blood to a series of diagnostic examinations for the investigation of the entire gastrointestinal tract (Table 1). The goal of the study is to demonstrate a difference of 50% in mortality from colorectal disease between the annually screened and the control group at a power $(1-\beta)$ of approximately 0.90. The annual mortality from cancer of the colon in the control group is assumed to be 0.001 (5). The duration of the study is 10 years (5 years of screening and 5 years of follow-up). The mortality basis for analysis allows for a reduction in the effects of the lead-time bias and length-biased sampling problems encountered with survival rate methods (1,2,4,11).

The evaluation of the usefulness of the Hemoccult technique as a screening device for large populations involves answers to several questions relating to modes of distribution and collection, participant compliance and acceptance, and optimum screening intervals. The Colon Cancer Control Study is designed to provide information which should be useful in approaching these questions. The study design requires a randomized group, screened on alternate years after the initial screen, to enable us to examine the interval question. Other aspects of the design provide for the study of critical factors in the use of the mails for large population screening and follow-up and the evaluation of methods of maximizing the various compliances (return of screening materials and surveys, agreement to accept diagnostic services at a designated facility, fidelity in follow-through with referrals for further consultation and treatment for gastrointestinal and other pathologies uncovered in the course of examination, etc.) required of participants.

TABLE 1. *General protocol: Colon Cancer Control Study, University of Minnesota*

1. Asymptomatic volunteers randomized to A-B-C

2.
   A. Screened biennially
      Surveyed annually
   B. Screened annually
      Surveyed annually
   C. Controls: surveyed annually

3. A and B complete 2 Hemoccult slides from each of 3 consecutive stools: 6 slides/screen.

4.
   i. At least 1 slide positive
   i. 6 negative slides
   ii. Return to cohort

5.
   ii. Diagnostic examination
      History and physical exam with lab studies
      Proctosigmoidoscopy
      Upper GI X-ray series
        (gastroscopy if indicated)
      Colonoscopy; air-contrast
        BE X-ray if indicated
      i. Fewer than 6 negative slides
      ii. Retest
      iii. Return to cohort

6.
   iii. Positive for pathology
   iv. Refer for treatment
   v. Return to cohort
   iii. Negative for pathology
   iv. Return to cohort

METHODS AND MATERIALS

Recruitment of volunteers between the ages of 50 and 80 years began in August 1975 and was completed in November 1977. All enrollees were to be residents of the State of Minnesota, admit to no history of colorectal cancer, and be asymptomatic for gastrointestinal problems at the time of enrollment. In one control and two experimental groups, 48,000 persons were randomized by age, sex, and geographic region of the state. Sample size requirements were calculated using the method of Taylor et al. (13) to be 45,000 persons with allowance for attrition. The date of entry into the project was taken as the date on which a properly completed, signed consent form was received by the study. The consent form contained complete information concerning the experimental nature of the study, its goals, and requirements for participation. Enrollees agreed to the detailed requirements of each of the proposed experimental groups since the specific group of allocation was not determined until after randomization. This agreement included annual or biennial submission of stool specimens for 5 years, prepared while observing the prescribed meat-free diet (8), follow-through with necessary diagnostic tests at the University of Minnesota Medical Center for the purpose of determining the cause of bleeding in the event of a positive test, and completion of annual health surveys for the testing and follow-up periods. Participants assigned to the third (control) group were asked to agree to the submission of annual health surveys (Table 1). The customary access, confidentiality, notification of personal physician, and discontinuance without prejudice statements were clearly stated.

Hemoccult slides used for the project are specially prepared from standard materials used for the manufacture of the usual commercial product. The "model" used throughout is the original (single-well) Hemoccult. However, the cover is distinctively printed ("University of Minnesota, Colon Cancer Control Study") to permit detection of slides submitted that may be of other than study origin. Sensitivity of slide lots (University of Minnesota—2557:1975 and 2587:1978) was determined at the time of manufacture to 2 to 3 mg of "added hemoglobin per gram of stool" (H. Wells, *personal communication*). Batch 2587 was characterized as giving "a more intense reaction." Interpretation of slides is based on the presence or absence of any blue color after the prescribed interval following application of the reagent (no scaling of reaction intensity is attempted) (9,10). Rehydration of slides prior to addition of the reagent was begun July 1977 per manufacturer recommendation (3,14,15).

Participants are asked to submit six slides prepared at the rate of two slides per stool for three consecutive stools (regardless of when they occur) commencing 24 hr after the diet begins. Slides are dated at use and returned in a postage-paid envelope. Persons submitting at least one positive slide are examined at the University of Minnesota Hospitals according to an examination protocol, consisting of complete history and physical examination, proctosigmoidoscopy, upper GI X-ray series (and gastroscopy if indicated), single-column barium enema (BE) X-ray, and colonoscopy. [This protocol recently has been modified to omit the single-column BE X-ray in favor of colonoscopy only (6), with double-contrast BE X-ray in cases in which the entire colon is not visualized (Table 1).] Patients found to have neoplasms not completely removed at biopsy are counseled relative to therapy. Decisions concerning treatment of malignancies found are made by the patient and his/her personal physician. Patients submitting six slides negative for occult blood are returned to cohort for continued screening. Persons returning fewer than six negative (no positive) slides are retested. Those persons whose conditions require therapy for malignancy or other serious disorder are returned to cohort for continued screening when therapy is completed and/or when resumption of screening is appropriate.

Slides of biopsied tissue and surgically removed tumors[b] are reviewed by the project pathologist and are stored in the project tissue registry. This same procedure is followed for tissue showing malignancy which is obtained at autopsy or from surgical procedure, for all cancer-related deaths occurring in the study population. A Death Review Committee (epidemiologist, oncologist, surgeon, and pathologist) determines the relationship of cancer of the colon and/or rectum (if involved) to the cause of death through examination of the history, pathology reports, autopsy findings, and tissue review. Reviewers have no knowledge of the screened/control group membership of the participant case.

TABLE 2. *Diagnostic findings for 2,160 patients submitting at least 1 guaiac-positive stool sample (Hemoccult) in series of 6 samples[a]*

	Examined U of M		Examined elsewhere[b]		Total	
	No.	(%)	No.	(%)	No.	(%)
Initial screen						
GI cancer	64	(8)	11	(9)	75	(8)
Polyp	260	(32)	13	(11)	273	(29)
Other[c]	491	(60)	93	(80)	584	(63)
Subtotal	815		117		932	
2nd and 3rd screens						
GI cancer	28	(3)	6	(3)	34	(3)
Polyp	231	(23)	15	(7)	246	(20)
Other	751	(74)	197	(90)	948	(77)
Subtotal	1010		218		1228	
All screens						
GI cancer	92	(5)	17	(5)	109	(5)
Polyp	491	(27)	28	(8)	519	(24)
Other	1242	(68)	290	(87)	1532	(71)
Total	1825	(84)	335	(16)	2160	

[a] Two from each of three consecutive stools, by initial vs second and third screens (to date) by examination site, April 1977–June 1979.
[b] Examination protocols of varying procedural content.
[c] "Other" includes breast, lung, prostate, and other non-GI malignancies as well as carcinoma *in situ* and atypias of varying degrees. Twenty-five percent of the "other" findings are cases in which no probable cause of bleeding was found.

RESULTS

Examination of 2,160 patients revealed 109 (5%) cases with one or more GI malignancies (including two pancreatic cancers with secondary bleeding in the colon) and 519 (24%) cases with one or more polyps (Table 2). Moreover, 60.5% (64/92) of the cases with GI malignancies found at the University of Minnesota and 64.7% (11/17) of those diagnosed at other facilities were the result of the initial screen. Initial screen cases accounted for approximately 44% of all University of Minnesota examined cases and 34% of all "elsewhere" examined cases reported in Table 2. Other findings (71%) included lung, breast, and prostatic cancers, diverticulosis, hemorrhoids, and hiatus hernia (often in combination), and "normal findings."

Table 3 displays the distribution of 94 cancers by the Dukes' (12) classification diagnosed in 90 (the pancreatic first-degree malignancies omitted) cases examined at the University of Minnesota. A similar distribution of 17 malignancies diagnosed in 17 patients examined at other facilities is also seen. Patients examined at the University of Minnesota undergo examination according to the uniform

TABLE 3. *Dukes' classification[a] of 94 GI malignancies found in 90 cases examined at the University of Minnesota (study protocol) and 17 cases examined elsewhere (various protocols), April 1977–June 1979*

Tumor location	No. of cases	Dukes' classification			
		A	B	C	D
Examined U of M					
Single colon or rectum	82	52	13	13	4
Two colon	1	2	—	—	—
Two colon	1	2	—	—	—
Colon and appendix	1	—	—	1(C)	1(Ap)
Colon and stomach	1	2	—	—	—
2° colon	1	—	—	—	1
Stomach	3	1	—	1	1
Total cancers	94	59	13	15	7
%/Class		63%	14%	16%	7%
Total cases[b]	90				
Examined elsewhere					
Single colon or rectum	5	5	—	—	—
Single colon or rectum	5	—	5	—	—
Single colon or rectum	4	—	—	4	—
Single colon or rectum	3	—	—	—	3
Total cancers	17	5	5	4	3
%/Class		29%	29%	24%	18%
Total cases	17				

[a] The Dukes classification used to classify the malignancies in this study is A = tumor confined to the tissues of the wall but not reaching the extramural tissues; B = tumor extending through the wall (or serosa of colon) and involving the extramural tissues, but without lymph node metastases; C = tumor penetrating through intestinal wall with positive nodes; D = adjacent organ invasion, peritoneal seeding, or metastases to distant sites.

[b] 92 cases are shown in Table 3. The 2 cases omitted here are pancreatic cancer cases with bleeding into the gut.

protocol established at the beginning of the project (Table 1). Patients examined elsewhere have been examined by protocols of varying procedural content. The frequency of multiple malignancies discovered at the University versus single tumors found by other protocols, and differences in the proportions of malignancies by the Dukes classification between the two groups (Table 3) may reflect the difference in protocols.

ACKNOWLEDGMENTS

This research is supported in part by Contract NCI NO1-CB-53862, National Cancer Institute, and the Fraternal Order of Eagles.

We gratefully acknowledge the scientific contributions of Joseph Patrick Horstmann, M.D., Department of Surgical Pathology, University of Minnesota Medical Center.

REFERENCES

1. Boyd, N. F. (1978): A preliminary appraisal of the effects of length biased sampling and observer variability of screening. In: *Screening in Cancer: A Report of a UICC International Workshop, Toronto, Canada, April, 1978*, edited by A. B. Miller, pp. 40–49. International Union Against Cancer, Geneva.
2. Breslow, L., Thomas, L., Upton, X. (1977): Mammography in screening for breast cancer: Group reports. Report of the National Cancer Institute Ad Hoc Pathology Working Group to Review the Growth and Microscopic Findings of Breast Cancer Cases in the HIP Study, 59:521–530.
3. Cholko, J. J. (1977): Modification in Hemoccult test. *Manufacturers Memorandum*. Smith-Kline Diagnostics, Sunnyvale, CA.
4. Enstrom, J. E., and Austin, D. F. (1977): Interpreting cancer survival rates. *Science*, 195:847–851.
5. Gilbertsen, V., Church, T., Grewe, F., Mandel, J., McHugh R., Schuman, L., and Williams, S. (1980): The design of a study to assess occult blood screening for colon cancer. *J. Chronic Dis. (in press)*.
6. Gilbertsen, V., Williams, S., Schuman, L., and McHugh, R. (1979): Colonoscopy in the detection of carcinoma of the intestine. *Surg. Gynecol. Obstet.*, 149:877–878.
7. Gray, N. (1978): Screening for colo-rectal cancer. In: *Screening in Cancer: A Report of a UICC International Workshop, Toronto, Canada, April, 1978*, edited by A. B. Miller, pp. 306–307. International Union Against Cancer, Geneva.
8. Greener, D. (1969): Detection of silent colon cancer in routine examination. *CA*, 19–20:332.
9. Ostrow, J. (1979): More on relative usefulness of two tests for occult blood in stool. *Clin. Chem.*, 25:338.
10. Ostrow, J., Mulvaney, V., Hansell, J., and Rhodes, R. (1973): Sensitivity and reproducibility of chemical tests for fecal occult blood with an emphasis on false-positive reactions. *Am. J. Dig. Dis.*, 18:930–940.
11. Prorok, P. (1980): Evaluation of programs for early detection of cancer. In: *Statistical Methods for Cancer Screening Studies*, edited by Richard Cornell. Marcel Dekker, New York *(in press)*.
12. Schottenfeld, D., Winawer, S., and Miller, D. (1978): Screening and early diagnosis of large bowel cancer. In: *Screening in Cancer: A Report of a UICC Workshop, Toronto, Canada, April, 1978*, edited by A. B. Miller, pp. 308–323. International Union Against Cancer, Geneva.
13. Taylor, W., and Fontana, R. (1972): Biometric design of the Mayo Lung Project for Early Detection and Localization of Bronchogenic Carcinoma. *Cancer*, 30:1344–1347.
14. Wells, H. (1978): Evaluation of tests for fecal occult Blood. *Clin. Chem.*, 24:2209.
15. Wells, H., and Pagano, J. (1977): Hemoccult™ test reversal of false negative results due to storage. *Gastroenterology*, 72:1148 (abst.).

Colorectal Cancer: Prevention, Epidemiology,
and Screening, edited by S. Winawer, D. Schottenfeld,
and P. Sherlock. Raven Press, New York © 1980.

Preliminary Report of Fecal Occult Blood Testing in Germany

F. W. Schwartz, H. Holstein, and J. G. Brecht

Zentralinstitut für die kassenärztliche Versorgung in der Bundesrepublik Deutschland,
Cologne, Federal Republic of Germany

In the Federal Republic of Germany, the early detection of cancer is now regulated by statute by the social health insurance which covers approximately 91% of the population. The law of 1971 provides that screening examinations for early detection of cancer shall be available to all women from the age of 30 and to all men from the age of 45. Participation is voluntary and free of charge. A committee formed jointly by representatives of doctors and the sickness insurance funds established details of the program. The committee decided to introduce the Hemoccult test into this program effective January 1, 1977 for both sexes over the ages of 45 (1–8).

In Table 1 (4), the participation by the population is listed: 36% of eligible women (6.4 million, including those under 45 years) took part in 1977 as did 18% of eligible men (1.5 million). The age distribution of the participants in relation to the age distribution of the eligible population showed that the degree of participation decreased with increasing age in both sexes, the reduction being greater for women.

Stool testing was carried out in nearly 98% of cases in the medical practices of several disciplines including surgeons, internists, urologists, general practitioners, and gynecologists. In order to obtain preliminary observations with the Hemoccult test, the physicians were requested (8) to enter results regarding the test on a general report form which has been used since 1975 but which has not yet been adapted to the Hemoccult. The test was completed by 2.5 million women, mostly over 45 years, and by almost one million men (Table 3).

TABLE 1. *Participation in cancer screening: Federal Republic of Germany, 1977[a]*

Sex	Persons eligible	Persons examined	
		No.	%
Women	17.98	6.42	35.7
Men	8.11	1.47	18.1

[a] All numbers given in millions.

TABLE 2. *Hemoccult studies*

Reference	No. tested	Lower age limit	Average age	% Positive tests (No.)	Cases investigated	% Colorectal carcinomas (No.)
			A. Up to 1976			
3	5,016	> 40	—	2.1 (136)	117	11.1 (13)[a]
14	1,400	> 45	—	3.3 (46)	—	10.9 (5)[b]
12	1,103	—	—	ca. 5 (—)	—	ca. 7.3 (4)[b]
9	1,082 W 580 M 502	27	W 65.7 M 61.4	3.0 (32)	All	25.0 (8)[b]
6	1,600 (Volun.)	—	—	2.4 (39)	37	8.1 (3)[a]
	6,400 (Patients)	—	—	3.8 (243)	181	16.0 (29)[a]
			B. After 1976			
11	821 (Only women)	21	> 50[e]	3.5 (29)	All	10.3 (3)[d]
15[c]	11,505	—	—	1 (—)	—	ca. 8.7 (10)[b]
10 (Poll)	30,858 (Practice)	—	—	1.53 (472)	—	11.7 (55)[b]
13	W 2.4m (Practice)	(30)	Median = 54.5	1.0 (22,237)	2,084[f]	4.7 (98)[a]
	M 1.1m (Practice)	(45)	Median = 57.9	1.5 (15,795)	2,178[f]	10.7 (234)[7,8]

[a] 100 = all clarified cases.
[b] 100 = all positive cases.
[c] Cited according to Goerttler (ed.) (5).
[d] Incomplete result.
[e] Estimated on basis of 10-year classes.
[f] Selection: all cases with documented result of clarification.

TABLE 3. *Participation in the Hemoccult test, 1977*

Sex	Persons examined	Hemoccult participants	
		No.	%
Women	6,417,564	2,419,421	37.7
Men	1,468,666	1,057,961	72.1

RESULTS

Results may be seen in Table 4. The test was positive in almost 1% of women and 1.5% of the men tested. The recommendation to our doctors is that all positive screened patients should undergo further testing based on rectoscopy, barium enema with air contrast, and if these are negative, colonoscopy.

Table 5 shows the results of diagnostic testing for all cases of documentation. Confirmed carcinomas were documented by the physicians in 4.7% of the positive tests among women, and in 10.7% of the positive tests among men. In this evaluation, it was not possible to confirm the presence of polyps or nonmalignant sources of bleeding.

There was no significant difference in the age distribution between the population entered and the cases with positive tests.

TABLE 4. *Result of the Hemoccult test, 1977*

Sex	Hemoccult participants	Hemoccult positive	
		No.	%
Women	2,419,421	22,237	0.92
Men	1,057,961	15,793	1.49

TABLE 5. *Result of investigated positive Hemoccult tests, 1977*

Sex	No. with confirmed test	Carcinomas confirmed	
		No.	%
Women	2,084	98	4.7
Men	2,178	234	10.7

COMMENT

Comparison with national and international studies of these first results obtained under purely practical mass screening conditions shows an adequate agreement in important parameters. The rate of positive test results was generally lower when testing was done outside hospitals than when testing was done with hospital patients. Our observations are only preliminary, but we consider them to indicate that the test is feasible for mass screening. From 1980 onwards, more extensive evaluations will be made as a result of the incorporation of a reporting system.

REFERENCES

1. Durst, J., Neumann, G., and Schmidt, K. (1976): Okkultes Blut im Stuhl—ein Feldversuch im Rahmen der Krebsfrüherkennung. *Dtsch. Med. Wochenschr.,* 101:440–443.
2. Frühmorgen, P., and Demling, L. (1978): Erste Ergebnisse einer prospektiven Feldstudie mit einem modifizierten Guajak-Test zum Nachweis von okkultem Blut im Stuhl. In: *Kolorektale Krebsvorsorge,* edited by K. Goerttler, pp. 68–72, 2nd ed. Nürnberg.
3. Frühmorgen, P. (1976): Okkultes Blut im Stuhl. *Dtsch. Med. Wochenschr.,* 101:872–873.
4. Gesetzliche Krankheits-Früherkennungsmaßnahmen-Dokumentation der Untersuchungsergebnisse (1977): Männer und Frauen—herausgegeben von den Spitzenverbänden der Krankenkassen und der Kassenärztlichen Bundesvereinigung.
5. Gnauck, R. (1978): Die Treffsicherheit des Haemoccult-Screening, *Kolorektale Krebsvorsorge,* edited by K. Goerttler, pp. 73–80, 2nd ed. Nürnberg.
6. Gnauck, R. (1977): Dickdarmkarzinom-Screening mit Haemoccult. *Leber Margen Darm,* 7:32–35.
7. Greegor, D. H. (1967): Diagnosis of large-bowel cancer in the asymptomatic patient. *J.A.M.A.,* 201:943–945.
8. Kassenärztliche Bundesvereinigung (1976): Schnelltest auf occultes Blut im Stuhl mittels Testbriefen (modifizierter Guajac-Test nach Greegor) im Rahmen der gesetzlichen Krebsfrüherkennungs-Maßnahmen. *Merkblatt Nr.* 13.
9. Kunz, O., Siegel, P. (1976): Suchtest für okkulte Blutungen aus dem Dickdarm. *Therapie d. Gegenwart,* 115:1040–1048.
10. Otto, P. H., Bunnemann, H. (1977): Erste Erfahrungen bei der klinischen Abklärung positiver Haemoccult-Tests im Rahmen der neuen kolorektalen Krebsvorsorge im ersten Halbjahr 1977. In: *Kolorektale Krebsvorsorge,* edited by K. Goerttler, pp. 102–109, 2nd ed. Nürnberg.
11. Riedel, H., et al. (1977): Haemoccult-Teststudie im Rahmen der gynäkologischen Vorsorgeuntersuchungen. *Geburtshilfe u. Frauenheilkunde,* 37:27–35.
12. Ross, T. H., Johnson, J. C. M. (1976): Detecting colorectal cancer. *Arizona Med.,* 38:445.
13. Schwartz, F. W., et al. (1977): Vorliegendes Referat (eigenes Zahlenmaterial, Bundesrepublik).
14. Warm, K., et al. (1977): Modifizierte Guajakprobe zur Früherkennung von Tumoren des Verdauungstraktes. *Münch. Med. Wochenschr.,* 119.
15. Winawer, S. J. (1977): Results of a screening program for the detection of early colon cancer and polyps using fecal occult blood testing. *Digestive Week,* Toronto.

Colorectal Cancer: Prevention, Epidemiology, and Screening, edited by S. Winawer, D. Schottenfeld, and P. Sherlock. Raven Press, New York © 1980.

Role of Diet in Screening with Fecal Occult Blood Tests

Kerry Goulston

Gastroenterology Unit, Repatriation General Hospital, Concord 2139, Australia

BACKGROUND

The action of hemoglobin in facilitating oxidation of the chromogenic substrate is nonspecific, and may be mimicked by naturally occurring peroxidases present in the diet. False positive reactions may be due to either hemoglobin or muscle peroxidase present in red meat, poultry, and fish, or plant peroxidases present in fruit and vegetables (11). The peroxidase activity of red meat, dark poultry (e.g., pheasant), and dark fish (e.g., salmon, sardines) persists after boiling. It has been stated that this peroxidase activity is not destroyed by passage through the gastrointestinal tract (10,11), yet the peroxidase activity of blood itself has been shown to decrease sixfold in transit through the gastrointestinal tract (9). This loss of peroxidase activity is due to conversion of hemoglobin in protoporphyrin (19) and is accelerated *in vitro* by pancreatic juice (3) and trypsin (7,10,20); with the exception of turnip and horseradish, most plant peroxidases are destroyed by heat (10,11). It has been recommended that raw fruit and vegetables should be omitted from the diet because they may cause false positive reactions (10). Not all authorities agree. Some advise patients to consume copious quantities of raw fruit and vegetables during testing.

Earlier reports on the effect of iron medications on chemical fecal occult blood testing have been well summarized by Irons and Kirsner (11). Recently a good study detailed that iron medications and also laxatives and barium sulfate failed to produce false positive reactions (15).

It has been recommended empirically that testing be performed on a high roughage diet to decrease colonic transit time and stimulate colonic lesions to bleed (4,22).

Interfering substances, particularly reducing agents, may cause false negative reactions. A patient has been described who was found to have negative Hemoccult tests while taking 1 to 2 g ascorbic acid daily. On withdrawal of the ascorbic acid, all tests became strongly positive (12).

OUR STUDIES

The incidence of false positive and false negative Hemoccult reactions was determined using fecal samples containing blood quantitated by chromium-51 red blood cell labeling (1). We obtained 225 fecal samples from 40 patients on a normal diet, and 115 samples from 20 patients on a restricted diet. A diet was formulated on the basis of *in vitro* Hemoccult testing of 40 different foods. A wide variety of cooked and uncooked foods was homogenized, plated immediately on two hemoccult slides, and read by an independent observer. A diet excluding red meat, red fish such as salmon and tuna, offal meats, and most fresh fruit and vegetables was devised. Also, a high fiber content—bran, whole-grain bread, and nuts—was included in the diet. All salicylates, nonsteroidal antiinflammatory agents, and vitamin C supplements were suspended throughout the test period.

A single Hemoccult test was performed on each sample, and fecal blood quantitated by chromium-51 red cell labeling. On a normal diet, 11% of samples with less than 1.5 mg Hb/g gave a positive Hemoccult result. This was in agreement with previous studies which found positive rates of 8% (20) and 12% (15) on a normal diet.

On a restricted diet, only 2 of 100 samples (2%) containing less than 1.5 mg Hb/g gave a positive Hemoccult result. Although this effect of diet on positive rates for Hemoccult testing of occult blood in feces was significant ($p < 0.01$), there was no significant difference with respect to individual patients. When the results were analyzed with respect to individual patients, 10 of 40 patients on a normal diet gave false positive reactions, whereas 1 of 20 on the restricted diet gave a false positive reaction. In contrast to Hemoccult, Hematest (Ames) has a false positive rate of 18 to 35%, even on a restricted diet (8,17).

COMMENT

False positivity in Hemoccult testing may not be related to red meat in the diet (21). In fact, we have been unable to produce false positive Hemoccult tests in normal volunteers by a diet rich in red meat (K. Goulston, *unpublished observations*). It has been suggested that elimination of a meat-free diet may increase patient compliance in fecal occult blood testing. Our findings in 4,000 patients do not support this, as a similar compliance rate has been found in asymptomatic patients on a normal diet and on a restricted diet (K. Goulston and H. Gallagher, *unpublished data*).

As pointed out in a recent Lancet editorial (13), "frequently, papers on diagnostic methods cite the false-positive or false-negative rate, but these terms are highly ambiguous." A false positive fecal occult blood test may mean false positive due to an organic lesion other than colorectal cancer (that is, falsely positive for cancer), false positive due to a dietary or other interfering agent, a positive result yet no significant fecal blood measured by chromium-51 techniques. A "false" positive reaction must therefore be defined carefully by investigators. In screening programs, a positive Hemoccult reaction may occur in subjects without colorectal cancer. Investigators may report this as being due to dietary interference or other (noncancer) lesions such as colonic diverticula or hemorrhoids. In mass surveys of asymptomatic people, overall positive Hemoccult rates of 0.3 to 6.0% have been described (2,5,6,14,22).

Positive Hemoccult rates in asymptomatic subjects have been higher when tested on a normal diet (16,18). In screening asymptomatic people over 40 years of age, we have found an overall positive rate of 4.2% on a restricted diet (2,418 patients) compared with an overall positive rate of 5.5% on a normal diet (1,411 patients) (K. Goulston and H. Gallagher, *unpublished data*).

Because of this, and because of the results of comparing Hemoccult with chromium-51 red blood cell labeling estimations of fecal occult blood, we currently test all patients and screened populations on a restricted diet. The diet is restricted to avoid red meat, dark fish, offal meats, and most fresh fruit and vegetables. A high fiber content—bran, whole-grain bread, and nuts—is included in the diet. All salicylates, nonsteroidal anti-inflammatory agents, and vitamin C supplements are suspended through the test period.

We have shown that dietary restriction significantly lessens the false positive rate of Hemoccult on single fecal samples. Such dietary restriction has not significantly altered the false positive rate of Hemoccult II in screening patients— reducing the overall positive rate from 5.5 to 4.2% in our hands. However, we agree with Winawer (21) that even this small reduction may be important in reducing the number of the screened population subjected to unnecessary investigations. Therefore, it is our current practice to use Hemoccult with subjects on a restricted diet.

REFERENCES

1. Bassett, M. L., and Goulston, K. J. (1980): False positive and negative hemoccult reactions on a normal diet and effect of diet restriction. *Aust. N.Z. J. Med.,* 10:1–4.
2. Bond, J. H., and Gilbertsen, V. A. (1978): Early detection of colonic carcinoma by mass screening for occult stool blood: Preliminary report. *Gastroenterology,* 72, A–8:1031.
3. Bramkamp, R. G. (1929): The benizidine reaction: Some observations relating to its clinical application. *J. Lab. Clin. Med.,* 14:1087.
4. Greegor, D. H. (1971): Occult blood testing for detection of asymptomatic colon cancer. *Cancer,* 28:131–134.
5. Hastings, J. B. (1974): Mass screening for colorectal cancer. *Am. J. Surg.,* 127:228–233.
6. Helfrich, G. B., Petrucci, P., and Webb, H. (1977): Mass screening for colorectal cancer. *J.A.M.A.,* 238:1502.
7. Hepler, O. E., Wong, P., and Pihl, H. D. (1953): Comparison of tests for occult blood in feces. *Am. J. Clin. Pathol.,* 23:1263–1272.
8. Humphrey, T. B., and Goulston, K. J. (1969): Chemical testing of occult blood in faeces: Haematest, Occultest and guaiac testing correlated with 51 chromium estimation of faecal blood loss. *Med. J. Aust.,* 1:1291–1293.
9. Huntsman, R. G., and Liddell, J. (1961): Paper tests for occult blood in faeces and some observations on the fate of swallowed red cells. *J. Clin. Pathol.,* 14:436–438.
10. Illingworth, D. B. (1965): Influence of diet on occult blood tests. *Gut,* 6:595–598.

11. Irons, G. V., and Kirsner, J. B. (1965): Routine chemical tests of the stool for occult blood: An evaluation. *Am. J. Med. Sci.,* 249:247–260.
12. Jaffe, R. M., Kasten, B., Young, D. S., and MacLowry, J. D. (1975): False-negative stool occult blood tests caused by ingestion of ascorbic acid (vitamin C). *Ann. Intern. Med.,* 83:824–26.
13. *Lancet* Editorial (1979): The value of diagnostic tests. *Lancet,* 2:809–810.
14. Miller, S. R., and Knight, A. R. (1979): The early detection of colorectal cancer. *Cancer,* 40:945.
15. Morris, D. W., Hansell, J. R., Ostrow, J. D., and Lee, C. S. (1976): Reliability of chemical tests for fecal occult blood in hospitalized patients. *Am. J. Dig. Dis.,* 21:845–852.
16. Norfleet, R. G., and Roberts, R. C. (1979): Hemoccult screening for colonic neoplasms: report of a pilot project. *Wisc. Med. J.,* 78:25.
17. Ostrow, J. D., Mulvaney, C. A., Hansell, J. R., and Rhodes, R. S. (1973): Sensitivity and reproducibility of chemical tests for fecal occult blood with an emphasis on false-positive reactions. *Am. J. Dig. Dis.,* 18:930–940.
18. Ross, T. H., and Johnson, J. C. M. (1976): Detecting colorectal cancer. *Ariz. Med.,* 33:445–448.
19. Steingold, L., and Roberts, A. (1961): Laboratory diagnosis of gastrointestinal bleeding. *Gut,* 2:75–81.
20. Stroehlein, J. R., Fairbanks, V. F., McGill, D. B., and Go, V. L. M. (1976): Hemoccult detection of fecal occult blood quantitated by radioassay. *Am. J. Dig. Dis.,* 21:841–844.
21. Winawer, S. J. (1976): Fecal occult blood testing. *Am. J. Dig. Dis.,* 21:885–888.
22. Winawer, S. J., Miller, D. G., Schottenfeld, D., Leidner, S. D., Sherlock, P., Befler, B., and Stearns, M. W. (1977): Feasibility of faecal occult blood testing for detection of colorectal neoplasia. *Cancer,* 40:2616–2619.

Colorectal Cancer: Prevention, Epidemiology,
and Screening, edited by S. Winawer, D. Schottenfeld,
and P. Sherlock. Raven Press, New York © 1980.

Selective Screening for Colorectal Tumors in the Tel-Aviv Area: Technique and Initial Results

Paul Rozen, Zvi Fireman, Reuven Terdiman, *Shlomo M. Hellerstein, Jacob Rattan, and Tuvia Gilat

*Gastroenterology Department, Municipal Governmental Medical Center, Ichilov Hospital; Tel-Aviv University Sackler School of Medicine, Tel-Aviv, Israel; and *Department of Internal Medicine, Kaplan Hospital, Rehovot, Israel*

The incidence of colorectal cancer in Israel is lower than that found in the United States: 31.8 cases compared to 54.2 in Connecticut per 100,000 females, ages 35 to 64 years, 1967–1971, and is similar to that of Europe (9,15). Initial analysis of more recent data on large bowel cancer in Israel has shown only a slight increase in incidence during 1972–75 (Table 1). Even so, in Israel, it is the most common malignancy after breast cancer in females and lung cancer in males. Notable is the fact that European-American born Israeli Jews are much more commonly afflicted by this disease than other immigrant groups (Table 1). This disparity in incidence probably reflects differences in dietary habits as well as possible genetic influences. Israeli Jews consume more carbohydrate and fiber and less fat and meat than the American population, whereas Ashkenazim (Jews of European and American origin) eat more meat, milk, and eggs than non-Ashkenazim who use more non-meat protein. Within the Israeli-born population, the differences in dietary habits between the ethnic groups become blurred, and the colon cancer rates for males approach those of the European-American born (9). The calculated colorectal cancer incidence in Tel-Aviv city for all ages, male and female, is 73.2 cases per 100,000, 1970–1973. This high figure is due to the large proportion, 67%, of elderly Ashkenazi Jews in this area.

The clinical pattern of the disease in Israel is classic with less than half the cases being diagnosed at the stage where the tumor is confined to the bowel. The overall 5-year survival rate for a group of 161 patients from the Tel-Aviv area studied retrospectively was only 37% (11). This low figure is partly explained by the 8 months average duration of symptoms before diagnosis. This is about twice as long as in other reported series and indicates a low level of patient-doctor alertness for the disease.

For these reasons we felt that a pilot screening program for detecting colon tumors was justified (17). However, considering the efforts and costs involved, it should be selective and aimed at those groups where we could expect a higher

TABLE 1. *Selected data on colorectal cancer in Israel and Tel-Aviv*

Population (males and females)	Ages	Years	Incidence/100,000
All Jews	35–64	1967–71	31.4[a]
" "	"	1972–75	35[b]
European–U.S.A. born	"	1967–71	34.2[a]
African–Asian born	"	" "	14.6[a]
Israel born	"	" "	27.3[a]
Tel-Aviv			
European–U.S.A. born	45–64	1970–73	25.4[b]
" " "	All ages	" "	73.2[b]

[a] From Katz and Steinitz (9).
[b] Unpublished figures.

than usual yield. The criteria for selecting these groups were based on the above mentioned high incidence of colon cancer in Tel-Aviv in general and specifically in European, U.S.A., and Israel born Jews together with the recognized importance of the family history of tumors especially colonic (1,3,12,13), past history of cured colon (4) or female genital tumors (13,17), or a history of inflammatory bowel disease (5).

The screening technique was based on the detection of fecal occult blood (7,16) and/or direct inspection of the colon (6,18). The latter was used when the risk of colorectal tumors was especially high, using usually flexible sigmoidoscopy which we believed would increase patient acceptability for the procedure and increase the yield of nonbleeding tumors (14,17).

During the last 12 months, the importance of the screening program was brought out by publicity in newspaper and radio programs devoted to medical topics and meetings of general and hospital physicians.

MATERIALS AND METHODS

Population Examined

This included a "control," asymptomatic population (group 1), and four "high-risk" groups (Table 2).

Group 1

Asymptomatic Jewish population aged 35 to 65 years born in Israel, Europe, or America. This included two volunteer groups: (a) Residents of Tel-Aviv city who visited the Gastroenterology Clinic or were hospitalized for noncolonic symptoms and did not have a known family history of colon cancer. (b) All the adult members of a long- and well-established kibbutz (communal farm), irrespective of their family history, whose members are mainly European born.

TABLE 2. *Screening protocol and tests performed*

Group	Hemoccult	Flexible sigmoidoscopy	Colonoscopy
1. a. Asymptomatic Tel-Aviv residents	Yes	Yes	Only if prior test(s) positive
b. Kibbutz members	Yes	No	"
2. Family history of colon cancer	Yes	Yes	"
3. History of colon tumor[a]	No	No	Yes
4. History of IBD[b]	No	No	Yes
5. History of female genital tumors[c]	Yes	Yes	Only if prior test(s) positive

[a] Polyp or colon cancer, Dukes' A or B_1.
[b] Ulcerative colitis or Crohn's disease.
[c] Clinically "cured."

Group 2

Adult, first-degree relatives of patients with colon cancer or polyps. Using the hospital, Gastroenterology Clinic, and Oncology Department records for the last 5 years, we sent a letter of explanation to the families. Changes in address, language difficulties, and deaths limited the response. Another important limiting factor was the large number of patients with no available family due to the destruction and dispersion of European Jewry during World War II.

Group 3

Patients with a history of colon polyps during the last 5 years or with colon cancer limited to the bowel wall (Dukes B_1) or having survived 5 years with no evidence of disease were recalled for examination. They were identified by using the hospital, Gastroenterology Clinic, and Oncology Department records.

Group 4

All patients with inflammatory bowel disease were entered into the study and some were recalled especially for this purpose.

Group 5

Patients with curable or "cured" breast, uterus, or ovarian cancer have been selected for examination using the hospital and Oncology Department records. They are now being recalled for colon tumor screening.

Screening and Diagnostic Techniques (Table 2)

Fecal occult blood tests were performed using Hemoccult or Hemoccult II; the standard method of 6 examinations over 3 days was used (17). The patients were given a high residue diet but no restriction was made on the eating of poultry which is the most commonly eaten meat; its kosher preparation makes it virtually blood-free. Aspirin and other ulcerogenic drugs were stopped. The completed tests were examined invariably on the fourth day by an experienced physician. This test was used for groups 1, 2, and 5 (asymptomatic controls, relatives of colon tumor patients, and women with a history of genital tumors).

Flexible sigmoidoscopy, using the Olympus TCF-1S or CF-MB, was also performed in groups 1a, 2, 5 (Asymptomatic controls living in Tel-Aviv city, relatives of colon tumor patients, and women with a history of genital tumors), because of their assumed higher risk of colon tumors.

Colonoscopy using the Olympus CF-LB or CF-LB3R was performed (after a double contrast barium enema) on groups 3 and 4 (past history of colon tumors or inflammatory bowel disease) and also whenever the Hemoccult test was positive or a tumor was detected by flexible sigmoidoscopy in any patient. Polyps were removed endoscopically, and lesions suspected to be malignant were biopsied and resected if necessary.

Data Recording and Analysis

All persons examined were interviewed by a physician or lay person instructed in the subject. The parameters recorded for computer input included identification number, country of birth (or of father for Israeli born) for epidemiological studies; family history of colon, other gastrointestinal, and nongastrointestinal tumors; and history of gallbladder disease, inflammatory bowel disease, colon tumors, rectal bleeding, and hemorrhoids.

The examining physician completed the computer forms with the results of the Hemoccult tests, sigmoidoscopy, barium enema, and colonoscopic examinations when performed. Similarly, the results of surgery and the pathology examination were recorded. The size and anatomical localization of all colon tumors were noted and all pathology specimens were personally reexamined.

The program for data processing was written in Basic language for a DEC-PDP 11/05 computer (with a 32 kw memory).

Results

During the last 12 months, 784 persons have been examined. This included 444 kibbutz members (out of 603 available adults) who have completed their Hemoccult examination (group 1b). Of the Kibbutz members, 9 had positive results (Table 3), and 5 had had their colonoscopic and roentgen examinations. Two patients with four colon tumors were found; one had a Dukes' A cancer, and the other tumors were benign polyps. Further data from this group (1b) are not yet available.

A further 340 persons have been examined. They included the following groups: group 1a, asymptomatic Tel-Aviv residents, 32.5%; group 2, family

TABLE 3. *Results of tumor screening*

Group	Hemoccult-positive, %	Polyps[a], %	Cancer[b], %	Tumors[c], %
1. a. Asymptomatic: Tel-Aviv	2.8	3	0.9	3
b. Kibbutz	2.0	0.7[d]	0.2[d]	0.5[d]
2. Family history of colon tumor	4	6	1.3	6
3. History of colon tumor	N.E.	51.6	12.9	61.3
4. History of IBD	N.E.	0	0	0

[a] Only having benign polyps.
[b] " " cancer.
[c] " " a benign polyp or cancer.
[d] Incomplete results.
N.E., not examined.

history of colon tumors, 45.2%; group 3, past history of colon tumors, 9.3%; group 4, past history of inflammatory bowel disease, 11.8%; group 5, past history of female genital tumors, 1.5%. This last group will not be considered further. The mean age was 48 years, the sexes were equally distributed, and 75.5% were born in Israel, Europe, or the United States (Table 4). The family history of one or more first-degree relatives with a colon tumor was positive in 47.6%; in those with other gastrointestinal tumors and nongastrointestinal tumors, family history was positive in 15.7% and 17.2%, respectively.

Hemoccult examination and flexible sigmoidoscopy were performed on 270 persons from groups 1a, 2, and 5 (Table 2). Six Hemoccult examinations were invariably performed and 10 persons had positive results. Flexible sigmoidoscopy to a mean depth of 48 cm $\pm$ 0.7 SE was carried out in the same persons. The number of tumor patients (cancer or polyps) found was 13, of whom almost two-thirds were detected only by flexible sigmoidoscopy (Table 5).

Colonoscopy was performed in 26.2% of the total population examined (Table 2). The tumor findings included 24 polyps less than 0.5 cm in diameter in 15 patients and 35 polyps greater than 0.5 cm in 16 patients. Histological examination of the 39 available polyps showed that 3 patients had hyperplastic polyps, 17 patients had 27 tubular adenomas, 9 patients had 10 mixed villotubular adenomas, and 2 had carcinoma *in situ*. Following surgery 2 patients were

TABLE 4. *Characteristics of population examined and of selected groups*

	Total population[a]	Controls[a]	Family history of colon tumors	History of colon tumors
Age (mean $\pm$ SE)	48 $\pm$ 0.7	51.1 $\pm$ 5.5	44.9 $\pm$ 8.6	59.2 $\pm$ 5.4
Males (%)	50.3	49.1	50.7	58.1
European–U.S.–Israel born (%)	75.5	75.9	78	74.2

[a] Excluding the kibbutz members (group 1b), whose data are not available.

TABLE 5. *Comparison of Hemoccult examination and flexible sigmoidoscopy in detecting rectosigmoid tumors*

No.[a]	Hemoccult-positive, %	Tumor[b] patients, %	Patients with tumors found by sigmoidoscopy, %	
			Hemoccult-pos.	-neg.
270	3.7	4.8	1.8	3.0

[a] This includes the asymptomatic controls and those with a family history of colon tumors and history of female genital tumors.
[b] Benign and malignant tumors.

shown to have Dukes' B_2, 1 had Dukes' C, and 2 had Dukes' D colon cancer.

The screened population was then reanalyzed as described below (Tables 3, 4, and 6).

Controls (Group 1a)

This consisted of 110 persons, none of whom had a known family history of colon tumors. However, 26% had a family history of non-colon cancer in a first-degree relative. Rectal bleeding was noted by 27%, whereas 38% believed they had hemorrhoids. The Hemoccult examination was positive in 2.8%. Five polpys were found in 4 patients, 4 were tubular adenomas and 1 was mixed villotubular. One Dukes' C cancer was detected.

Group with Family History of Colon Tumor (Group 2)

This consisted of 156 persons, 8 of whom had a history of colon polyps in their immediate family; the others having had colon cancer. There were no proven cases of familial polyposis. There were 71 further first- and second-

TABLE 6. *Tumor findings*

	Controls	Family history of colon tumors	History of colon tumors
No. examined	110	156	31
Polyps			
<0.5 cm	2	5	16
>0.5 cm	3	11	20
Hyperplastic		1	1
Tubular	4	6	17
Villotubular	1	5	4
Cancer			
Carcinoma *in situ*		2	
Dukes' A			
B_1			
B_2			2
C	1		
D			2

degree relatives with 78 non-colon cancers in the patients' families. Rectal bleeding was noted by 19%, whereas 39% believed they had hemorrhoids. Hemoccult examination was positive in 4%. In 11 patients 16 polyps were found. Histological examination showed that 1 was hyperplastic, 6 tubular, 6 mixed villotubular, and 2 had carcinoma *in situ.*

Group with a History of Colon Polyps or Cancer (Group 3)

These 31 patients were significantly older than those in the previous two groups, 59.2 years, and males predominated (58%); 74% were European-United States-Israel born. One-third had a prior history of supposedly cured colon cancer (Dukes' A or B_1) and two-thirds a previous colon polyp. The lesions had been treated a mean of 3.6 years and 2 years, respectively, before recall. Colonoscopy was performed in all cases and 36 polyps were found in 16 patients. Histological examination showed that 1 was hyperplastic, 17 tubular, and 4 mixed, villotubular. Cancer was found in 4 patients, and laparotomy showed that 2 were Dukes' B_2 and 2 were Dukes' D. Over 60% of this group had a benign or malignant tumor detected.

Group with Inflammatory Bowel Disease (Group 4)

This included 39 patients, 70% of whom had ulcerative colitis, and the remainder had Crohn's disease. The extent of the disease involved more than the rectum and sigmoid in half the cases. The mean duration of disease was 6.5 years $\pm$ 1.2 SE. Colonoscopy and multiple biopsies were performed in all cases, and no evidence of malignancy was found in any patient.

DISCUSSION

In this pilot project we attempted to answer two questions. First, is such a screening program feasible in the Tel-Aviv area and second, were our criteria for selective screening valid? It would appear that an affirmative response to both questions is correct, but with some reservations.

In order to extend this pilot trial into the field of preventive medicine, a suitable body—whether governmental, municipal, or the local cancer society—must accept responsibility for organizational and financial details. The administrative and medical staff and facilities required for a preventive medical service are not within the province of a busy general hospital. However, it is possible to use existing facilities after work hours or those of self-sufficient rural communities (8) or large industrial complexes if finances are available for staff, equipment, and administrative expenses. We expect that after further experience, firm recommendations can be made regarding the future of this program.

Our selection of persons to be examined would seem to be justified. This is reflected in the positivity rate for the Hemoccult test in the kibbutz group, which is the usual 2%, but higher in the asymptomatic Tel-Aviv residents of

European origin and even higher in the colon tumor families. This is also reflected in the 3% and 6% tumor rates found, respectively. These rates are higher than would be expected from random screening (17).

We did learn that it is difficult to find adult members of colon tumor families because of the large number of cancer patients without available adult relatives. The age group aimed at was low starting from 35 years, in order to find and remove premalignant polyps (6). The response of the 30- to 40-year-olds was encouraging (Table 4), but the more suitable ages, 45 to 55, were not available and/or were unwilling to enter a preventive medical program.

The high tumor yield in patients with a previous history of treatable colon tumors reconfirms that this group must remain under constant medical supervision based on direct inspection of the total colon (4). In contrast, as we have already found, inflammatory bowel disease in Israel is associated at present with a low incidence of malignant changes (5). However, we will continue to keep this group under close supervision looking for premalignant changes in routine yearly biopsies.

As known, a significant number of rectosigmoid tumors are found in Hemoccult-negative patients by routine sigmoidoscopy (16). By using flexible sigmoidoscopy we obtained excellent patient compliance, increased significantly the area examined, and increased the tumor yield in the Hemoccult-negative population. By reaching the descending colon almost routinely, it is possible to examine the area that has at least 50% of the colon tumors (14). Hopefully, the Hemoccult examination helps detect bleeding tumors above this area (16). At present, in our framework, flexible sigmoidoscopy is practical only in selected persons due to the costs and efforts involved. Criteria for selection in our area would be the higher risk age group with a positive genetic and ethnic background.

The screening technique of careful patient selection, Hemoccult tests, and flexible sigmoidoscopy examination would seem to have increased the tumor yield significantly, thereby reducing costs. This has been described as "enrichment" (10) and may be applicable to other geographic areas of low and medium colon tumor incidence.

The tumor yield was mainly premalignant polyps of significant size. Notable is the low number of hyperplastic polyps, and this will require further confirmation. The number of cancers found was small, but the proportion of early and resectable cancers was higher than expected in Tel-Aviv. The cancer yield could probably be increased by searching for, and examining, an older population whom it is assumed would have a shift from benign to malignant tumors with increasing age. Even so, the usefulness of polypectomy in cancer prevention has been well established (6), and when the population at risk is identified, they can be kept under routine surveillance.

SUMMARY

In this pilot study of colon tumor screening involving 784 persons selected by using the epidemiological markers of age, geographic origin, family and/or past history of colon tumors, we obtained a high tumor yield. The screening method of Hemoccult examination was markedly improved by the routine use of flexible sigmoidoscopy. Our results are encouraging enough to warrant a further continuation of the program.

ACKNOWLEDGMENTS

Dr. T. Gilat is an Established Investigator of the Chief Scientist's Office, Ministry of Health, Israel; Dr. J. Rattan is a Recipient of a Canadian-Israel Cancer Research Fellowship. We express our appreciation to Mrs. Z. Samuels and the nursing staff of Kibbutz Givat Brenner for their assistance and to Drs. Katz and Steinitz of the Israel Cancer Registry for their help in calculating recent data.

REFERENCES

1. Anderson, D. E., and Romsdahl, M. M. (1977): Family history: A criterion for selective screening. In: *Genetics of Human Cancer,* edited by J. J. Mulvihill, R. W. Miller, and J. F. Fraumeni, Jr., pp. 257–262. Raven Press, New York.
2. Bavly, S. (1972): *Levels of Nutrition in Israel 1968/69.* Central Bureau of Statistics, Special Services No 368, Jerusalem.
3. Bussey, H. J. R., Veale, A. M. D., and Morson, B. C. (1978): Genetics of gastrointestinal polyposis. *Gastroenterology,* 74:1325–1330.
4. Gabrielsson, N., Granqvist, S., and Ohlsén, H. (1976): Recurrent carcinoma of the colon in the anastomosis diagnosed by roentgen examination and colonoscopy. *Endoscopy,* 8:47–52.
5. Gilat, T., Zemishlany, Z., Ribak, J., Benaroya, Y., and Lilos, P. (1974): Ulcerative colitis in the Jewish population of Tel-Aviv-Yafo. II. The rarity of malignant degeneration. *Gastroenterology,* 68:933–938.
6. Gilbertsen, V. A., and Nelms, J. M. (1978): The prevention of invasive cancer of the rectum. *Cancer,* 41:1137–1139.
7. Gnauk, R. (1978): Hemoccult screening (letter to the editor). *Am. J. Dig. Dis.,* 23:569.
8. Heeb, M. A., and Ahlvin, R. C. (1978): Screening for colorectal cancer in a rural area. *Surgery,* 83:540–541.
9. Katz, L., and Steinitz, R. (eds.) (1977): *Cancer in Israel, Facts and Figures.* State of Israel Publication, Jerusalem.
10. Kristein, M. M. (1979): A model of the cost effectiveness of screening with fecal occult blood testing. Proceedings of the International Symposium on Colorectal Cancer, New York.
11. Krotowski, M. (1976): Factors affecting prognosis in patients with carcinoma of the colon and rectum. Thesis, Sackler School of Medicine, Tel-Aviv, Israel.
12. Lynch, H. T., Brodkey, F. D., Lynch, P., Lynch, J., Maloney, K., Rankin, L., Kraft, C., Swartz, M., Westercamp, T., and Guirgis, H. A. (1976): Family risk and cancer control. *JAMA,* 236:582–584.
13. Lynch, H. T., Harris, R. E., Lynch, P. M., Guirgis, H. A., Lynch, J. F., and Bardawil, W. A. (1977): Role of heredity in multiple primary cancer. *Cancer,* 40:1849–1854.
14. Rhodes, J. B., Holmes, F. F., and Clark, G. M. (1977): Changing distribution of primary cancers in the large bowel. *JAMA,* 238:1641–1643.
15. Waterhouse, J. A. H., Muir, C. S., Correa, P., and Powell, J. (eds.) (1976): *Cancer Incidence in Five Continents, Vol. III.* IARC Scientific Publications, Lyon.
16. Winawer, S. J., Miller, D. G., Schottenfeld, D., Leidner, S. D., Sherlock, P., Befler, B., and Stearns, Jr., M. W. (1977): Feasibility of fecal occult-blood testing for detection of colorectal neoplasia. *Cancer,* 40:2616–2619.
17. Winawer, S. J., Sherlock, P., Schottenfeld, D., and Miller, D. (1976): Screening for colon cancer. *Gastroenterology,* 70:783–789.
18. Woolf, W. I., and Shinya, H. (1974): Earlier diagnosis of cancer of the colon through colonic endoscopy (colonoscopy). *Cancer,* 34:912-931.

Colorectal Cancer: Prevention, Epidemiology,
and Screening, edited by S. Winawer, D. Schottenfeld,
and P. Sherlock. Raven Press, New York © 1980.

Computer Models and the Evaluation of Colon Cancer Screening Programs

David M. Eddy

Engineering-Economic Systems, Terman Engineering Center, Stanford University,
Stanford, California 94305

THE PROBLEM

As physicians and policy makers, we constantly face difficult questions concerning the use of medical procedures. The case of colon cancer screening is typical. Should we recommend that all persons over 50 have an annual Hemoccult test? What is the health impact and what are the costs of such a program? Would it be preferable to recommend a different initial age or frequency? If a proctosigmoidoscopy were added, how would this change our recommendations? Should a flexible proctosigmoidoscope be used instead of the rigid model? What research should be done to help answer these questions? And what should we do in the interim, before the research results are available?

One way to estimate the most effective and efficient screening program is trial and observation. It would be ideal to have information from randomized clinical trials (RCTs) of each program option in each clinical setting, and to count empirically the costs and benefits in each case. But this is clearly impossible. Such research is expensive and time consuming, and our observations would be made obsolescent by any changes in the technology of screening, diagnosis, or treatment. There is simply neither the time nor the money to conduct 10- to 15-year multimillion dollar RCTs on all the interesting clinical options. To make today's decisions and to design today's research, it will be necessary to analyze all the information and insights we now have so as to understand the structure and behavior of the problem. We must use this information to design interim policies and to set research priorities that strike at the most important points of uncertainty.

AN APPROACH

One way to do this is to use a mathematical model that integrates and generalizes the lessons of clinical research and clinical judgment. The basic steps are to define the main components of the problem, identify the relationships between the components, and translate those relationships into quantitative terms. Many sources supply good information about different components of the problem. By constructing a unifying analytical framework, it is possible to explore the relative importance of each factor, to estimate the costs and effectiveness of various screening program options given today's information, and to determine the value of collecting better information. The model is a planning tool. It does not generate answers. It generates insights and understanding, which, when combined with existing research results and clinical experience, can help rationalize the design of future research programs and clinical policies.

A MODEL OF COLON CANCER SCREENING

A model of colon cancer screening has been constructed. It allows one to trace the expected fate of a patient under various program options, or, alternatively, it can be viewed as tracing the fates of a large population of patients. It is programmed on a computer with which health planners can interact, specifying patient characteristics, program options, and other important factors, and receiving information about the effectiveness and costs of the selected program. The following is a brief description of the model and some of the main assumptions. A complete description is available in Eddy (2).

Clinical Dynamics

The clinical dynamics of screening for cancer of the colon are extremely complicated. There are four main features that must be incorporated in any model of this disease if it is to be realistic.

1. Three screening tests can be offered: a digital examination of the rectal area, a sigmoidoscopy, and a test for occult blood in the stool. This means that there are four ways that a malignant lesion can come to clinical attention in a screening program: through one of the three tests at a screening session, and through self-referral by the patient for symptoms in the interval between sessions.

2. Two types of lesions must be analyzed. It seems undeniable that some invasive carcinomas of the colon come from adenomatous polyps. It is also undeniable that some invasive lesions are not preceded by a polypoid stage, but rather arise *de novo* from the mucosa. The mathematical model must be able to analyze the impact of screening given different assumptions about these two sources of invasive cancers.

3. The screening tests search different areas of the colon. A digital examination can reach 7 to 10 cm up the rectum, depending on the technique of the examiner. A sigmoidoscopy can potentially examine the distal 25 cm of the large bowel. Occult blood tests can be positive if there is bleeding anywhere in the colon, or elsewhere in the gastrointestional tract for that matter, at the time of testing.

4. Lesions do not occur at the same frequency in all regions.

Screening Scenarios

To understand fully the complexity forced by these features, consider the following scenario. It is August 3, and an asymptomatic 60-year-old man is about to be screened. His records reveal that on August 3, three years ago, he had a benign polyp discovered by sigmoidoscopy and removed, the area examined having been 25 cm. On August 3, two years ago, he had a negative test for occult blood in the stool. And on October 3, ten months ago, his family physician performed a rectal examination and found nothing. To analyze the value of various screening programs we must be able to estimate many numbers. For example, what is the chance that a digital examination today will reveal a polyp or an invasive lesion, and, if a lesion is discovered, how far advanced will it be? To calculate these the following facts must be taken into account: (a) the distal 25 cm was negative 3 years ago to a sigmoidoscopic examination, which has a certain effectiveness in detecting malignant lesions; (b) 2 years ago there was no occult bleeding as determined by the Hemoccult test, which has its own effectiveness; (c) a digital examination, again with its own effectiveness, was negative 10 months ago; and (d) the patient, whose biological and psychological behavior has given him a certain propensity to delay in seeking care, has not sought care for symptoms or signs of colon cancer.

Put another way, (a) the rectal region (last 10 cm) was screened by a digital examination 10 months ago, by a sigmoidoscope 3 years ago, by an occult blood test 2 years ago, and by the patient himself today; (b) the region from 25 cm to 10 cm was screened by a sigmoidoscope 3 years ago, by an occult blood test 2 years ago, and by the patient himself today; and (c) the area of the colon higher than 25 cm was screened by an occult blood test 2 years ago, and by the patient himself today. If the practitioner's digital examination is negative today and sigmoidoscopic examination is done, the probability of a true positive result will depend on the same facts, except that the timing of the last negative rectal examination has changed; it was negative an instant ago. Notice that the sigmoidoscope might still detect a lesion in the rectum, because this test may have a different occult interval than the digital examination. Now suppose that the sigmoidoscopy is negative and that 8 months from now an occult blood test is performed. These scenarios are complicated, but they are reasonable, and mathematical formulas have been developed to analyze them.

DESCRIPTION OF THE COMPUTER MODEL

Model Inputs

The model integrates information about the following inputs.

1. Patient age and sex
2. Patient relative risk category

3. Age- and sex-specific colon cancer incidence rates
4. Age- and sex-specific mortality rates from other causes of death
5. Complication rates of diagnostic and therapeutic procedures (e.g., the perforation rate of a proctosigmoidoscopy)
6. The effectiveness of a Hemoccult test
7. The effectiveness of a digital rectal examination
8. The effectiveness of a sigmoidoscopy
9. The effectiveness of therapy
10. Assumptions about the proportion of invasive malignant lesions that come from polyps
11. Assumptions about the proportion of polyps that will eventually become malignant
12. Assumptions about the proportion of malignant lesions that develop in the three main regions: the distal 10 cm, 25 to 10 cm from the anus, and the region proximal to 25 cm from the anus
13. The times of previous applications of each screening test
14. The planned schedule of future digital rectal examinations
15. The planned schedule of future Hemoccult tests
16. The planned schedule of future sigmoidoscopies

Model Outputs

Given any values for these inputs, we can obtain estimates of the following clinical information. This list is not exhaustive.

1. The probability that the patient will be diagnosed as having colon cancer in any given year in the future
2. The probability that the patient will be a surviving colon cancer patient during any year in the future
3. The probability that the patient will die of colon cancer in any year
4. The probability that the patient will die of other causes in any year. From the above we can calculate the 5, 10, 15 . . . -year survival rates, and the patient's life expectancy.
5. The probability that a patient will have a malignant lesion detected by a digital examination, an occult blood test, a sigmoidoscopy, or the patient himself in any given interval of time in the future
6. The survival rates (1 year, 5 year, 10 year, . . . any year) of patients given that their lesions were detected by any of these tests, or the patient himself, given any screening schedule
7. The probability that the patient will have a biopsy in any year
8. A comparison of the mortality rate of a lesion detected at a screening session with the mortality rate of that lesion if the patient postponed the screening appointment or waited until the lesion became symptomatic

If one prefers population statistics, these data can easily be presented in that form. For example, given a population of 100,000 50-year-old average-risk women, we can estimate the expected number of them who will be diagnosed as having colon cancer, and so forth.

Cost Model Inputs

This model can generate information to enable a health planner to evaluate the costs of a program. By assigning costs to any of the events, he can calculate the probability that any cost will be incurred in any interval of time. Inputs to the cost model are listed below:

1. Financial costs. To study the costs of the screening program options, a health planner can enter estimates for the financial costs of the following events:
   a. Digital examination of the rectum by a practitioner
   b. Hemoccult test
   c. Sigmoidoscopy
   d. Differential diagnosis of detected lesions
   e. Initial treatment of colon cancer
   f. Continuing care of a colon cancer patient (an annual cost)
   g. Terminal care of a patient dying of colon cancer
   h. Terminal care of a patient dying of other causes
   i. Death
2. Intangible costs. We can designate any units for the intangible costs of any of the events described above. These costs are extremely difficult to measure. We do not attempt to solve this problem here. But if we want to explore the intangible costs of a program, the model will generate the necessary data.
3. Discount rates. To find the present value of a time stream of future costs and benefits, a health planner can designate a discount rate. Any rate can be chosen and different rates can be assigned to different events.

Cost Model Outputs

These include the following:

1. The total expected cost of any of the events discussed above
2. The present value of the costs

These are only the most obvious cost calculations. The model generates a large amount of information about the probabilities of various events. This information can be tapped to help calculate the cost of virtually any situation in which a decision-maker is interested.

Some Specific Assumptions

This model has been used to estimate the costs and effectiveness of various screening programs. The estimates given in the tables to follow were based on the following main assumptions.

1. Seventy-five percent of invasive colon cancers come from polyps.
2. The duration of the premalignant polyp stage averages 7 years with a minimum of 1 month and a maximum of 14 years.
3. Five percent of all adenomas eventually become malignant.
4. About one-third of malignant lesions are within reach of a digital examination, and about two-thirds are within reach of a sigmoidoscope, but are not revealed.
5. Estimates of the effectiveness of the Hemoccult test are based on data from the University of Minnesota and Memorial Sloan-Kettering Cancer Center (1, 3; V. A. Gilbertsen, *personal communication*).
6. The false positive rate of the Hemoccult test is 1%.
7. The costs of some items are as follows:
   a. Hemoccult test—$2
   b. Sigmoidoscopy—$35
   c. Differential diagnosis—$350
   d. Initial therapy of colon cancer—$6,000
   e. Terminal care of colon cancer patient—$17,000
   f. Terminal care of patient dying of other causes—$10,000

Other data were obtained from standard sources (e.g., incidence rates were obtained from the Third National Cancer Survey).

SOME RESULTS

Costs and Effects of Various Programs

This model has been used to estimate some of the cost and effectiveness measures of colon cancer screening programs. Values of some of the outcome measures for various screening policies for a 50-year-old, average-risk woman are shown in Table 1. The results for males show slightly less effectiveness at slightly higher costs, because the mortality rates for other diseases are higher for men than they are for women, and the relative importance of colon cancer is lower. The two most important assumptions behind the data in Table 1 are that the false positive rate of the occult blood test is 1%, and that 75% of cancers come from adenomas. The importance of these assumptions will be discussed below. The estimated effectiveness of the occult blood test is based on an analysis of two controlled trials using a particular brand of occult blood test, the Hemoccult test.

The first and second columns of Table 1, labeled "Frequency of tests," define

TABLE 1. Values of outcome measures for various screening policies for a 50-year-old, average-risk woman

Frequency of tests (e.g., every x years)		Decrease in probability of diagnosis of colon cancer (%)	Increase in life expectancy (days)	Decrease in lost earnings (dollars)	Present value of program costs (dollars)	Difference (dollars)
Guaiac	Scope					
1	1	2.82	83.83	178.17	553.14	374.97
1	2	2.66	81.37	169.38	244.69	75.31
1	3	2.55	78.84	164.48	145.08	−19.40
1	4	2.43	76.71	160.34	98.60	−61.74
1	5	2.29	74.54	156.25	74.09	−82.16
1	never	.09	26.69	57.66	71.86	14.20
5	5	1.65	53.27	111.14	45.09	−66.05
2	4	1.68	64.80	135.06	77.63	−57.43

the screening program analyzed in each row. The entries give the number of years between screening tests. For example, entries "1, 2" designate a program consisting of an annual occult blood test and a biennial sigmoidoscopy. For brevity's sake, the term "scope" refers to a sigmoidoscopy and "guaiac" refers to an occult blood test. The third column shows the decrease in the probability that a patient will ever be diagnosed as having colon cancer. In the absence of a screening program, a 50-year-old female has about a 5% chance of ever being diagnosed as having colon cancer. Since a major benefit of screening is the removal of adenomas before they become malignant, and since it is assumed in this example that 75% of all colon cancers are preceded by an adenoma, the data in this column show a major decrease in morbidity from cancer. The fourth column shows the increase in life expectancy in days for all women who are screened. The savings in lost earnings are given in column 5. By postponing the time of death, the screenees have a longer productive life; this is reflected by a decrease in the amount of earnings lost due to premature death. Notice that this program concerns a 50-year-old female, and that the expected decrease in lost earnings for a male would be considerably higher. The present value of the financial costs of the screening program (discounted at 3%) is found in column 6; the "difference" is column 6 minus column 5.

In Fig. 1 the increases in life expectancy are compared to the present values of the screening program financial costs. With an annual occult blood test and a sigmoidoscopy every 5 years, about 89% of the increase in life expectancy is obtained at about 13% of the cost, compared with an annual occult blood test and a sigmoidoscopy every year.

Age to Initiate Screening

To determine the age at which screening with a sigmoidoscope should begin, let us view the problem from the standpoint of a 45-year-old woman who is

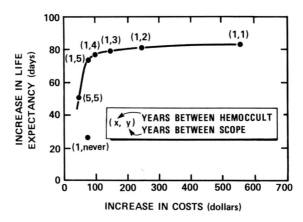

FIG. 1. Effect of screening a 50-year-old average-risk woman for colon cancer: life expectancy versus total program costs for different screening policies.

receiving an annual occult blood test and who must decide whether to begin receiving sigmoidoscopies now or wait to begin receiving this examination when she is 50 or 55 years old. Let the program consist of an annual occult blood test and a sigmoidoscopy every 5 years. If she never enters the program, the probability she will eventually be diagnosed as having colon cancer is about 5.06%. Table 2 shows the impact on some cost-effectiveness measures of starting the sigmoidoscopy at various ages.

This example assumes that the woman is receiving an occult blood test annually from age 45 on. The effect of starting this test at different ages could also be examined.

Some Sensitivity Analyses

Many factors affect the structure of a colon cancer screening program. Let us consider three important ones: the false positive rate of the occult blood test, the proportion of malignant lesions that come from polyps, and the costs of screening.

False Positive Rates

The false positive rate of the occult blood test has its main effect on the risks, pain, and costs of screening. For example, let us focus on the financial costs. The expense of tracking down a hidden source of bleeding can be great. In the literature, estimates of the proportion of people who do not have cancer or adenoma, but who do have positive tests, range from less than 1% to 10%. Among other things, this depends on the type of test used, the diet followed by the patient, and the circumstances of the study. There is evidence that with the Hemoccult test and with careful patient instruction, false positive rates can be kept in the range of 0.5 to 2%. The importance of a low false positive rate is shown in Table 3, which gives the life expectancy and present value of screening costs for a 50-year-old, average-risk woman under different assumptions about the proportion of noncancer patients who have positive Hemoccult tests. The screening program in this example is an annual Hemoccult test and a sigmoidoscopy every 5 years.

The importance of the false postive rate is obvious from this table.

Role of Adenomatous Polyps

Another important factor affecting screening is the role of adenomas in the genesis of malignant lesions. The results given above are based on the assumption that 75% of malignant lesions come from adenomas. However, as discussed above, there is considerable uncertainty about this number. One value of this screening theory is that we can examine the impact of different assumptions. For example, if only 25% of malignant lesions come from adenomatous polyps and 75% come directly and rapidly from the mucosa, we would expect to

TABLE 2. *Age to initiate sigmoidoscopy: cost-effectiveness measures, 45-year-old, average-risk woman*

Age to start sigmoidoscopy	Decrease in probability get cancer (%)	Increase in life expectancy (days)	Decrease in lost earnings (dollars)	Present value of program costs (dollars)	Difference (dollars)
45	2.34	81.80	194.58	109.40	−85.18
50	1.92	75.76	166.72	86.08	−80.64
55	1.82	67.96	137.10	71.73	−65.37

TABLE 3. *Effect of Hemoccult false positive rate: cost-effectiveness measures, 50-year-old, average-risk woman*

False positive rate (%)	Life expectancy (days)	Increase in cost of differential diagnosis (dollars)	Increase in present value of screening costs (dollars)
1	74.54	66.81	74.09
5	74.41	330.11	337.44
10	74.25	659.23	666.63

observe cost-effectiveness measures such as those in Table 4. These results are for a 50-year-old, average-risk woman who receives (a) an annual Hemoccult (with a false positive rate of 1%) and sigmoidoscopy, or (b) a Hemoccult annually and sigmoidoscopy every 5 years.

The changes in life expectancy and changes in program costs associated with these different assumptions about the Hemoccult false positive rate and the role of polyps are shown in Figs. 2 and 3. The points marked by squares are the points associated with different false positive rates (FP); the points marked by triangles are points generated by assuming that most malignant lesions (75%) arise *de novo* from the mucosa.

Financial Costs

The model generates information that can be used to explore the importance of uncertainty about the financial costs of different events. As an example, let us consider the present value of the cost of screening a 50-year-old, average-risk woman with an annual Hemoccult and a sigmoidoscopy every 5 years.

The first column of Table 5 gives the main events that have financial costs. "Hemoccult" refers to all the occasions that a Hemoccult test is given. "Scope" refers to the times a woman undergoes sigmoidoscopy. "Diff. diagnosis" refers to the occasions when a woman is worked-up for a positive finding at screening. This may represent either a true positive or false positive test result. The other three terms refer to the costs of delivering initial care to a patient who has colon cancer, of delivering terminal care to a patient who is dying of colon cancer, and of delivering terminal care to a patient who is dying of other causes. The second column of Table 5, labeled "Cost per unit," gives the cost for each event that was assumed when the results of Tables 1 through 4 were generated. The third column gives the present value of the expected financial cost of each event. The total of this column is the present value of the total expected cost of screening and treating a patient.

For example, the first item in this column says that $37.61 is the expected present value of delivering all the Hemoccult tests (at $2 per test) to a woman annually until she is either found to have colon cancer or dies. The fourth

TABLE 4. *Effect of different polyp/cancer assumptions: cost-effectiveness measures, 50-year-old, average-risk woman*

Frequency of tests (e.g., every x years)		Decrease in probability get cancer (%)	Increase in life expectancy (days)	Decrease in lost earnings (dollars)	Present value of program costs (dollars)	Difference (dollars)
"Hemoccult"	Scope					
1	1	1.19	72.84	153.09	627.27	474.70
1	5	0.59	48.15	103.01	166.79	63.78

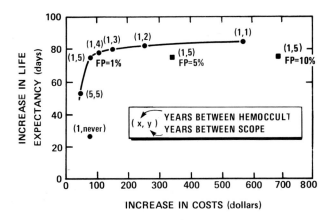

FIG. 2. Effect of screening a 50-year-old average-risk woman for colon cancer: life expectancy versus total program costs for different screening policies. Impact of Hemoccult false-positive rate.

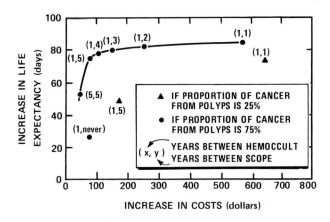

FIG. 3. Effect of screening a 50-year-old average-risk woman for colon cancer: life expectancy versus total program costs for different screening policies. Impact of different assumptions about the role of adenomatous polyps.

TABLE 5. *Costs of screening a 50-year-old, average-risk woman, annual Hemoccult test and sigmoidoscopy every 5 years*

Event	Cost per unit	Cost
Hemoccult	$2	$ 37.61
Scope	$35	$146.33
Diff. diagnosis	$350	$ 68.62
Early Ca Rx	$6,000	−$ 73.94
Term Ca Rx	$17,000	−$178.37
Other term Rx	$10,000	$ 73.84
Total expected cost		$ 74.09

item in this column says that an expected present value of $73.94 will be saved per patient by reducing the cost of initial therapy, because some polyps will be found and removed before they become malignant, and therapy is less expensive. Notice that all the costs and savings add up to the total expected cost of the program ($74.09) as given in the fifth row, sixth column of Table 1.

To explore the impact of different estimates of the financial costs of events, one starts with the second column of Table 5. For example, if a health planner believes that a sigmoidoscopy can be delivered for $20, which is 47% of the assumed cost of $35, then the entry in the third column can be changed to be 47% of $146.33, which is $83.62, and the revised third column added to get $11.38 as the total present value of the screening program. If a health planner believes that the cost of performing differential diagnosis on a patient who has a positive test result is $500, or 143% of the assumed value of $350, then the entry in the third column ($68.62) can be multiplied by 1.43 to get $98.13, and the revised third column added to get $103.60 as the total present value of the program. Thus, by examining Table 5 one can learn how each of the events that has financial costs contributes to the total financial cost of the program.

This discussion pertained to the costs of screening a 50-year-old, average-risk woman with an annual Hemoccult and a sigmoidoscopy every 5 years. A comparison with other policies (e.g., a sigmoidoscopy every year) requires that costs be reanalyzed for each policy; tables similar to Table 5 are available for doing this. When all the policies are reanalyzed, Tables 1 through 4 can be rewritten. These types of changes are reflected as shifts in the curves shown in Figs. 1, 2, and 3. It is interesting that different assumptions about costs may stretch or contract these curves, or move them to the right or left, but the basic shapes are unchanged—the bend always occurs near the point (1,5).

ACKNOWLEDGMENTS

The preparation of this report was supported by a grant from the Kaiser Family Foundation. Some of the work was performed for the Blue Cross/Blue Shield Association and the National Cancer Institute under Contract No. N01-CN-65371.

REFERENCES

1. Bond, J. H., and Gilbertsen, V. A. (1977): Early detection of colonic carcinoma by mass screening for occult stool blood: Preliminary report. *Gastroenterology,* 72:A-8/1031.
2. Eddy, D. M. (1980): *Screening for Cancer: Theory, Analysis and Design.* Prentice-Hall, Englewood Cliffs, N.J.
3. Winawer, S. J., Leidner, S. D., Miller, D. G., Schottenfeld, D., Befler, B., Kurtz, R. C., Sherlock, P., and Stearns, M., Jr. (1977): Results of a screening program for the detection of early colon cancer and polyps using fecal occult blood testing. *Gastroenterology,* 72:A-127/1150.

Colorectal Cancer: Prevention, Epidemiology, and Screening, edited by S. Winawer, D. Schottenfeld, and P. Sherlock. Raven Press, New York © 1980.

Issues of Patient Compliance

*M. Snyder Halper, **S. Winawer, **R. S. Brody, *M. Andrews, **D. Roth, and **G. Burton

*Preventive Medicine Institute-Strang Clinic, New York, New York 10016; and **Memorial Sloan-Kettering Cancer Center, New York, New York 10021*

The "Detection of Early Colon Cancer" program is a controlled trial of screening for colorectal cancer jointly sponsored by the Memorial Sloan-Kettering Cancer Center and Preventive Medicine Institute–Strang Clinic. In addition to undergoing rigid sigmoidoscopy, a segment of the Strang Clinic patient population has fecal occult blood testing as part of their comprehensive examination. They are asked to prepare six Hemoccult smears while on a meat-free, high fiber diet, and to bring them in on the day of their examination.

A part of this ongoing control trial is an investigation of factors related to patient compliance with fecal occult blood testing. An understanding of compliance is important from a cost-benefit viewpoint. Low compliance is incompatible with an efficient and cost-effective study. Noncompliant patients cannot benefit from screening procedures, and efforts to retrieve them are both costly and inefficient.

Patient compliance with the Hemoccult slide test, therefore, raises an essential issue: How can a reference population be motivated to participate in a colon cancer screening program? It is to address this issue and those of cost and efficiency that investigators of the Colon Cancer Screening Program felt a responsibility to study patient compliance. Our aim was not merely to monitor the rate of patient compliance, but rather also to try to begin to understand what causes compliance and noncompliance. In pursuit of this aim, we sought to identify major characteristics of those patients in our population who complied with Hemoccult slide preparation and those who did not and to compare these groups. We postulated that these data could help us comprehend the complex phenomenon of compliance and possibly improve it. The data also could be used to design effective and efficient guidelines for subsequent colon cancer screening programs, so that screening participation would be high and cost and efficiency maintained. Moreover, inasmuch as this program can be viewed as a possible prelude to larger efforts involving substantial segments of the general population, we hoped that our data could help shape strategies with an impact far beyond the confines of our limited project.

Until now, only three programs have addressed the issue of Hemoccult slide compliance. A recent American Cancer Society sponsored Lieberman Study evaluated the willingness of the public to perform the slide test. Using a variety of methods to distribute the slides to a randomly selected adult population, investigators found the average return rate for all methods to be only 15%. Even going into the home and leaving slides yielded a low 20% return rate (10). On the other hand, dealing with a well-motivated, self-selected population, enrolled in a clinical trial, Gilbertson *(this volume)* reported that 85% returned slides sent to them by mail. Similarly, our own program has reported overall compliance rates of 85% when patients were asked to prepare slides as part of their Strang examination (16).

Previous studies have indicated that compliers and noncompliers have different and identifiable characteristics. However, these studies showed that no single demographic variable was definitively linked with compliance (3,9). What seemed to emerge, though, was that patient perception is a crucial variable in explaining compliance. In particular, perceptions of symptoms, diseases, body sites, and regimens produce different emotional responses which seem to effect compliance (4,6–8).

A subsample of the study population was designated for a more in-depth analysis of their compliance beliefs and practices. In addition to a set of Hemoccult slides, this compliance population was asked to complete a special self-administered questionnaire relating to their perceptions of health behavior in general, and Hemoccult slide preparation in particular.

HEALTH BELIEF MODEL

Multiple factors are thought to determine whether a given individual follows a recommended health procedure, including health beliefs, socioeconomic status, age, family history, medical history, and media cues. And although no health or social science discipline has built an all-embracing body of theory to explain health behavior, several models and hypotheses are available as a means of understanding various health behaviors. Perhaps the best known and most widely respected is the Health Belief Model (1). Developed by Rosenstock (14) and based on some of the work of Lewin et al. (12), it seeks to explain health behaviors, including compliance, by relating the individual's perceptions to the likelihood of his taking action. The model hypothesizes that a decision to undertake a health action will not be made unless the individual is psychologically ready to take it. It tries to fit different factors related to health decision making into a sensible framework or "model" which summarizes items and explains compliance by highlighting the interactive or synergistic impact of the variables. Researchers using the model postulate that individuals or groups might be principally motivated by different combinations of variables, and it is in unlocking these combinations that behaviors, like compliance, can be better understood and possibly manipulated.

The following broad indices are commonly associated with the Health Belief

Model: general health motivation (i.e., concern about one's health and a sense of efficacy about one's capacity to improve it, belief in asymptomatology, past health practices), perceived susceptibility to disease, perceived severity of disease, perceived benefits from recommended health action, confidence in physicians and medical care, and perceived barriers to compliance (Table 1). Although no one factor is considered to be perfectly predictive of compliance, related variables in combination are thought to be capable of influencing individuals to be more ready or likely to comply with a recommended health action.

Researchers using the Health Belief Model report substantial evidence of its utility in explaining and predicting health action. In addition, the reliability of Health Belief measures has been validated by that research (13). Recently, for example, a study conducted to assess the construct convergent validity of the Health Belief Model variables indicated that they can be measured using a Likert scale or multiple choice questionnaire (5). By modifying these indices to the specific requirements of our own research on Hemoccult slide compliance, we were able to construct a compliance questionnaire using a five-point scale, multiple choice design.

DATA COLLECTION AND METHODOLOGY

The compliance study population was a subsample drawn from almost 22,000 Strang Clinic patients enrolled in the ongoing "Detection of Early Colon Cancer" program. This essentially well educated, middle class population was about 85% white and 15% black. Their decision to have the Strang examination can be taken as an indication of their high level of motivation. The compliance study subsample included all patients 40 years and older who presented themselves for the first time at Strang Clinic for a comprehensive physical examination from July 1978, through January 1979. This sample of 1,143 patients was sent the self-administered compliance questionnaire based on the Health Belief Model, as part of their regular appointment package.

Along with this questionnaire, patients were also sent the Strang Clinic health history questionnaire, instructions to prepare for the examination, six Hemoccult slides, sticks, and instructions to follow a special no-meat, high fiber bulk diet for the slide preparation. These instructions asked that the stool specimens be smeared with sticks onto the treated slide. Two smears were to be taken from different parts of the same bowel movement for three days for a total of six slides. Instructions stated simply that the slide test was "being evaluated by the National Cancer Institute as a method for the early detection of tumors of the colon." Both the compliance questionnaire and the Hemoccult slides were to be completed and brought with the patient on the day of his examination. For purposes of our analysis, we defined compliance as the completion of at least four out of six slides. Patients who had not been able to complete their slides in time for their examination were asked to mail them to us.

The compliance questionnaire consisted of 84 multiple choice questions. The

TABLE 1. *Health belief model*

Individual perceptions (level of readiness to take recommended action)	Modifying factors	Outcome
Motivation a. Belief in asymptomatology b. Perceived control over health matters c. Attitude and faith in medical care d. General health concern **Value of threat reduction** a. Perceived severity of disease b. Perceived susceptibility c. Belief in interference of disease with aspects of daily life **Probability of action reducing the threat** a. Belief in benefit of the action b. Perceived efficacy of test, regimen c. Belief in modern medicine	**General** a. Demographic variables b. Psychosocial variables c. Personal and family history d. Experiences with disease in question (site) e. Past experience with medical care f. Access to medical care Readiness to take recommended health action **Cues to action** a. Mass media campaign b. Symptoms c. Peer group pressure d. Letters or phone calls from medical facility e. Illness or death of family member or friend f. Newspaper or magazine article	Likelihood of compliance with a. Learning and changing attitudes and beliefs about risks and disease b. Following medical advice c. Changing risk-reducing behaviors

Adapted from Becker et al. and Kirscht (2,11).

five broad indices derived from the Health Belief Model that we included in the questionnaire were general health motivation, perceived susceptibility, perceived severity, perceived benefits, and perceived barriers to the Hemoccult slide preparation (Table 2). Other items included demographic information, personal history of illness, and family history of cancer and/or colon-related conditions. The following is a brief description of the five major indices and their subindices:

1. General health motivation. Questions were asked to determine health beliefs and motivation about health in general. Subindices under this broad category include health practices, locus of control and belief in asymptomatology. Recently, locus of control questions—e.g., how much control does an individual perceive he has over his health? does he view his health fatalistically?—have emerged as especially important guides in discerning general health motivation.

2. Perceived susceptibility. Perceiving oneself as susceptible to a disease that is related to a recommended health action is normally considered necessary if the patient is to be in a state of readiness to act. Usually, however, this perception is not sufficient in itself to induce the action.

3. Perceived severity. Susceptibility does not touch the question of whether the patient perceives the disease in question to be serious enough to warrant taking the recommended action. This requires that the investigator inquire as to the perception of the disease's severity by asking how life disrupting the patient believes the illness would be.

4. Perceived benefits. Questions were asked to ascertain patients' general faith in medical care, as well as their belief in the efficacy of treatment for certain ailments. Generally, it is believed that the patient must perceive that physicians or medical care can confer benefits in the course of treating an illness before he will take steps to prevent or treat it.

5. Perceived barriers of the Hemoccult slide test. From the patient's viewpoint, we tried to determine how difficult he considered the regimen, how time consuming he believed it to be, and how much he felt it would interfere with his routine.

FINDINGS

An initial analysis was done to compare the response rate between compliers and noncompliers. It is important to note that these preliminary results are not free from bias. Further analysis will be necessary to determine if the differences found were explicable on the basis of age and personal history, for example. Our tentative findings, however, may suggest deeper trends or relationships or provoke future analysis, and thereby clearly are worth sharing with the professional community.

Of the 1,143 subjects sent questionnaires, 55 were deemed ineligible for the screening study because of age or mistakes in initial status, and were therefore

TABLE 2. Compliance questionnaire items by index

All questions require multiple choice answers from "not at all" to "very much" along a five point scale.

1. General health motivation

Health motivation in general
- How concerned are you about your own health?
- How concerned are you about the possibility of getting sick?
- How easily would you say you get sick?
- How much would you say you worry about getting sick?

Health practice
- How often do you visit the doctor, even when you're well?
- How much do you exercise each week?
- How much special care do you take to maintain a healthy diet?

Locus of control
How much do you agree with the following:
- Most of what happens to my health is a matter of chance
- There are many things one can do to be healthy and avoid illness
- Most of the time I think preventing illness is in my own hands

Asymptomatology
How much do you agree with the following:
- A person can have a serious illness without knowing it
- Certain medical tests can lead to the discovery of a problem I did not know I had

2. Perceived susceptibility

Here is a list of illnesses people sometimes get. How much chance do you think there is that you could ever get . . . ?
- high blood pressure   · diabetes
- a heart problem   · cancer
- a broken bone   · arthritis
- a stroke   · a stomach ulcer
- pneumonia   · back pain

3. Perceived severity

If you got any of the following illnesses, how much do you think your daily routine or life-style would be interrupted?
- high blood pressure   · diabetes
- a heart problem   · cancer
- a broken bone   · arthritis
- a stroke   · a stomach ulcer
- pneumonia   · back pain
- How worried would you be if you were bleeding from the rectum?
- How much would you agree with the following:
- I seem to get the kind of illnesses that worry me a lot

4. Perceived benefits

How much do you feel that doctors can help these illnesses?
- high blood pressure   · diabetes
- a heart problem   · cancer
- a broken bone   · arthritis
- a stroke   · a stomach ulcer
- pneumonia   · back pain
- In general, thinking about things that doctors have told you to do when you were ill, how much would you say those things helped you to get well?
- How long would you wait to see a doctor if you had a cold?
- How long would you wait to see a doctor if you had a cough?
- How long would you wait to see a doctor if you were dizzy?
- How long would you wait to see a doctor if you were coughing or spitting up blood?
- How long would you wait to see a doctor if you were bleeding from the rectum?

- How important do you think it is to go to a doctor or a clinic for a health check-up even when you feel okay?
- How much do you agree with the statement:
- If I wait long enough, I will get over most illnesses
- I find that old-fashioned remedies are still sometimes better than the things doctors tell me to do
- I seem to get the kind of illnesses that doctors can't do much for
- In general, I have been satisfied with the care that I have received from doctors or clinics in the past

5. Perceived barriers

- How much would you say that staying on the special diet to prepare the stool slides interferes with your normal activities?
- How much would you say that staying on the special diet could cause you any harmful side effects?
- How much would you say that the stool slide test *instructions* helped you to prepare the slides?
- In preparing the stool slides, how much did you worry about the possible odor?
- How much did you worry about your ability to actually get a part of the stool from the toilet onto the slide?
- How much did you worry about the ability of the sticks provided to help you get the stool sample onto the slides?
- Did the two different diets present any conflict for you?
- How well would you say you understood the reason for the preparation of the stool slide test?
- How likely is it that the stool slide test could lead to the discovery of a problem that you do not know you have?

eliminated from the compliance population. Our total population, therefore, consisted of 1,088 individuals.

The compliance questionnaire was fully completed by approximately three-quarters of the population. Questionnaire responses and compliance status were coded and entered for computer analysis. (For a list of question items included in the questionnaire, see Table 2.)

Questions that were thought to measure various aspects of the Health Belief Model were analyzed to determine their internal consistency through the covariance approximation form, using the Spearman-Brown formula (14). Of those indices which were composed of more than 10 items, five of five had greater reliability than 0.69 (general health motivation, susceptibility, severity, benefits, and faith in medical care). Measures of internal consistency or reliability are indicators of the degree to which individual observations on a presumed set of variables are affected by random variation. Measures with high reliability indicate that a large proportion of the variance is determined by the variability specific to each item and in common with the other variables. Individual scores on a single item have limited utility as an indicator of an attribute of interest.

A set of items of high reliability is essential for assuring the credibility of a measured variable and will further increase the probability of detecting the differences between subgroups of the population being studied.

Of the 1,088 study patients, 953 or 86% complied with Hemoccult slide test whereas 153 or 14% did not comply. Of these, 95% completed all six Hemoccult slides.

Demographics

The following demographic variables were measured: age, sex, religion, ethnicity, education, marital status, and income. It was not expected that comparative analysis of single variables on the issue of compliance in this homogeneous population would yield statistically major differences, and, except for the age variable, they did not. The noncompliers appear to be younger than the compliers. Of the noncompliers, 41% are under the age of 50, as compared with only 30% of the compliers. Otherwise, we can report merely remarkably similar population profiles regarding the other six demographic variables.

General Health Motivation

The only question measuring motivation about health in general that revealed a difference between compliers and noncompliers was, "How concerned are you about your own health?" Of the noncompliers, 44% responded affirmatively, as compared with only 37% of the compliers, producing the surprising conclusion that noncompliers seem more concerned about their health than compliers. Answers to other questions in this category, however, disclosed no further differences between compliers and noncompliers.

Questions about health practices, including preventive measures, revealed no differences between compliers and noncompliers. But a major difference was observed in answer to the question, "How much do you visit the doctor, even when you are well?" More than 50% of the noncompliers replied, "not at all," whereas only one-third of the compliers fell into that category.

Looking at responses to the set of locus of control questions in combination, 91.3% of the compliers indicated a moderate or greater level of perceived control to at least two out of three locus of control questions, as compared with 86.3% of the noncompliers.

Perceived Susceptibility

The questionnaire lists several diseases and conditions: high blood pressure, diabetes, a heart problem, cancer, a broken bone, arthritis, a stroke, a stomach ulcer, pneumonia, and back pain. It then asks, "How much chance do you think there is that you could ever get [the above]?" Compliers and noncompliers answered in similar ways.

Perceived Severity

The same diseases and conditions were listed to measure the perceived severity of the affliction, and the question was asked, "If you got any of the following illnesses, how much do you think your daily routine or lifestyle would be interrupted?"

Again, compliers and noncompliers answered in similar ways to most of the illnesses listed, with one notable exception, cancer. An important difference was observed between compliers' and noncompliers' answers to the life-disrupting perceptions of cancer, the noncompliers seeing the disease as substantially more disruptive. Nearly 60% of the noncompliers answered "very much" to the question, "if you got cancer, how much would your daily routine or liberty be interrupted," as compared with only 41% of the compliers. Also, differences were observed concerning the perceived severity of stroke, and a modest difference was observed between compliers' and noncompliers' answers to the question, "How worried would you be if you noticed that you were bleeding from the rectum?" Noncompliers seem more worried about strokes but less worried about rectal bleeding than compliers.

Perceived Benefits

Questions were asked to ascertain patients' general faith in medical care, as well as their belief in the efficacy of treatment for certain ailments. Concerning high blood pressure, diabetes, broken bones, heart problems, arthritis, stroke, stomach ulcer, pneumonia, and back pain, compliers and noncompliers were in general agreement. But, again, modest differences can be seen between compliers' and noncompliers' answers to perceived benefits from cancer treatments. Nearly 10% of the noncompliers answered "not at all" to the question, "How much can doctors help cancer?" as compared with only 4% of the compliers.

Other questions designed to measure faith in medical care revealed no differences between compliers and noncompliers.

Perceived Barriers

Although it might be predicted that a self-selected fairly homogeneous population would reveal few major differences in the areas of demographics and general health beliefs, the same could not be argued when looking at perceived barriers. Direct questions about the very health action that the noncompliers failed to perform, therefore, were expected to yield sizable differences. It is important to note that a lower percentage of both compliers and the noncompliers responded to the slide questions, and in particular noncompliers were often nonrespondents.

Major differences were observed in four of ten questions, specifically, in items measuring the belief that staying on the special diet interferes with the patient's normal activities, the belief in the helpfulness of the stool slide test instructions, the perception of possible conflict of diets for proctoscopy and Hemoccult, and the perceived importance of the special Hemoccult diet for the accurate preparation of the stool slide test. Noncompliers, as expected, were more likely to feel that the diet was an interference, that the instructions were not helpful, and that the special diet was not important to the accurate preparation of the slides.

Compliers and noncompliers gave a similar distribution of answers to the questions measuring the belief that staying on the special diet to prepare the stool slides could cause harmful side effects, the concern about possible Hemoccult odor, the concern about their ability to get a part of the stool from the toilet onto the slide, the concern about the utility of the sticks provided to help get the stool sample onto the slides, the level of understanding about the reasons for the preparation of the stool slides, and the perceived likelihood that the stool slide test could lead to the discovery of a problem that would otherwise go undetected.

Personal History

Patients were asked whether they had had any of the conditions and illnesses that had been listed previously in the susceptibility, severity, and benefits sections of the questionnaire. Compliers reported more illness experience with high blood pressure, heart problems, broken bones, stomach ulcers, pneumonia, strokes, diabetes, cancer, arthritis, and back pain than did noncompliers. However, differences in reported history of broken bones, stroke, and cancer were slight.

Individuals were also asked if they had had a check-up in the past 3 years.

Not surprisingly, compliers answered "yes" 10% more often than did noncompliers.

Specific questions about colon-related medical history included questions about polyps, diverticulosis, rectal problems, and colon problems. In every case compliers reported more colon-related illnesses than did noncompliers.

DISCUSSION

It is too early in our efforts to discuss patterns of compliance differences with much authority. Moreover, observed differences in the areas of locus of control, perceived severity of cancer, perceived benefits of cancer treatment, and reported past health practices may well be explained on the basis of age and personal history differences. There are three areas, however, that already seem worthy of special mention and further research.

First, there appears to be an important difference in past medical practices of compliers and noncompliers. Although both groups elected to have Strang Clinic examinations, they reported differing attitudes toward check-ups. Three questions stand out: noncompliers seemed more reluctant to visit a doctor, particularly when they were well, fewer noncompliers had had a check-up in the past 3 years, and noncompliers reported less illness than did compliers. Even though reported illness may merely reflect more frequent physician visits associated with their greater age, compliers may well see themselves as more likely to be ill than do noncompliers.

Second, differences in beliefs between compliers and noncompliers concerning cancer cannot be ignored. Screenees were told in their instructions for preparing the Hemoccult slides that the slides were an early detection test for tumors of the colon. Although cancer is not specifically mentioned, it clearly was implied by these instructions. Noncompliers, viewing cancer as more severe and disruptive than compliers, may have been partially immobilized by this greater fear. Or, having been less confident in their physicians' ability to treat the disease, noncompliers may have been influenced by a deeper fatalism. Or perhaps the fear and fatalism interacted to discourage compliance.

Third, noncompliers were both more likely to view the special diet as an intrusion into their lives that may not have been necessary for accurate slide preparation and more critical of the test's instructions. Whether these response scores could be improved by a more sophisticated presentation of the test remains an open question. For although these criticisms may seem genuine enough to the respondents, they may in truth merely constitute rationalizations of deeper psychological forces (like fear or denial) that may actually be governing behavior.

FUTURE ANALYSIS AND RESEARCH

This chapter has reported results from our first stage of analysis, in which only simple comparative procedures were used. Once the number of items has been reduced through the method of principal components, future multivariate analysis will be conducted to test specific hypotheses pertaining to differences between compliers and noncompliers. All this, we trust will add to our explanatory and predictive capacity.

Future research, it seems to us, might profitably be directed at two areas. First, although the Health Belief Model posits a causal relationship between certain beliefs and certain behaviors, it is possible that the beliefs themselves are chiefly the product of certain preexisting psychological variables, such as fear and denial. Cancer, after all, is apt to be viewed as a life-threatening illness of unique horror, and the emotional reactions it provokes may well be decisive in shaping related beliefs as to empirical matters. This emotional reaction, in turn, presumably grows out of the patient's life situation—his prior psychological history, his age and physical condition, his ties to his family and community— since his mind could hardly encounter cancer as a *tabula rasa.* Yet only a pedant would hold that this recognition requires analysis regressing to infancy. A more practical approach would be to identify the key psychological variables, and determine their association with prior life situation variables, subsequent belief variables, and end-stage dependent compliance variables. For if psychological variables emerge as more potent causative factors than belief variables, compliance strategies might well consider aiming their fire at this deeper level.

Second, more extensive analysis of Hemoccult testing procedures might reveal that a more sophisticated presentation would have led to higher rates of compliance. Presumably, presentations tailored to the individual patient and his peculiar needs and problems would be most effective. Yet the cost of this method might render it unfeasible. If the patient population could be pre-tested and categorized, however, several alternative approaches could be devised to deal with the different kinds of patients.

SUMMARY

Eleven hundred and forty-three initial Strang patients who were in the Colon Cancer Screening Study were sent self-administered questionnaires based on the Health Belief Model. Indices measured were general health motivation, perceived susceptibility, perceived severity, perceived benefits, and perceived barriers, particularly regarding the Hemoccult slide test. The purpose of this study was to ascertain which factors were related to compliance behavior. Questionnaire data are currently undergoing analysis, and although no pattern of health beliefs can at this stage with certainly be linked to compliance, areas of heuristic value can be identified as including past practice of physician visits, beliefs concerning cancer, and attitudes toward the slide test itself.

More analysis is needed to reduce present variables to those major indices which may affect compliance outcomes. Future research is indicated to answer questions of the impact of fear and denial that may prove central to slide test compliance.

ACKNOWLEDGMENTS

This study has been partially supported by the National Cancer Institute's Grant CA15429–07. The authors would also like to express appreciation to Strang Clinic staff member, Barbara Kallini, for her technical assistance, and to Dr. David Schottenfeld, Chief of Epidemiology, Memorial Sloan-Kettering Cancer Center/New York Hospital-Cornell, for his support and guiding interest.

REFERENCES

1. Becker, M. (ed.) (1974): The health belief model and personal health behavior. *Health Educ. Monogr.*, 2:324–474.
2. Becker, M. H. (1974): The health belief model and sick role behavior. *Health Educ. Monogr.*, 2:409–419.
3. Blackwell, B. (1973): Patient compliance. *N. Engl. J. Med.*, 289:249–253.
4. Cobb, B., Clark, R., McGuire, C., and Howe, C. (1954): Patient-responsible delay of treatment in cancer. *Cancer*, 7:920–926.
5. Cummins, M., Jette, A., and Rosenstock, I. (1978): Construct validation of the health belief model. *Health Educ. Monogr.*, 6:394–405.
6. Davis, M. (1966): Variations in patients' compliance with doctors' orders: analysis of congruence between survey responses and results of empirical investigations. *J. Med. Educ.*, 41:1037–1048.
7. Goldsen, R., Gerhardt, P., and Handy, V. (1957): Some factors related to patient delay in seeking diagnosis for cancer symptoms. *Cancer*, 10:1–7.
8. Green, L. (1976): Site and symptom-related factors in secondary prevention of cancer. In: *Cancer: The Behavioral Dimensions,* edited by J. W. Cullen, B. H. Fox, and R. N. Isam, pp. 45–61. Raven Press, New York.
9. Haynes, R., and Sackett, D. (1974): *An Annotated Bibliography on the Compliance of Patients with Therapeutic Regimens.* McMaster University Health Sciences Center, Ontario, Canada.
10. James, W. (1977): Motivation for participation in cancer screening programs. Annual meeting, American Cancer Society of Preventive Oncology, February 4 and 5, New York.
11. Kirscht, J. P. (1974): The health belief model and illness behavior. *Health Educ. Monogr.*, 2:387–408.
12. Lewin, K., Dembo, T., Festinger, L., and Sears, P. (1944): Level of aspiration. In: *Personality and the Behavior Disorders: A Handbook Based on Experimental and Clinical Research,* edited by J. M. Hunt, pp. 333–378. The Ronald Press, New York.
13. Maiman, L., Becker, M., Kirscht, J., Haefner, D., and Drachman, R. (1977): Scales for measuring health belief and model dimensions: a test of predictive value, internal consistency, and relationships among beliefs. *Health Educ. Monogr.*, 5:215–230.
14. Rosenstock, I. (1966): Why people use health services. *Milbank Mem. Fund Q.*, 44:94–127
15. Tryon, R. (1957): Reliability and behavior domain validity: Reformation and historical critique. *Psychol. Bull.*, 54:229–249.
16. Winawer, S., Miller, D., Schottenfeld, D., Leidner, S., Sherlock, P., Belter, B., and Stearns, M. (1977): Feasibility of fecal occult blood testing for detection of colorectal neoplasia. *Cancer*, 40:2616–2619.

Colorectal Cancer: Prevention, Epidemiology, and Screening, edited by S. Winawer, D. Schottenfeld, and P. Sherlock. Raven Press, New York © 1980.

Early Detection of Colorectal Cancer with a Modified Guaiac Test—A Screening Examination in 6,000 Humans

P. Frühmorgen and L. Demling

Department of Medicine, University of Erlangen, Nürnberg, D-5852, Erlangen, West Germany

Whereas in 1953 16 of every 100,000 inhabitants of the Federal Republic of Germany died of a colorectal carcinoma, in 1975 this figure had risen to 36 per 100,000 inhabitants, that is, 22,302 people (Fig. 1). With respect to mortality, carcinoma of the colon had become the most frequent cancer in man. Moreover, as a result of improved roentgenological (double-contrast technique) and endoscopic (colonoscopy) methods, and the fact that the potential malignancy of adenomas (70% of all colonic polyps) has been confirmed, colorectal carcinoma moved into the foreground of medical and health political interests. Only early diagnosis and timely therapy can, at the present time, improve the poor prognosis of colorectal carcinoma.

This question should be clarified in a prospective study: Is the search for occult blood in the stools within the framework of a screening examination (high degree of accuracy, great sensitivity, fast and easy to perform) a suitable method for the selection of patients for subsequent X-ray and endoscopic examinations?

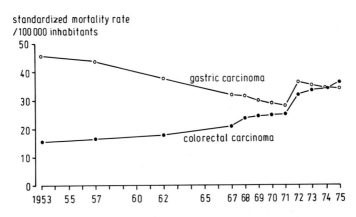

FIG. 1. Incidence of colorectal and gastric carcinomas in the Federal Republic of Germany.

METHOD

In a prospective field study, we investigated the efficacy of a modified guaiac test (Hemoccult) in 6,007 people over 40. The evaluation was carried out at room temperature, 30 sec after the application of a few drops of the stabilized developer solution. Whenever an occult blood test was positive, the patient was subjected to a thorough diagnostic work-up on an inpatient basis (rectal digital palpation, rectosigmoidoscopy, double-contrast enema, colonoscopy, esophagogastroduodenoscopy). Every participant in the study was given three "test envelopes." Dietary measures were limited to the avoidance of raw and half-cooked meat for 3 days prior to carrying out the test and also for the 3 days of the test, on each of which a little stool was applied to one of the test envelopes.

RESULTS

Of 6,007 participants, each of whom had been provided with three test envelopes, 5,016 (83.5%) returned evaluable test envelopes, so that a total of 15,048 envelopes were evaluated. In 136 (2.7%) of the people taking part, one, two

TABLE 1. *Detection of a source of bleeding in patients with occult bleeding (117 patients)*

Certain or probable source of bleeding	69[1]
	29[2]
	5[3]
	2[4]
Improbable sources of bleeding	9[1]
No source of bleeding	3

TABLE 2. *Pathological findings in patients with occult bleeding (117 patients)*

Finding		No. of patients
Carcinomas		13
Radical surgery	8	
Palliative surgery	2	
Inoperable	3	
Polyps		83
Adenomas	49	
Adenomas with severe atypia	2	
Hyperplastic	25	
Pseudopolyps	7	
Polyposis coli		3
Hemorrhoids (7/13 cancer)		83
Miscellaneous		
Colon		69
Upper GI tract		65

TABLE 3. *Positive findings*

	No. of carcinomas
+ 86 (63.9%)	3 (1/29)
++ 36 (26.5%)	6 (1/6)
+++ 14 (10.3%)	5 (1/3)

TABLE 4. *Comparison of diagnostic methods*

Method	Carcinomas (*N* = 13)	Polyps (*N* = 83)
Rectal digital	0	0
Rectosigmoidoscopy	8	21/83 (25%)
Double-contrast enema	8 (+2)	42/83 (51%)
Colonoscopy	13	82/83 (99%)

or three positive findings were established. Then 117 of these people with demonstrated occult bleeding subjected themselves to an inpatient examination.

In 90% of these cases, one or two certain or probable sources of bleeding were found in the colon after an intensive search (Table 1). The diagnostic yield was astonishingly high. In addition to other pathological findings, we were able to diagnose 13 carcinomas, 2 adenomas with severe cellular atypia (so-called focal carcinomas), and 83 polyps (49 adenomas) (Table 2).

The probability of finding a carcinoma increased markedly with the number of positive test results (Table 3). A comparison of the diagnostic methods has shown that none of the polyps and none of the carcinomas were detected by rectal digital palpation. The high degree of diagnostic reliability of colonoscopy is obvious (Table 4).

DISCUSSION

Since no marked improvement in the prognosis of colorectal carcinoma can be expected from surgical methods, early detection is of considerable importance. This is important since the surgical treatment of colorectal carcinoma in Dukes' A stage has a 5-year survival rate of approximately 90%, and the rigorously applied removal of colonic polyps may significantly reduce the incidence of carcinoma.

When endoscopic and roentgenological examination techniques are employed, colonic carcinoma may be found at a curable state in every case, and this also applies to initially benign but later malignant polyps (adenomas). The latter can, moreover, be removed during the primary diagnostic endoscopic examination in the same session without the need for conventional surgical intervention. Colonoscopic polypectomy not only represents an initial diagnostic method, but also permits true carcinoma prophylaxis, i.e., preventive care. It is also adequate therapy for adenomas with severe cellular atypia (so-called focal carcinoma), or for adenomas with invasive carcinoma showing grade I or grade II malignancy, provided the local removal can be effected together with surrounding healthy tissue. The mortality rate of the radical surgical operation exceeds the 3% risk of lymphatic metastases in adenoma with invasive adenocarcinoma present at the time of polypectomy. Considering the expenditure needed for staff and equipment, colonoscopy and X-ray examination are not suitable as screening methods. An alternative is selection of high-risk groups. Our study has shown that demonstration of occult blood in the stools provides a high degree of selection for healthy persons, who may then be subjected to the proper diagnostic methods.

The percentage of positive test results in our group (2.7%) is also confirmed approximately by others workers, although the sensitivity of the test envelopes is not uniform (2–6). A comparison of the costs of various preventive examinations shows that there is a low cost for a carcinoma discovered on the basis of the demonstration of occult blood. (Table 5).

The limitations of the method for the detection of occult blood in the stools are indicated by the number of false negative and false positive results and by the fact that accuracy is obtainable only in cases of bleeding from the large bowel. Our experience points to some 10% "false positives" and some 20 to 30% "false negatives" in the case of carcinoma; for polyps, the figures are about 30 to 50%, depending on the size of the polyp. False negative findings are also observed after the oral intake of ascorbic acid (7).

In addition, the time interval between the sampling of the stools and the evaluation of the test envelopes—in particular in borderline concentrations of blood—is of great importance. Thus 21 days after preparation of the test envelopes, we obtained negative results in a number of stools containing unknown concentrations of blood. In quantitative examinations, we established negative results in all cases with a blood concentration of 0.1%, and in some cases with a blood concentration of 0.6%, from the 3rd day after sampling. Concentrations of blood of 1.0% were all positive up to and including the 21st day.

On the basis of these facts, we recommend that no ascorbic acid be ingested for 3 days prior to, and then for the duration of, the test, and that the test envelopes be examined within 14 days.

False positive findings simulated by foodstuffs containing hemoglobin or myo-

TABLE 5. *Mass screening examinations (costs)*

Finding	Cost
1 Positive gynecological-cytological finding	DM 15,000–16,000
1 Confirmed cancer, neck of the uterus	DM 40,000–80,000
1 Cancer confirmed at rectoscopy	DM 45,000–50,000
1 Cancer detected with Hemoccult (Erlangen study)	DM 9,000–12,000

globin are possibly of only secondary importance. Feifel et al. (1) were able to show that in test subjects under the age of 45, no positive findings were seen, either with a normal diet or with a "provocative diet" (salami, raw beef, peanuts).

The search for occult blood in the stools (provided the test instructions are complied with), colonoscopy routinely carried out in selected persons, and endoscopic polypectomy will premit us to take a considerable step forward in our efforts to provide prophylactic measures and establish an early diagnosis in colorectal carcinoma.

SUMMARY

Because of the considerable requirements for staff and equipment and also the costs involved, endoscopy and radiology are not suitable for use in screening examinations. Thus the only effective alternative is the selection of high-risk groups in the population.

In a prospective study, the demonstration of occult blood in the stools has been shown to be an effective method for the selection of patients from among apparently healthy people who can then be subjected to the more complicated (expensive) diagnostic measures. This situation has been clarified in a screening examination within the framework of a prospective study involving 6,007 people. In 117 of 136 persons with demonstrated occult bleeding, we found, among other things, 13 carcinomas, 2 adenomas with severe cellular atypia, and 83 polyps.

REFERENCES

1. Feifel, G., Männer, C., and Liebe, S. V. (1978): Der Haemoccult-Test ohne diätetische Einschränkung. In: *Kolorektale Krebsvorsorge,* edited by K. Goerttler. Wachholz, Nürnberg.
2. Glober, G. A., and Peskoe, S. M. (1974): Outpatient screening for gastrointestinal lesions using guaiac-impregnated slides. *Am. J. Dig. Dis.,* 19:399.
3. Gnauck, R. (1974): Okkultes Blut im Stuhl als Suchtest nach kolorektalem Krebs und präkanzerösen Polypen. *Z. Gastroenterol.,* 12:239.
4. Gnauck, R. (1977): Dickdarmkarzinom-Screening mit Haemoccult. *Leber Magen Darm,* 7:32.
5. Greegor, D. H. (1971): Occult blood testing for detection of asymptomatic colon cancer. *Cancer,* 28:131.
6. Hastings, J. B. (1974): Mass screening for colorectal cancer. *Am. J. Surg.,* 127:228.
7. Jaffe, R. M., Kasten, B., Young, D. S., and Maclowry, J. D. (1975): False-negative stool occult blood tests caused by ingestion of ascrobic acid (vitamin C). *Ann. Intern. Med.,* 83:824.

Colorectal Cancer: Prevention, Epidemiology, and Screening, edited by S. Winawer, D. Schottenfeld, and P. Sherlock. Raven Press, New York © 1980.

Commentary

David H. Greegor

The principal point of controversy in fecal occult blood testing seems to be the actual percentage of false negatives. Any test with many false negatives would hardly qualify as a screening test. Therefore it would behoove all of us to study carefully our false negatives before they go to surgery. We need to see the effect of various diets on known cancer cases—what encourages them to bleed and what seems to prevent it.

With occult blood immunological methods, it may be possible to detect quantitatively very small amounts of human blood in fecal material. Since this test does not detect upper GI tract bleeding, it may be possible by combining it with Hemoccult to be able to determine whether the bleeding source is above or below the cecum.

The problem of false positive tests and the resultant high cost of complete diagnostic follow-up is important. It is understandable how any physician and his asymptomatic patient can be frustrated by a $500.00 work-up disclosing absolutely nothing. Large-scale studies must be completed in order to furnish necessary statistics and guidelines.

Colorectal Cancer: Prevention, Epidemiology,
and Screening, edited by S. Winawer, D. Schottenfeld,
and P. Sherlock. Raven Press, New York © 1980.

Introduction: Inflammatory Bowel Disease— Considerations of Etiology and Pathogenesis

Joseph B. Kirsner

Department of Medicine, University of Chicago, Chicago, Illinois 60637

The etiology and pathogenesis of ulcerative colitis and Crohn's disease of the small and/or large intestine remain obscure, despite the increasing familiarity with these disorders (6,7). The similar clinical features and course of inflammatory bowel disease (IBD) everywhere in the world, despite differing ethnic populations, environmental circumstances, dietary habits, and sociocultural customs is noteworthy. The rising incidence of Crohn's disease, apparently worldwide, is of particular interest and suggests involvement of environmental agents in its pathogenesis (5,9). Attempts to clarify the nature of ulcerative colitis and Crohn's disease on the basis of discernible tissue and cellular reactions, as determined by light, scanning, and electron microscopy and histochemical and immunologial reactions, are informative and undoubtedly significant, but interpretation of such observation is limited by questions as to the constancy and specificity of the observed changes, by the influences of antibacterial, adrenocortical steroids and other therapeutic agents, nutritional state, by individual differences in host response, and by the likelihood that both the small and the large intestine have a limited repertoire of tissue reactions regardless of the inciting etiologic mechanism (11). The large number and the variety of the local and systemic complications of IBD are unique to these disorders. Since they almost invariably are secondary to the bowel inflammation, they direct attention to the diseased bowel as the likely source of various systemic diseases, and as a prime area for further research—as, for example, in the study of the systemic complications of jejunoileal bypass operations.

More directly, numerous experimental attempts to reproduce human IBD by diverse procedures thus far have failed (9). A variety of enteric and colonic inflammatory bowel diseases are found among various animal species, including an ileitis in pigs, a granulomatous enteritis in horses, and a colitis in Boxer dogs, but these "natural" animal states have not been investigated thoroughly and their possible relationship to human inflammatory bowel disease is not known. Psychogenic disturbances, although clinically important in the course of IBD, remain to be clarified, especially in terms of their specificity, their pathophysiological effects on the bowel, and their capacity for inducing a tissue reaction such as IBD. This approach may become more attractive in view of the recently demonstrated fact that cells widely dispersed in the neuraxis and the gastrointestinal system share the ability to secrete the same or similar peptide messengers. Microbiological causes thus far have eluded extensive investigations. Currently, intestinal anaerobes, *Yersinia enterocolitica,* pathogenic forms of *Escherichia coli,* and bacterial endotoxins and other metabolites are of particular interest. The considerable information now accumulated on the apparent "transmissibility" of Crohn's disease (and ulcerative colitis) suggests a viral etiology, but the evidence remains inconclusive; and improved virological techniques will be required to clarify this hypothesis (1). The systemic location of granulomas (face, muscle, bone, epiglottis) noted occasionally is of interest in this connection. Substantial gaps remain in our knowledge of the gut microflora, the mechanisms of bacterial adherence and nonadherence to the intestinal epithelium, the role of the gastrointestinal secretory immune system (e.g., IgA), and the local lymphoid cells in the protection of the bowel wall against microbiological, viral, and immunological injury, and the dynamics of immune competence and possible immune weakness at the bowel mucosal surface (5,10,13).

Consideration of immunological mechanisms in IBD includes experimental immunological attempts to reproduce either ulcerative colitis or Crohn's disease (thus far unsuccessful), the nonspecific colon "autoantibodies," circulating antigen-antibody immune complexes, cell-mediated immune responses including the respective roles of T and B lymphocytes, the possible significance of circulatory lymphocyte cytotoxicity for colonic epithelial cells, the as yet incompletely defined immunologic resources and immunologic functions of the gastrointestinal tract, the possible role of the gastrointestinal lymphoid tissue including intraepithelial lymphocytes, and the possible role of the gastrointestinal secretory immune system, especially secretory IgA (but including IgG, IgM, and IgE) in the evolution of the IBD tissue reaction (2,3,4,12,16). Present incidence, demonstrating the local accumulation of immunoglobulins and various components of complement (Clq, C_3, for example), in addition to B lymphocytes, though yet incomplete, suggests a significant immunologically mediated reaction in the bowel wall, in both Crohn's disease and ulcerative colitis.

The diminished response of circulating lymphocytes to various mitogens, especially in Crohn's disease but also in ulcerative colitis, has suggested to some observers the presence of an immunodeficiency state in Crohn's disease, but the evidence is inconclusive. Lymphocyte responses are variable and possibly capricious, and reactions may be dispersed in a wide variety of circumstances including undernutrition, advancing age, operations such as cholecystectomy, and also by cellular inhibitory factors circulating in the blood of patients with IBD (5). Possible genetic influences, facilitating the development of IBD—including immune defects (e.g., selective immunoglobulin deficiency, selective complement deficiency) associated with particular histocompatibility haplotypes (e.g., C_2 deficiency associated with the $A_{10} B_{18}$ haplotype)—in addition to the already emphasized association between ankylosing spondylitis and the HLA-B_{27} haplotype deserve more study. With regard to "familial IBD" (8,11), the possible role of a common and prolonged exposure of families living in the same household to an environmental agent (possibly a "slow virus") is suggested perhaps by the increased incidence of lymphocytotoxic antibodies (LCA) among some IBD families, but the evidence for such a mechanism remains insufficient; and improved methods of demonstrating significant viral exposure (possibly via the use of interferon) are needed.

Although the etiology and the pathogenesis of ulcerative colitis and of Crohn's disease remain elusive, the "nonspecific" inflammatory bowel diseases have emerged as very important clinical problems and also as "rosetta stones," facilitating clarification of both gastrointestinal and nongastrointestinal disorders, through the application of basic scientific knowledge, the increasingly sophisticated study of the immunocellular features of the IBD tissue reaction in the bowel, the study of local and systemic problems so unique to IBD, and the investigation of host defenses and genetic-immunological interactions (16). Significant advances can be anticipated in the immediate future, progress which hopefully will clarify the nature of nonspecific inflammatory bowel disease and provide the solution to this challenging medical problem.

Few precancerous conditions offer as many intriguing opportunities for the investigation of human cancerogenesis as ulcerative colitis. The circumstances of a younger than usual age group at increased risk and the lengthy induction period (7 years and longer) enhance whatever mechanisms are involved in the neoplastic transformation of erstwhile normal colonic and intestinal epithelial cells. The unique tissue reaction of ulcerative colitis, characterized in part by pronounced cellular infiltration with lymphocytes, plasma cells, and eosinophils in addition to polymorphonuclear leukocytes, the intense vascular congestion, loss of the basement membrane of the epithelial cells, disorganization of the ground substance of the connective tissue, decreased tissue alkaline phosphatase among other enzymes such as succinic dehydrogenase, the reduced number of argentaffin cells but increased numbers of Paneth and mast cells, the increased concentrations of substances such as prolylhydrolase, norepinephrine, and various prostaglandins, each pose interesting biological questions in relation to the integrity of the bowel wall and to crypt cell kinetics. Lipkin, for example, utilizing tritiated thymidine, has demonstrated increased DNA synthesis in the superficial colonic epithelium in experimental colon cancer in the presence of a colonic microflora.

The studies of Morson and others (9) have demonstrated an interesting and apparent precancerous tissue phase, epithelial dysplasia, antedating the development of overt cancer; resembling the precancer of the skin, the cervix, the stomach, and other organs. The epithelial dysplasia may involve any part of the colon and rectum, may be patchy or diffuse, and, indeed, may be absent despite the presence of carcinoma, a series of events obviously requiring further study.

Adapting the concept of "external" environmental carcinogenic influences in colon cancer to the vulnerable ulcerative colitis population suggests up-to-date studies of both the aerobic and anaerobic bowel microflora, in relation not only to the intake of animal fat and protein but also to changes in the micorflora associated with the disease itself, including the presence of narrowed segments of the bowel, a situation promoting stasis and bacterial overgrowth, In this regard, the increased frequency of cancer of the small bowel in Crohn's disease patients with stenosed or bypassed loops is noteworthy. Extending the "environmental" concept also suggests measurements of normal and abnormal steroids in the bowel content, excessive quantities of bile salts and bile acid metabolites, as well as *N*-nitroso compounds, and other precarcinogens and mutagens resulting from anaerobic bacterial action.

Alterations in the immune status of IBD patients (ulcerative colitis, and especially Crohn's disease) attributable not only to the disease *per se* but also to the associated undernutrition, the large number of circulating inhibitors of lymphocyte and other cellular defenses in IBD, intensified perhaps by the therapeutic use of immunosuppressive drugs (6-mercaptopurine, azathioprine), and the additive radiation effect of repeated X-ray examinations of IBD patients (11,12), together with the increasingly important role of immunoregulatory mechanisms in cancer vulnerability and cancer resistance, all indicate the need for further investigation of immune aberrations among IBD patients, those with and those without bowel cancer.

The immune status of the gastrointestinal tract *per se* (especially the small intestine and the colon) also deserves continuing scrutiny. There is now sufficient evidence to implicate immunological mechanisms in the tissue reaction of both ulcerative colitis and Crohn's disease; as evidenced in part by the increased number of B lymphocytes, immunoglobulins (especially IgG, IgA, and IgM), and the recent demonstration within the diseased bowel of C_{1q} and C_3 components of complement. Alterations in either or both the systemic and the local GI immune defense systems conceivably may be a factor in the origin of carcinoma in IBD.

The familial occurrence of IBD in 15 to 20% of patients with ulcerative colitis or Crohn's disease (8) introduces yet another important mechanism into the IBD-cancer relationship: the genetic factor, recognized in a wide variety of human neoplasms including cancer of the colon. Since immune regulations and immune defense involve genes located at the I, K, and D regions of the major histocompatibility complex (MHC), the interrelationships between individual vulnerability to IBD and to colorectal cancer are especially intriguing.

This brief overview of potential research opportunities for studies of the evolution of cancer of the colon and rectum in inflammatory bowel disease thus encompasses many of the currently identified conceptual areas for cancer research generally. Intensified efforts in these directions should bring rewards in new knowledge and understanding of cellular biology and neoplastic processes, extending far beyond the limits of the gastrointestinal tract.

REFERENCES

1. Beeken, W. L., Mitchell, D. N., and Cave, D. R. (1976): Evidence of a transmissible agent in Crohn's disease. *Clin. Gastroenterol.,* 5:289–302.
2. Bull, D. M., and Bookman, M. A. (1977): Isolation and functional characterization of human intestinal mucosal lymphoid cells. *J. Clin. Invest.,* 59:966–974.
3. Ferguson, A. (1976): Models of intestinal hypersensitivity. *Clin. Gastroenterol.,* 5:271–278.
4. Hodgson, H. J. F., Potter, B. J., and Jewell, D. P. (1977): Immune complexes in ulcerative colitis and Crohn's disease. *Clin. Exp. Immunol.,* 29:187–196.
5. Katz, D. H. (1977): *Lymphocyte Differentiation, Recognition and Regulations.* New York, Academic Press.
6. Kirsner, J. B. (1969): Clinical observations on inflammatory bowel disease. *Med. Clin. N. Am.,* 53:1195–1217.
7. Kirsner, J. B. (1970): Ulcerative colitis—1970. *Scand J. Gastroenterol.,*
8. Kirsner, J. B. (1973): Genetic aspects of inflammatory bowel disease. *Clin. Gastroenterol.,* 2:557–575.
9. Kirsner, J. B. (1976): Observations on the etiology and pathogenesis of inflammatory bowel disease. In: *Gastroenterology 4th Ed., Vol. 2,* edited by H. L. Bockus, pp. 521–539. W. B. Saunders Co., Philadelphia.
10. Kirsner, J. B. (1978): Inflammatory bowel disease—considerations of etiology and pathogenesis. *Am. J. Gastroenterol.,* 69:253–271.
11. Kirsner, J. B., and Shorter, R. G. (1975): *Inflammatory Bowel Disease,* Lea and Febiger, Philadelphia.
12. Kraft, S. C., and Kirsner, J. B. (1976): Immunology in gastroenterology. In: *Gastroenterology, Vol. 4,* edited by H. L. Bockus, pp. 601–628. Philadelphia, W. B. Saunders Co.
13. Levin, M. J., and Zaia, J. A. (1977): Immunosuppression and infection—progress? *(Editorial) N. Engl. J. Med.,* 296:1406–1408.
14. Perlmann, P., Lagercrantz, R., and Hammarström, S. (1976): Lower gastrointestinal system: ulcerative colitis and Crohn's disease (regional enteritis). In: *Textbook of Immunology, Vol. 2,* edited by P. A. Mischer and H. J. Muller-Eberhard. Grune and Stratton, New York.
15. Schachter, H., and Kirsner, J. B. (1975): Definitions of inflammatory disease of unknown etiology. *Gastroenterology,* 68:591–600.
16. Walker, W. A., and Isselbacher, K. J. (1977): Intestinal antibodies. *N. Engl. J. Med.,* 297:767–773.
17. Whorwell, P. J., and Wright, R. (1976): Immunological aspects of inflammatory bowel disease. *Clin. Gastroenterol.,* 5:303–321.

Colorectal Cancer: Prevention, Epidemiology, and Screening, edited by S. Winawer, D. Schottenfeld, and P. Sherlock. Raven Press, New York © 1980.

Risk of Cancer in Inflammatory Bowel Disease

Ghislain Devroede

Departement de Churugie, Unité de Recherche Gastrointestinale, Université de Sherbrooke, Sherbrooke, Quebec, Canada J1h 5n4

The risk of cancer in ulcerative colitis has long been recognized (2,3), but its magnitude has been the object of major controversy (Fig. 1).

STATISTICAL CONSIDERATIONS

Most of the discrepancies between various reports simply result from the chosen statistical approach. When a patient is exposed to a risk which is not limited to a specific time period, but remains constantly present, it is quite meaningless to speak of a "percentage" of patients developing the said complication. For instance, in the subject at hand, ulcerative colitis, the longer the duration of follow-up, the more cancers are likely to develop. Also, as time elapses the number of patients available for study diminishes. Some are simply lost, because it is difficult to follow a homogeneous population for long periods of time. This is particularly so with a mobile population, or if the study comes from a center recruiting its patients from a wide geographic area. Furthermore, although some patients with ulcerative colitis may be known to be alive and well, they become *ipso facto* immune from colon cancer if they have undergone proctocolectomy. Such patients should be deleted from the population at risk as soon as they undergo surgery. Finally, prospective clinical studies were not fashionable 20 years ago. Thus, in most studies, some of the patients were only recently diagnosed and should either be excluded if the risk is known to begin after several years, or included only to the extent of the duration of their follow-up. The arguments explain why the "percentage" of patients with colitis developing cancer is a fraction whose numerator increases with the duration of follow-up, while its denominator decreases with time (Fig. 2).

The duration of follow-up is also crucial if the risk is not present from the beginning of the disease. In ulcerative colitis, it appears to be nil for the first 5 years and minimal for the following 5 years. Studies with follow-ups of less than 5 years will thus automatically show no incidence of cancer.

Another important statistical aspect deals with the time chosen as the beginning of follow-up. Ideally this should be the onset of symptoms rather than the time of diagnosis. The appearance of bloody diarrhea is fortunately striking

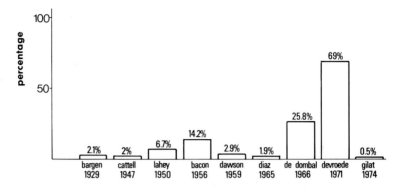

FIG. 1. Risk of cancer complicating ulcerative colitis, expressed as a percentage of the group, is widely evaluated. From this method, no acceptable conclusion can be drawn.

enough to permit a rather precise dating of the beginning of disease in ulcerative colitis. But if the time of diagnosis is chosen as time zero, one would expect a higher incidence of cancer, at an earlier time, because of prior existence of the disease.

Finally, details of treatment should be recorded since they may affect the natural history of disease.

The use of actuarial methods in this type of problem is not new (9,18), and such methods have been extensively discussed (12–15). For each period of follow-

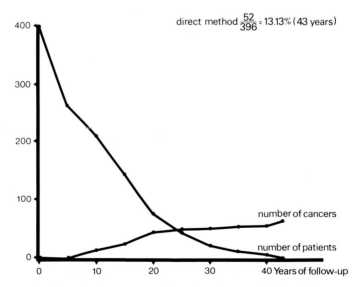

FIG. 2. Cancer risk in children with ulcerative colitis. The longer the follow-up of patients, the more cancers. It would be meaningless to express this risk as a "percentage" of the group, disregarding duration of the study. From Devroede et al. (15).

up in the retrospective actuarial method, one assumes that patients are lost uniformly with time and the mathematics of the method take this into account. The prospective "generalized" actuarial method has been devised because most studies on cancer risk in colitis originate from referral centers which only see "survivors" of larger groups of unknown size and fate. Some data suggest that the use of a "classic" actuarial analysis tends to underestimate risks, at least during the first few years of the study (12). The principle of the "generalized" method is relatively simple, and patients are assumed to enter also uniformly during each period of the study.

These statistical considerations may appear awesome to the clinician who deals with a colitic patient at risk of cancer, but it is essential to understand them if one is to take a critical look at the misleading literature on the subject.

AVAILABLE STUDIES IN ULCERATIVE COLITIS

A number of studies now available use an appropriate statistical analysis. They have shown some undisputable facts, reproducible from center to center. The risk of cancer in ulcerative colitis is considerable, (9,15,18), particularly in extensive ulcerative colitis. It is obvious after 10 years of history (9,15,28,33) and keeps increasing with time (Fig. 3). Patients may develop invasive carcinoma after 5 to 10 years of disease (8,9,15,33,39–41), but the risk is only around 3% and some authors did not find any for the first decade (1,28,35). However, severe mucosal dysplasia—or carcinoma *in situ*—may develop even during the first 5 years of disease (40). Four different centers have now published data showing a roughly similar cancer risk. One of these studies dealt exclusively

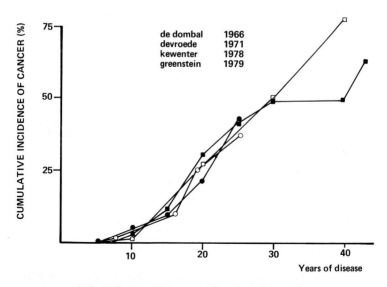

FIG. 3. Cancer risk in extensive ulcerative colitis.

with all patients residing in a single city (33). From this one may conclude that the high risk of cancer is not related to the type of center reporting on such patients.

Cancer may occur in patients with left-sided colitis (7,18,22), but the risk in extensive disease is greater (15). However, most long-term studies began before the era of colonoscopy. Barium enemas notoriously underestimate the extent of disease (Fig. 4) (15,36). To date, no study has been published on the risk in left-sided colitis, as defined by colonoscopy and biopsy. One study defined it as disease distal to the mid-transverse colon as seen on barium enema, but this was confirmed at colonoscopy or colectomy only in some patients (28). It showed that patients with left-sided colitis tended to remain cancer free about

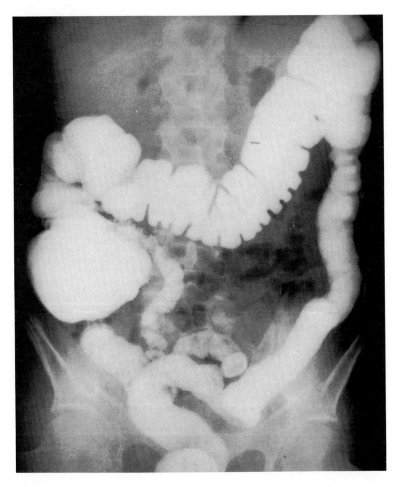

FIG. 4. Barium enema in this patient with universal colitis on colonoscopy fails to demonstrate disease in the right part of the bowel.

10 years longer than those with extensive disease. For example, the probability of cancer after 30 years was 50% for patients with extensive disease but only 20% for those with left-sided disease ($p < 0.01$). Moreover, once the risk began, the incidence paralleled that of patients with extensive colitis. Because of the limitations imposed by a diagnosis made at barium enema in the above study, there may have been an overestimation of the size of the population with left-sided colitis, some of them having a radiologically left-sided disease but in fact having unrecognized right-sided disease as well. Such overestimation could have produced an underestimation of the cancer incidence since the numerator of the incidence ratio includes only proven left-sided cases while the denominator includes other cases as well. Overall, one may speak of a risk of cancer of 20% per decade, beginning at 10 years after onset of disease for patients with extensive colitis and at 20 years for those with left-sided colitis.

The risk of cancer in patients with ulcerative colitis limited to the rectum is much lower than in those with more extensive disease. In a study (15) defining this former group as having a diseased rectum as seen at endoscopy associated with a normal barium enema, the risk began in the third decade after onset of disease and then paralleled the other groups. The difference was statistically significant ($p < 0.01$). However, classification of the patients was done at onset of the disease, and with the actuarial analysis, it was not possible to identify those patients initially having proctitis and then progressing to a more extensive disease, therefore falling into groups with a higher risk of large bowel cancer. To date, only 3 patients have been reported as suffering simultaneously of carcinoma and disease limited to the rectum and sigmoid (21,41,48). The probability of pure chance association has not been calculated, and thus the risk of cancer in patients with ulcerative proctitis is not known while appearing minimal.

Age at onset of disease has long been said to be a factor of risk, younger patients being more exposed to carcinoma (17,18,38,46). All these studies, however, failed to take into account the shorter lengths of follow-up for older patients. Four studies (9,15,28,33) reported roughly the same incidence of cancer in extensive colitis even though one of them (15) was limited to a follow-up of children younger than 14 years. This suggests that age *per se* is not an important factor, although children aged 5 to 9 at onset of disease possibly run a slightly greater risk (15). In one study dealing specifically with this question, the patient-years of follow-up were obtained for each decade and age-specific incidences calculated. There was no tendency for a greater risk among younger patients with either extensive or left-sided colitis (28). The same was found in a homogeneous population (33). If one now considers a different statistical parameter, namely, the much higher ratio of observed-to-expected cancer incidence in children with ulcerative colitis (27), it simply reflects the fact that colorectal cancer is rare among young people in the general population. But, as compared to cancer risk in older colitis patients, early age at onset of colitis does not appear to exert any independent influence on cancer risk, except for leading to a longer duration of disease.

The severity of the first episode of colitis is said to be another factor increasing cancer risk in ulcerative colitis (18). The sustained chronicity may also increase the risk as contrasted to intermittent disease (18). There has been no actuarial analysis of these findings. Moreover, it may be hazardous to define severity of the disease, however careful and precise this definition. A mild course of disease does not exclude cancer risk, several patients contracting it after years of remission (15,27).

Surgical treatment reduces the incidence of cancer in ulcerative colitis (Fig. 5).

Total colectomy associated with ileorectal anastomosis does not protect against rectal cancer (38). This is not surprising in view of the uniform distribution of cancer throughout the large bowel. In a large series of patients followed for long periods of time after successful ileorectal anastomosis, the cumulative risk of rectal cancer was found to be nil at 10 years, 6% at 20 years, 15% at 30 years, and 32% at 43 years (1). This risk is reduced as compared to that of patients who remain at risk with their entire large intestine (Fig. 5). One can speculate that the mechanism of reduced risk is that surgery reduces the

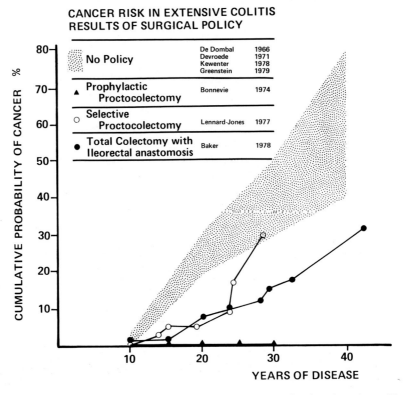

FIG. 5. Surgical therapy alters the incidence of cancer complicating ulcerative colitis.

surface of bowel at risk. In addition, if an ileostomy is performed but part of the large bowel remains *in situ,* cancer may still develop in the defunctionalized portion (4). This suggests that luminal factors do not play a major role in the genesis of cancer complicating ulcerative colitis.

The most radical approach, proctocolectomy, improves survival as compared to medical treatment (15) and is followed by a survival similar to that of the general population (5,15,50), once the operation has been performed with success. When prophylactic proctocolectomy is performed in all patients with 10 years of history of disease (5) (Fig. 5), cancer is not reported to occur.

Another approach has been to single out for radical surgery those patients at greater risk. When cancer occurs in patients with ulcerative colitis, it is frequently associated with or preceded by mucosal dysplasia elsewhere in the large bowel or in the rectum (39). This finding has been confirmed by many centers (7,11,20,31,40,41,44,45,53). Patients with mild dysplasia appear to be immune from cancer, although the risk increases as dysplasia progresses from moderate to severe (35). Grading the dysplasia is, however, a source of interobserver variation. It is not known either for what degree of severity of dysplasia surgery is best indicated. Moreover, not all patients with carcinoma and ulcerative colitis have rectal dysplasia (16,20,33,41,44,45,53). As compared with the natural history of disease, cancer risk appears lowered through individual assessment of cancer risk by clinical and histological criteria (35). This means that some patients underwent surgery for dysplasia before rather than after they developed carcinoma. For these patients, one can speak of selective prophylaxis.

Whether, over the next decades, performing proctocolectomy only in patients identified by their dysplasia can reduce both the incidence of surgery and that of cancer remains to be seen. To date, no long-term actuarial analysis has been done simultaneously on cumulative incidence of cancer and cumulative performance of surgery. One could theorize that cumulative performance of surgery is high with no cancer incidence in the hands of those advocating prophylactic proctocolectomy (5), low with high cancer incidence in the hands of those without fixed policy (9,15,28,33), and intermediate in the hands of those advocating selective proctocolectomy (35,36) or partial resection of the bowel (1). If protecting some subjects from unnecessary surgery is not acquired at the cost of an increased mortality from cancer, the value of selective proctocolectomy will have been demonstrated.

No random trial has been done to compare prophylactic proctocolectomy after 5 to 10 years of disease with selective proctocolectomy on the basis of dysplasia. For emotional and practical reasons, it is doubtful it will ever be done. Finally, is the quality of life of a patient living with a constant sword of Damocles over his head—the threat of cancer, undergoing frequent biopsies, having repeated colonoscopies, running higher risk of death, and living with the symptoms of colitis—any better than that of a patient living with an ileostomy?

Cancers complicating ulcerative colitis are different from those occurring in the general population (1,11,18,27,44,45). They are more undifferentiated, more often multiple and distributed uniformly throughout the large bowel rather than concentrated in the cecum and rectosigmoid area. The clinical diagnosis is difficult (11) because the only features distinguishing cancer from colitis are an abdominal mass and obstruction (27), and these are late findings. There are conflicting data on survival after these cancers develop as compared to that after *de novo* cancer. Some studies demonstrated a much lower survival for patients with colitic cancer (7,11,47). Other studies, however, demonstrated somewhat similar survival (25,27,29,30). Poor prognosis is partly due to delayed diagnosis (11,27), and improvement should be expected with the recognition of mucosal dysplasia (35,36). The undifferentiated nature and multiplicity of neoplasia should not be expected to be altered, however, by this approach.

AVAILABLE STUDIES IN CROHN'S DISEASE

There is only one actuarial study of cancer risk in the colon or rectum in Crohn's disease. After 20 years of history, it is only 2.8%, which is much lower than in ulcerative colitis but 20 times that of the general population (51). Other reports are only anecdotal (22,23,32,42,43). Some of the statistical considerations discussed above apply even more in Crohn's disease. For instance, the onset of disease is often not as clear-cut as in ulcerative colitis, and vague abdominal symptoms may precede by many years the establishment of a firm diagnosis. There is also a diagnosis difficulty in Crohn's colitis. Colonic involvement, although recognized in 1953, was universally accepted only 10 years ago, and the differentiation of Crohn's colitis from ulcerative colitis is the subject of controversy (10,34). It is not known whether the lower risk in Crohn's colitis results from the frequently fecal involvement of the colon.

Cancer of the small bowel may also complicate Crohn's disease (22,24,52). Although it was not studied by actuarial methods, this mere occurrence is striking because of the low incidence of cancer at this site in the general population. A study used the ratio of observed to expected cases, and despite the limitations of statistics, demonstrated that the risk of cancer complicating Crohn's disease was in excess for the small intestine and pancreas (23). In contrast to its occurrence in the general population, cancer develops in the distal small intestine in this group (37) and may be multifocal (6,26,49). Bypassing of involved bowel predisposes to cancer in the excluded segment (26,37,49).

OTHER FORMS OF COLITIS

No data have been produced to establish whether cancer occurs more often in patients with schistosomiasis (19).

REFERENCES

1. Baker, W. N. W., Glass, R. E., Ritchie, J. K., and Aylett, S. O. (1978): Cancer of the rectum following colectomy and ileorectal anastomosis for ulcerative colitis. *Br. J. Surg.,* 65:862–868.

2. Bargen, J. A. (1928): Chronic ulcerative colitis associated with malignant disease. *Arch. Surg.,* 17:561–576.
3. Bargen, J. A. (1929): Complications and sequellae of chronic ulcerative colitis. *Ann. Intern. Med.,* 3:335–352.
4. Beauregard, G., and Devroede, G. J. (1974): Cancer risk in ulcerative colitis: its independence of luminal factors. *Can. J. Surg.,* 17:313–315.
5. Bonnevie, O., Binder, V., Anthonisen, P., and Riis, P. (1974): The prognosis of ulcerative colitis. *Scand. J. Gastroenterol.,* 9:81–91.
6. Clemmensen, T., and Johansen, A. A. (1972): A case of Crohn's disease of the colon associated with adenocarcinoma extending from cardia to the anus. *Acta Pathol. Microbiol. A Scand.* [A], 80:5–8.
7. Cook, M. G., and Goligher, J. C. (1975): Carcinoma and epithelial dysplasia complicating ulcerative colitis. *Gastroenterology,* 68:1127–1136.
8. Dawson, I. M., and Pryse-Davies, J. (1959): The development of carcinoma of the large intestine in ulcerative colitis. *Br. J. Surg.,* 47:113–128.
9. de Dombal, F. T., Watts, J. McK., Watkinson, G., and Goligher, J. C. (1966): Local complications of ulcerative colitis: Stricture, pseudopolyposis and carcinoma of colon and rectum. *Br. Med. J.,* 1:1442–1447.
10. Devroede, J. G. (1974): Differential diagnosis of colitis. *Can. J. Surg.,* 17:369–374.
11. Devroede, G. J., Dockerty, M. B., Sauer, W. G., Jackman, R. J., and Stickler, G. B. (1972): Cancer of the colon in patients with ulcerative colitis since childhood. *Can. J. Surg.,* 15:369–374.
12. Devroede, G. J., and Taylor, W. F. (1976): On calculating cancer risk and survival of ulcerative colitis patients with the life table method. *Gastroenterology,* 71:505–509.
13. Devroede, G. J., Taylor, W. F., Greenstein, A. J., and Janowitz, H. D. (1979): Comment calculer l'histoire naturelle d'une maladie? *Gastroenterol. Clin. Biol.,* 3:259–266.
14. Devroede, G. J., Taylor, W. F., Greenstein, A. J., and Janowitz, H. D. (1979): Natürlicher Verlauf einer Krankheit: Berechnungen und Fehlermöglichkeiten. *Chirurg.* 50:297–307.
15. Devroede, G. J., Taylor, W. F., Sauer, W. G., Jackman, R. J., and Stickler, G. B. (1971): Cancer risk and life expectancy of children with ulcerative colitis. *N. Engl. J. Med.,* 285:17–21.
16. Dobbins, W. O., Stock, M., and Ginsberg, A. L. (1977): Early detection and prevention of carcinoma of the colon in patients with ulcerative colitis. *Cancer,* 40:2542–2548.
17. Edling, N. P. G., and Ecklöf, O. (1961): Distribution of malignancy in ulcerative colitis. *Gastroenterology,* 41:465–466.
18. Edwards, F. C., and Truelove, S. C. (1964): The course and prognosis of ulcerative colitis. IV. Carcinoma of the colon. *Gut,* 5:1–22.
19. El-Afifi, S. (1964): Intestinal bilharziasis *Dis. Colon Rectum,* 7:1–13.
20. Evans, D. J., and Pollock, D. J. (1972): In situ and invasive carcinoma of the colon in patients with ulcerative colitis. *Gut,* 13:566–570.
21. Farmer, R. G., and Brown, C. H. (1967): Ulcerative colitis confined to the rectum and sigmoid flexure: Report of 124 cases. *Dis. Colon Rectum,* 10:177–182.
22. Farmer, R. G., Hawk, W. A., and Turnbull, R. B., Jr. (1971): Carcinoma associated with mucosal ulcerative colitis and with transmural colitis and enteritis (Crohn's disease). *Cancer,* 28:289–292.
23. Fielding, J. F., Prior, P., Waterhouse, J. A., and Cooke, W. T. (1972): Malignancy in Crohn's disease. *Scan. J. Gastroenterol.,* 7:3–7.
24. Ginzburg, L., Schneider, K. M., Dreizin, D. H., and Levinson, C. (1956): Carcinoma of the jejunum occurring in a case of regional enteritis *Surgery,* 39:347–351.
25. Goldgraber, M. B., and Kirsner, J. B. (1964): Carcinoma of the colon in ulcerative colitis. *Cancer,* 17:657–665.
26. Goldman, L. I., Bralow, S. P., Cox, W., and Peale, A. R. (1970): Adenocarcinoma of the small bowel complicating Crohn's disease. *Cancer,* 26:1119–1125.
27. Greenstein, A. J., Sachar, D. B., Pucillo, A., Vassiliades, G., Smith, H., Kreel, I., Geller, S. A., Janowitz, H. D., and Aufses, A. H., Jr. (1979): Cancer in universal and left-sided ulcerative colitis: Clinical and pathological features. *Mt. Sinai J. Med. N.Y.* 46:25–32.
28. Greenstein, A. J. Sachar, D. B., Smith, H., Pucillo, A., Papatestas, A. E., Kreel, I., Geller, S. A., Janowitz, H. D., and Aufses A. H. (1979): Cancer in universal and left-sided ulcerative colitis: Factors determining risk. *Gastroenterology,* 77:290–294.
29. Hinton, J. M. (1966): Risk of malignant change in ulcerative colitis. *Gut,* 7:427–432.

30. Hughes, P. G., Hall, T. J., Block, C. E., Levin, B., and Moossa, A. R. (1978): The prognosis of carcinoma of the colon and rectum complicating ulcerative colitis. *Surg. Gynecol. Obstet.,* 146:46–48.
31. Hulten, L., Kewenter, J., and Ahren, C. (1972): Precancer and carcinoma in chronic ulcerative colitis. *Scand. J. Gastroenterol.,* 7:663–669.
32. Jones, J. H. (1969): Colonic cancer and Crohn's disease. *Gut,* 10:651–654.
33. Kewenter, J., Ahlman, H., and Hulten, L. (1978): Cancer risk in extensive ulcerative colitis. *Ann. Surg.,* 188:824–828.
34. Kirsner, J. B. (1975): Problem in the differentiation of ulcerative colitis and Crohn's disease of the colon: the need for repeated diagnostic evaluation. *Gastroenterology,* 68:187–191.
35. Lennard-Jones, J. E., Morson, B. C., Richie, J. K., Shove, D. C., and Williams, C. B. (1977): Cancer in colitis: assessment of the individual risk by clinical and histological criteria. *Gastroenterology,* 73:1280–1289.
36. Lennard-Jones, J. E., Parrish, J. A., Misiewicz, J. J., Ritchie, J. K., Swarbrick, E. T., and Williams, C. B. (1974): Prospective study of outpatients with extensive colitis. *Lancet,* 1:1065–1067.
37. Lightdale, C. J., Sternberg, S. S., Posner, G., and Sherlock, P. (1975): Carcinoma complicating Crohn's disease. Report of seven cases and review of the literature. *Am J. Med.,* 59:262–268.
38. MacDougall, I. P. M. (1964): The cancer risk in ulcerative colitis. *Lancet,* 2:655–658.
39. Morson, B. C., and Pang, L. S. C. (1967): Rectal biopsy as an aid to cancer control. *Gut,* 8:423–434.
40. Myrvold, H. E., Kock, N. G., and Ahren, C. H. R. (1974): Rectal biopsy and precancer in ulcerative colitis. *Gut,* 15:301–304.
41. Nugent, F. W., Haggitt, R. C., Colcher, H., and Kutterhuf, G. C. (1979): Malignant potential of chronic ulcerative colitis. Preliminary report. *Gastroenterology,* 76:1–5.
42. Parrish, R. A., Karsten, M. B., McRae, A. T., and Moretz, W. H. (1968): Segmental Crohn's colitis associated with adenocarcinoma. *Am. J. Surg.,* 115:371–375.
43. Perrett, A. D., Truelove, S. C., and Massarella, G. R. (1968): Crohn's disease and carcinoma of the colon. *Br. Med. J.,* 2:466–468.
44. Riddell, R. H. (1976): The precarcinomatous phase of ulcerative colitis. *Curr. Top. Pathol.,* 63:179–219.
45. Riddell, R. H., and Morson, B. C. (1979): Value of sigmoidoscopy and biopsy in detection of carcinoma and premalignant change in ulcerative colitis. *Gut,* 20:575–580.
46. Rosenquist, H., Ohrling, H., Lagercrantz, R., and Edling, N. (1959): Ulcerative colitis and carcinoma coli. *Lancet,* 1:906–908.
47. Slaney, G., and Brooke, B. N. (1959): Cancer in ulcerative colitis. *Lancet,* 2:694–698.
48. Sparberg, M., Fennessy, J., and Kirsner, J. B. (1966): Ulcerative proctitis and mild ulcerative colitis: a study of 220 patients. *Medicine (Baltimore),* 45:391–412.
49. Tyers, C. F. O., Steiger, E., and Dudrick, S. J. (1969): Adenocarcinoma of the small intestine and other malignant tumors complicating regional enteritis: case report and review of the literature. *Ann. Surg.,* 169:510–518.
50. Watts, J. McK., de Dombal, F. T., Watkinson, G., and Goligher, J. C. (1966): Long-term prognosis of ulcerative colitis. *Br. Med. J.,* 1.1447–1453.
51. Weedon, D. D., Shorter, R. G., Ilstrup, D. M., Huizenga, K. A., and Taylor, W. F. (1973): Crohn's disease and cancer. *N. Engl. J. Med.,* 289:1099–1103.
52. Wyatt, A. P. (1969): Regional enteritis leading to carcinoma of the small bowel. *Gut,* 10:924–927.
53. Yardley, J. H., and Keren, D. F. (1974): "Precancer" lesions in ulcerative colitis: a retrospective study of rectal biopsy and colectomy specimen. *Cancer [Suppl.],* 34:835–844.

Colorectal Cancer: Prevention, Epidemiology, and Screening, edited by S. Winawer, D. Schottenfeld, and P. Sherlock. Raven Press, New York © 1980.

Risk of Colon Cancer in Ulcerative Colitis in Low Incidence Areas—A Review

T. Gilat and P. Rozen

Department of Gastroenterology, Ichilov Hospital and Tel-Aviv University Sackler School of Medicine, Tel-Aviv, Israel

It has been well documented that the risk of colon cancer in patients with ulcerative colitis is higher than in the general population. This fact is not in dispute. The question we want to raise is whether this risk is universally equal, irrespective of genetic, dietary, environmental, and other geographic variables; i.e., that if a physician is located in Warsaw or Hong Kong, can he still base his treatment of patients with ulcerative colitis on cancer incidence figures competently calculated in Rochester, Minnesota, and London? In theory, many data suggest that the presumptive answer should be negative. In animal studies the effect of various carcinogens can be altered markedly by additional variables such as the amount of fat or bran in the diet (Zedeck, *this volume*). There is no *a priori* reason to expect that the carcinogenic factor(s) in ulcerative colitis should behave differently. In practice, numerous data suggest that the incidence of cancer of the colon in ulcerative colitis does vary among various populations in different geographic locations. In the following pages, we present and review these data.

COLON CANCER IN ULCERATIVE COLITIS IN SEVERAL GEOGRAPHIC LOCATIONS

The risk of colon cancer is related to the extent of colon affected by ulcerative colitis and the duration of the disease. In many large series of ulcerative colitis, these data are not precisely given, thus precluding exact comparisons. Nevertheless, since most large series include a mixture of cases with distal as well as extensive colonic involvement and a range of years of follow-up, it is not surprising that considerable similarities become apparent. Thus, in eight of the larger series from the United States and England (2,4,6,7,11,12,15,17), the prevalence of colon cancer (percentage) was as follows: 2.5, 2.9, 3.5, 2.9, 3, 3.3, 3.6, and 3.8. A study performed in Madrid (13) showed a comparable prevalence of 3.5%.

In contrast, data from several other countries showed quite different results. In Israel (10), a study of 504 patients with ulcerative colitis revealed only 3 cases of colon cancer (0.6%). One of the cases had ulcerative colitis for only 3 years and only the rectosigmoid was affected, making it questionable whether the two diseases were causally related. The follow-up in this series by Gilat et al. (10) was from 1 to 46 years, with a mean of 7.54 years. One-hundred-six cases were followed for more than 12 years. Only 36 of the 504 cases were operated, some with preservation of the rectum; therefore, little bias can be attributed to the operation rate.

Another study from Israel by Dinai (5) found a somewhat higher rate (1.4%) of colon cancer in Jewish patients with ulcerative colitis. This study of 645 patients diagnosed during the years 1955 through 1966 and followed until 1975 was, however, based on hospitalized cases only from the whole of Israel; whereas the study of Gilat et al. (10) was a population study of patients living in the Greater Tel-Aviv area between the years 1961 and 1970. This area comprises about one-third of the population of Israel. Thus, the series of Dinai (5) is a more selected group of more severe cases requiring hospitalization. Also, out of their 9 cases with carcinoma of the colon, at least in three cases (cases 2, 8, 9—Table 41) the relation to ulcerative colitis is problematic. For instance, in case 9 after several months of diarrhea with a nondiagnostic sigmoidoscopy, a tumor was found in the sigmoid colon. At autopsy numerous ulcerations were found in the colon. Without these 3 cases, the incidence of colon cancer would be 0.9%. Considering this and the more selective nature of the series, it can be said that both studies from Israel found a low incidence of colon cancer in Jewish patients with ulcerative colitis.

Several series of ulcerative colitis with particularly low incidences of colon cancer are listed in Table 1. The series from Ankara (1) is small and has a short follow-up; therefore, it is not representative. The series from Copenhagen (3) would seem to provide a facile explanation for the nonexistence of colon cancer among the 332 cases with ulcerative colitis. The authors regarded "the existence of symptoms for more than 10 years, with extensive radiologic changes" as an indication for surgery, especially in cases starting in childhood. However, on closer examination it becomes apparent that: more than 10% of the patients had had the disease for 11 to more than 30 years at time of admission to the study; only 12 of 56 operated patients had the rectum removed at first operation; even after the final operation about half of the 56 patients had preservation of

TABLE 1. *Colon cancer in ulcerative colitis*

Location	No. of cases	% with colon cancer	Reference
Prague	645	0.5	Nedbal and Maratka (14)
Ankara	60	0	Aktan et al. (1)
Tel-Aviv	504	0.6	Gilat et al. (10)
Copenhagen	332	0	Bonnevie et al. (3)
France	200	1.0	Terris and Hillemand (18)

TABLE 2. *Excess risk of colon cancer in patients with ulcerative colitis*

Location	Enhanced risk	Reference
Rochester, Minn.	× 20	Sedlack et al. (16)
London	× 25–30	MacDougal (12)[a]
Tel-Aviv	× 3.3	Gilat et al. (10)

[a] Cases with distal colitis excluded.

the rectal stump. All surgical and fatal cases had histologic examination of the colon. Under these circumstances a zero incidence of colon cancer is remarkable.

The series from Prague (14) consists of 645 cases with a particularly long follow-up; 21.2% followed for more than 20 years, and another 31.6% followed for 10 to 19 years. The operation rate was low, especially for the older, longer followed patients (7.5%). Only 3 cases of cancer of the colon were found among the 645 patients (0.5%). The series from France (17) is representative of many European series with a cancer incidence of 1%.

A comparison of overall cancer incidence rates in patients with ulcerative colitis is a crude measurement. It was made mandatory by the fact that in most series more exact measurements were not performed. However, several authors have calculated the actual versus expected colon cancer incidence in their patients, thus allowing an estimate of the increased risk in ulcerative colitis. The data are given in Table 2. They show that the risk of colon cancer in patients with ulcerative colitis is much higher in London and Rochester, Minnesota, than in Tel-Aviv.

COMMENT

More studies are needed to quantify exactly the cancer risk in patients with ulcerative colitis in various ethnic and geographic groups. Only then will the picture become clearer permitting more definite conclusions.

However, assuming that *prima facie* evidence is available for the existence of differences, what could the explanation be? A considerable body of evidence based mainly on studies of migrant populations indicates that cancer of the colon in man is determined mainly by environmental factors. Several colonic carcinogens were identified in animal studies, the human carcinogen(s) having not yet been determined. Diet, especially animal fat and protein, may be important as a primary or contributing factor. Genetic factors may be paramount in some, especially familial cases.

The cause of ulcerative colitis and inflammatory bowel disease (IBD) in general is unknown. The failure to identify an infectious or causative agent has shifted medical attention to the search for endogenous causes, again without success. Recently, epidemiological evidence has accumulated indicating the importance and possible predominance of environmental factors in the causation of IBD (8,9). This evidence is based in part on the study of migrant populations (mainly Ashkenazi Jews) and in part on the increasing incidence of IBD in defined populations (9). The putative environmental factor(s) have not been identified, and genetic factors may coexist.

It is thus apparent that the development of colon cancer in patients with ulcerative colitis may be subject to the influence of numerous factors, mostly exogenous, partly endogenous, all of them as yet unidentified. It is therefore conceivable that the incidence of colon cancer in patients with ulcerative colitis may vary considerably depending on the particular combination of environmental and genetic factors prevailing in a given population. We were unable to find an obvious correlation between the prevalence of colon cancer in the general population and its prevalence in patients with ulcerative colitis in several geographic locations.

More and more precise data are urgently needed on the risk of colon cancer in patients with ulcerative colitis in various parts of the globe. These data may contribute to our understanding of both disease processes. In the meantime, our above mentioned colleague from Warsaw or Hong Kong should read the excellent studies from Rochester, Minnesota, but would be well advised to supplement them with local data. An automatic and uncritical extrapolation of data may not be in the best interests of his patients.

ACKNOWLEDGMENTS

T. Gilat is an Established Investigator of the Chief Scientist's Bureau, Ministry of Health, Israel.

REFERENCES

1. Aktan, H., Paykoc, Z., and Erian, A. (1970): Ulcerative colitis in Turkey. *Dis. Colon Rectum,* 13:62–65.
2. Bargen, J. A., and Gage, R. P. (1960): Carcinoma and ulcerative colitis: Prognosis. *Gastroenterology,* 39:385–393.
3. Bonnevie, O., Vibeke Binder, Anthonisen, P., and Riis, P. (1974): The prognosis of ulcerative colitis. *Scand. J. Gastroenterol.,* 9:81–91.
4. Dawson, I. M. P., and Pryse-Davies, J. (1959): The development of carcinoma of the large intestine in ulcerative colitis. *Br. J. Surg.,* 47:113.
5. Dinai, Y. (1976): Epidemiological and clinical aspects of ulcerative colitis in Israel. M. D. Thesis, Tel-Aviv University, Sackler Medical School, Tel-Aviv, Israel.
6. Edwards, F. C., and Truelove, S. C. (1964): The course and prognosis of ulcerative colitis. Part IV. Carcinoma of the colon. *Gut,* 5:15–22.
7. Fennessy, J. J., Sparberg, M. B., and Kirsner, J. B. (1968): Radiological findings in carcinoma of the colon complicating chronic ulcerative colitis. *Gut,* 9:388–397.
8. Gilat, T. (1979): Etiology of inflammatory bowel disease. *J. Clin. Gastroenterol.,* 1:299–300.
9. Gilat, T., and Rozen, P. (1979): Epidemiology of Crohn's disease and ulcerative colitis: Etiologic implications. *Isr. J. Med. Sci.,* 15:305–308.
10. Gilat, T., Zemishlany, Z., Ribak, J., Benaroya, Y., and Lilos, P. (1974): Ulcerative colitis in the Jewish population of Tel-Aviv Yafo. II. The rarity of malignant degeneration. *Gastroenterology,* 67:933–938.

11. Goligher, J. C., deDombal, F. T., Watts, J. McK. et al. (1968): *Ulcerative Colitis,* p. 365. Balliere Tindall & Cassell, London.
12. MacDougal, J. P. M. (1964): The cancer risk in ulcerative colitis. *Lancet,* 2:655–658.
13. Mogena, H. G., Melero Calleja, E., Bueno, G., et al. (1972): Colitis ulcerosa. *Rev. Clin. Esp.,* 126:277–288.
14. Nedbal, J., and Maratka, Z. (1968): Ulcerative colitis in Czechoslovakia. *Am. J. Proctol.,* 19:106–113.
15. Nefzger, M. D., and Acheson, E. D. (1963): Ulcerative colitis in the United States Army in 1944. Follow-up with particular reference to mortality in cases and controls. *Gut,* 4:183–192.
16. Sedlack, R. E., Nobrega, F. T., Kurland, L. T. et al. (1972): Inflammatory colon disease in Rochester, Minnesota, 1935–1964. *Gastroenterology,* 62:935–941.
17. Slaney, G., and Brooke, B. N. (1959): Cancer in ulcerative colitis. *Lancet,* 2:694–698.
18. Terris, G., and Hillemand, B. (1970): Recto-colite ulcero-hemorragique. *Encycl. Med.-Chir. (Paris),* 9059:A10.

Colorectal Cancer: Prevention, Epidemiology,
and Screening, edited by S. Winawer, D. Schottenfeld,
and P. Sherlock. Raven Press, New York © 1980.

Cancer in Crohn's Disease: Memorial Hospital Experience and Review of the Literature

Charles J. Lightdale and Paul Sherlock

Memorial Sloan-Kettering Cancer Center, New York, New York 10021

Whereas the association between ulcerative colitis and adenocarcinoma of the colon has been solidly established (19,20), it was assumed for some time that Crohn's disease of the colon was not premalignant (22,23,31,34). In fact, in cases of inflammatory bowel disease, the occurrence of a carcinoma was considered by some to be diagnostic of ulcerative colitis (51). There is increasing evidence, however, that Crohn's disease is associated with the development of adenocarcinoma in both the small and large intestine, although the risk is not quantitatively as great as with ulcerative colitis (1,3–5,7,8,10–18,21,24,25,27–30,33,35,36,38,40,42–50,52–58). At Memorial Sloan-Kettering Cancer Center, we have encountered 5 cases of carcinoma of the colon complicating Crohn's colitis, which are reviewed here in the context of 30 additional cases that we could find in the literature.

PATIENTS

At Memorial Sloan-Kettering Cancer Center, we have observed 5 patients who were diagnosed at surgery as having both Crohn's disease involving the colon and colonic adenocarcinoma. The surgical pathology was reviewed, and clinical data were analyzed for age, sex, duration of diarrheal complaints, clinical features of Crohn's disease, presentation of carcinoma, and survival.

RESULTS

In our 5 patients, review of the surgical pathology confirmed the presence both of typical Crohn's colitis and of adenocarcinoma in an area of the bowel affected by the inflammatory process. All 5 cases of Crohn's colitis were clearly separable from ulcerative colitis by clinical and pathological criteria (Table 1). In 3 of the 5 patients, granulomas were present in areas of inflamed colon, and in all 5 patients, the inflammation was transmural. Skip areas typical of Crohn's were present in 4 of 5 of our cases. Ileal disease characteristic of Crohn's was present to a varying degree in all patients, and fistulae typical of Crohn's

TABLE 1. *Inflammatory findings in 5 patients with Crohn's colitis and cancer*[a]

Patient	Granulomas	Transmural disease	Rectal involvement	Skip areas	Small bowel disease	Fistulae
1	2+	2+	1+	1+	2+	2+
2	2+	2+	0	1+	1+	2+
3	0	2+	0	1+	2+	0
4	2+	2+	0	1+	2+	0
5	0	2+	1+	1+	1+	0

[a]0, not present; 1+, occurs but not prominent or distinctive; 2+, distinctive or prominent feature.

disease were present in 3 of 5. Rectal involvement is much more characteristic of ulcerative colitis than Crohn's disease in American patients, and was not a prominent feature in any of our patients.

The age of our patients when they developed colon carcinoma averaged 39 years. Three of the 5 patients were under age 35 (Table 2). Symptoms of long-standing diarrhea were present in all, with an average of 16 years of chronic symptoms (Table 2). If the splenic flexure is used to separate proximal from distal colon, 4 of 5 patients had cancer that occurred in the more proximal colon including the ascending and transverse colon (Table 3).

Presenting symptoms of colonic cancer were partial obstruction and abdominal mass in 2 patients (Table 3). In 2 other patients, chronic cutaneous fistulae

TABLE 2. *Clinical features of patients with cancer and Crohn's disease*

Patient	Age	Sex	Post-corticosteroids	Post-bowel surgery	Chronic symptoms (years)
1	50	F	+	+	30
2	30	M	0	+	15
3	25	M	+	0	13
4	56	M	+	0	9
5	34	M	0	0	15

TABLE 3. *Characteristics of cancers in Crohn's disease*

Patient	Cancer presentation	Colon cancer location	Postoperative survival
1	Nodule in fistula	Sigmoid	2 years—died, metastases
2	Increased fistula drainage	Transverse	16 months—died, amyloidosis
3	Partial obstruction	Splenic flexure	Living > 7 years
4	Incidental surgical finding	Transverse	Living > 6 years
5	Partial obstruction	Transverse	4 months—died, metastases

became involved by carcinoma. One presented with nodular carcinomatous tissue in the tract, and the other with increased fistula drainage. In another patient, a small cancer was found incidentally on pathological examination of the resected colon removed for severe inflammation and intractable bleeding.

We are able to follow all 5 patients after the diagnosis of cancer at surgery (Table 3). Two patients developed metastatic cancer. One died of amyloid kidney disease 16 months postoperatively with no evidence of cancer at autopsy. Two others have survived longer than 5 years, and presumably are free of cancer, although both continue to suffer from Crohn's disease.

DISCUSSION

In all 5 of the cases reported here, review of the clinical course and the surgical pathology confirmed the presence both of typical Crohn's disease and of adenocarcinoma in an area of bowel affected by the inflammatory process (15,26,37,39). Including these patients, our search of the literature has disclosed 35 such cases in all (3,14,18,28,30,33,44,45,53,54). The problem of assessing the risk of large bowel cancer in Crohn's disease is hazardous in retrospect, since Crohn's disease has been recognized to affect the colon for only approximately 20 years and some previous cases were probably misdiagnosed as ulcerative colitis (39). Thayer (51) has pointed out that failure to recognize cancer of the colon in Crohn's disease may have been due to a reluctance to classify a case of inflammatory bowel disease as Crohn's disease if a malignant tumor was found. In a report from the Mayo Clinic, Weedon and colleagues (53) showed that in 356 patients who had Crohn's colitis diagnosed before age 21, 8 developed colorectal cancer (2.2%). The risk of developing carcinoma of the colon was 20 times greater than in age- and sex-matched controls. Perrett and colleagues from the Radcliffe Infirmary (45) reported 3 cases of colonic carcinoma in a series of 82 patients with Crohn's disease affecting the colon (3.7%). The results of these studies conflict with other reports, however, and further studies of populations with Crohn's colitis will be needed to develop a better understanding of the magnitude of the risk (22,23). In our 5 patients with Crohn's colitis and colon carcinoma, 4 had onset of disease before age 21, and they had a history of symptoms from 9 to 30 years (average 16 years) before developing a cancer.

Since colon carcinoma is relatively common in western societies, it is possible that the apparent association with Crohn's colitis is due to chance. Using incidence and prevalence data from Britain in 1973, Darke et al. (18) estimated the chance occurrence of colon carcinoma in a patient with Crohn's disease to be one in 10 million $(1:10^7)$. On the basis of reported figures alone, even assuming bias, the number of instances of colon carcinoma occurring in patients with Crohn's far exceeds chance. Although an observed association between these diseases does not prove a causal relationship (2,6,9,41), there are two other points which suggest a relationship of carcinoma to Crohn's disease. For one, carcinoma superimposed on Crohn's disease appears more frequently in younger patients than would be expected. In general, the incidence of *de novo* colon cancer increases steadily with age, but there is a significant increase in frequency beginning only in the fifth decade. In 19 of the 35 reported cases of Crohn's disease, adenocarcinoma developed in patients under 40 years of age. Our 5 patients had an average age of 39. Secondly, the carcinomas reported superimposed on Crohn's occur in the colon in a distribution similar to that of the inflammatory disease rather than to *de novo* colon carcinoma. Although there has been some trend for *de novo* carcinomas to occur more proximally, approximately 70% occur from the splenic flexure to the anus. In Crohn's colitis, the majority of reported cancers (21 of 35 including this series) have occurred in the proximal or transverse colon, similar to the distribution seen in inflammatory disease.

The risk of developing carcinoma of the colon in Crohn's colitis appears to be considerably less than in ulcerative colitis, but the possibility of this occurrence should still be kept in mind. The risk is not large enough in magnitude to consider prophylactic colectomy. The signs and symptoms of carcinoma—such as weight loss, anorexia, abdominal mass, obstruction, bleeding, and fistuliza- tion—can be mimicked by Crohn's disease making early diagnosis difficult. Re- section of the carcinoma at an early stage (patients 3 and 4) can be curable. Although in most cases of carcinoma complicating Crohn's disease surgery has been required for diagnosis, the use of colonoscopy with biopsy and cytology to supplement radiological studies may help to detect carcinoma earlier in suspect patients (32). Biopsy and cytology evaluation of suspicious changes in chronic fistulae can be obtained (patients 1 and 2). Although the precise risk has not been defined, an awareness of the possibility of carcinoma complicating Crohn's disease on the part of the physician and surgeon may allow for a more favorable outcome in more patients.

REFERENCES

1. Almond, C. H., Neal, M. P., and Moedl, K. R. (1960): Regional ileitis with coincidental ileal carcinoma. *Mo. Med.,* 57:452.
2. Almy, T. P., and Sherlock, P. (1966): Genetic aspects of ulcerative colitis and regional enteritis. *Gastroenterology,* 51:757.
3. Atwell, J. D., Duthie, H. L., and Goligher, J. C. (1965): The outcome of Crohn's disease. *Br. J. Surg.,* 52:966.
4. Beachley, M. C., Loebel, A., Lankan, C. A., Rothman, D., and Boldi, A. (1973): Carcinoma of the small intestine in chronic regional enteritis. *Am. J. Dig. Dis.,* 18:1095.
5. Ben Asher, H. (1971): Adenocarcinoma of the ileum complicating regional enteritis. *Am. J. Gastroenterol,* 55:391.
6. Berkson, J. (1946): Limitations of the application of four-fold table analyses to hospital data. *Biometrics,* 2:47.
7. Berman, L. G., and Prior, J. T. (1964): Adenocarcinoma of the small intestine occurring in a case of regional enteritis. *Mt. Sinai J. Med. (N.Y.),* 31:30.
8. Bersack, S. R., Howe, J. S., and Rehak, E. N. (1958): A unique case with roentgenological evidence of regional enteritis of long duration with histological evidence of diffuse adenocarci- noma. *Gastroenterology,* 34:703.

9. Bisordi, W., and Lightdale, C. J. (1976): Identical twins discordant for ulcerative colitis with colon cancer. *Am. J. Dig. Dis.*, 21:71–73.
10. Brown, N., Weinstein, V. A., and Janowitz, H. D. (1970): Carcinoma of the ileum twenty-five years after bypass for regional enteritis: a case report. *Mt. Sinai J. Med. (N.Y.)*, 37:675.
11. Bruni, H., Lilly, J., Newman, W., and McHardy, G. (1971): Small bowel carcinoma as a complication of regional enteritis. *South. Med. J.*, 64:577.
12. Buchanan, D. P., Huebner, G. D., Woolvin, S. C., North, R. L., and Novack, T. D. (1959): Carcinoma of the ileum occurring in an area of regional enteritis. *Am. J. Surg.*, 97:336.
13. Cantwell, J. D., Kettering, R. F., Carney, J. A., and Ludwig, J. (1968): Adenocarcinoma complicating regional enteritis: report of a case and review of the literature. *Gastroenterology*, 54:599.
14. Clemmersen, T., and Johansen, A. (1972): A case of Crohn's disease of the colon associated with adenocarcinoma extending from cardia to the anus. *Acta Pathol. Microbiol. Scand.*, 80:5.
15. Cook, M. G., and Dixon, M. F. (1973): An analysis of the reliability of detection and diagnostic value of various pathological features in Crohn's disease and ulcerative colitis. *Gut*, 14:255.
16. Crohn, B. B., and Yarnis, H. (1958): *Regional Ileitis*, p. 74. Grune & Stratton, New York.
17. Crohn, B. B., and Yarnis, H. (1966): Granulomatous colitis: an attempt at clarification. *Mt. Sinai J. Med. (N.Y.)*, 33:503.
18. Darke, S. G., Parks, A. G., Grogano, S. L., and Pollock, D. N. (1973): Adenocarcinoma and Crohn's disease. A report of two cases and analysis of the literature. *Br. J. Surg.*, 60:169.
19. Devroede, G. J., Taylor, W. F., Sauer, W. G., Jackman, R. J., and Stickler, G. B. (1971): Cancer risk and life expectancy of children with ulcerative colitis. *N. Engl. J. Med.*, 285:17.
20. Edwards, F. C., and Truelove, S. C. (1964): The course and prognosis of ulcerative colitis. IV. Carcinoma of the colon. *Gut*, 5:15.
21. Farmer, R. G., Hawk, W. A., and Turnbull, R. B. (1970): Carcinoma associated with regional enteritis: a report of two cases. *Am. J. Dig. Dis.*, 15:365.
22. Farmer, R. G., Hawk, W. A., and Turnbull, R. B., Jr. (1971): Carcinoma associated with mucosal ulcerative colitis, and with transmural colitis and enteritis (Crohn's disease). *Cancer*, 28:389.
23. Fielding, J. F., Prior, P., Waterhouse, J. A., and Cooke, W. T. (1972): Malignancy in Crohn's disease. *Scand. J. Gastroenterol.*, 7:3.
24. Frank, J. D., and Shorey, B. A. (1973): Adenocarcinoma of the small bowel as a complication of Crohn's disease. *Gut*, 14:120.
25. Ginzburg, L., Schneider, K. M., Dreizin, D. H., and Levinson, C. (1956): Carcinoma of the jejunum occurring in a case of regional enteritis. *Surgery*, 39:347.
26. Glotzer, D. J., Gardner, R. C., Goldman, H., Hinrichs, H. R., Rosen, H., and Zetzel, L. (1970): Comparative features and course of ulcerative and granulomatous colitis. *N. Engl. J. Med.*, 232:582.
27. Goldman, L. I., Bralow, S. P., Cox, W., and Peale, A. R. (1970): Adenocarcinoma of the small bowel complicating Crohn's disease. *Cancer*, 26:1119.
28. Hardy, D. G., and Youngs, G. R. (1972): Crohn's disease and carcinoma of the rectum. *Int. Surg.*, 57:504.
29. Hoffert, P. W., Weingarten, B., Friedman, L. D., and Morecki, R. (1963): Adenocarcinoma of the terminal ileum in a segment of bowel with coexisting active ileitis. *N.Y. State J. Med.*, 63:1567.
30. Hywel Jones, J. (1969): Colonic cancer and Crohn's disease. *Gut*, 10:651.
31. Jones, J. H. (1969): Colonic cancer and Crohn's disease. *Gut*, 10:651.
32. Katz, S., Sherlock, P., and Winawer, S. J. (1972): Rectocolonic exfoliative cytology: A new approach. *Am. J. Dig. Dis.*, 17:1109.
33. Kipping, T. A., and Rowntree, T. (1970): Crohn's disease of the colon with carcinoma of the rectum. *Proc. R. Soc. Med.*, 63:753.
34. Kirsner, J. B. (1970): Ulcerative colitis 1970—Recent developments. *Scand. J. Gastroenterol.* [*Suppl.*], 6:63.
35. Kornfeld, P., Ginzburg, L., and Adlersberg, D. (1957): Adenocarcinoma occurring in regional jejunitis. *Am. J. Med.*, 23:493.
36. Lear, P. E. (1958): The physiological basis for the surgical management of regional enteritis. *Surg. Clin. North Am.*, 38:545.
37. Lewin, K., and Swales, J. D. (1966): Granulomatous colitis and atypical ulcerative colitis. Histological features, behavior, and prognosis. *Gastroenterology*, 50:211.

38. Lightdale, C. J., Sternberg, S. S., Posner, G., and Sherlock, P. (1975): Carcinoma complicating Crohn's disease. *Am. J. Med.*, 59:263–268.
39. Lockhart-Mummery, H. E., and Morson, B. C. (1961): Crohn's disease (regional enteritis) of the large intestine and its distinction from ulcerative colitis. *Gut*, 2:189.
40. Magnes, M., and DeBell, P. (1969): Carcinoma associated with terminal ileitis. *J. Med. Soc. N.J.*, 66:573.
41. Mainland, D. (1963): *Elementary Medical Statistics*, p. 111. W. B. Saunders Co., Philadelphia.
42. Morowitz. D. A., Block, G. E., and Kirsner, J. B. (1968): Adenocarcinoma of the ileum complicating chronic regional enteritis. *Gastroenterology*, 55:397.
43. Papp, J. P., and Pollard, H. M. (1971): Adenocarcinoma occurring in Crohn's disease of the small intestine. *Am. J. Gastroenterol.*, 56:149.
44. Parrish, R. A., Kansten, M. B., McRae, A. T., and Moritz, W. H. (1968): Segmental Crohn's colitis associated with adenocarcinoma. *Am. J. Surg.*, 115:371.
45. Perrett, A. D., Truelove, S. C., and Massarella, G. R. (1968): Crohn's disease and carcinoma of the colon. *Br. Med. J.*, 2:466.
46. Rha, C. K., and Wilson, J. M., Jr. (1971): Adenocarcinoma of the ileum with coexisting regional enteritis. *Arch. Surg.*, 102:630.
47. Schofeld, P. F. (1972): Intestinal malignancy and Crohn's disease. *Proc. R. Soc. Med.*, 65:783.
48. Schuman, B. M. (1970): Adenocarcinoma arising in an excluded loop of ileum. *N. Engl. J. Med.*, 283:136.
49. Sheil, F. O., Clark, C. G., and Goligher, J. C. (1968): Adenocarcinoma associated with Crohn's disease. *Br. J. Surg.*, 55:53.
50. Steele, D. C., and McNeely, D. T. (1960): Adenocarcinoma arising in a site of chronic regional enteritis. *Can. Med. Assoc. J.*, 83:379.
51. Thayer, W. R., Jr. (1970): Crohn's disease (regional enteritis): A look at the last four years. *Scand. J. Gastroenterol. [Suppl.]*, 6:165.
52. Tyers, G. F. O., Steiger, E., and Dudrick, S. J. (1969): Adenocarcinoma of the small intestine and other malignant tumors complicating regional enteritis. *Ann. Surg.*, 169:510.
53. Weedon, D. D., Shorter, R. G., Ilstrup, D. M., Huizenga, K. A., and Taylor, W. F. (1973): Crohn's disease and cancer. *N. Engl. J. Med.*, 289:1099.
54. Wein, M. A., Spector, N., and Robinson, H. M. (1964): Regional ileitis complicated by adenocarcinoma. *Am. J. Gastroenterol.*, 41:58.
55. Weingarten, B., Parker, J. G., Chazen, E. M., and Jacobson, H. G. (1959): Adenocarcinoma of the jejunum in non-specific granulomatous enteritis. *Arch. Surg.*, 78:483.
56. Weingarten, B., and Weiss, J. (1960): Malignant degeneration in chronic inflammatory disease of the colon and small intestine. *Am. J. Gastroenterol.*, 33:203.
57. Wyatt, A. P. (1969): Regional enteritis leading to carcinoma of the small bowel. *Gut*, 10:924.
58. Zisk, J., Shore, J. M., Rosoff, L., and Friedman, N. B. (1960): Regional ileitis complicated by adenocarcinoma of the ileum. A report of two cases. *Surgery*, 47:970.

Colorectal Cancer: Prevention, Epidemiology, and Screening, edited by S. Winawer, D. Schottenfeld, and P. Sherlock. Raven Press, New York © 1980.

Use of Dysplasia as an Indicator of Risk for Malignancy in Patients with Ulcerative Colitis

B. C. Morson

St. Mark's Hospital, London, EC1V 2PS England

PATIENT AT RISK

Since the first reports of carcinoma of the large intestine occurring in patients with ulcerative colitis, there have been many attempts to estimate the risk of malignant change (1,4,22). There have been difficulties in defining the population of patients at risk because different hospitals study samples which are influenced by variations in methods of selection (20). For example, the incidence of carcinoma in ulcerative colitis in medically managed patients is lower than in those treated surgically. Despite these difficulties, there is general agreement that the incidence lies between 3 and 5% of all cases (5).

The next step has been to show how this increased risk varies with length of history and the clinical type of colitis. Here again there is general agreement that the risk of malignant change begins when the patient has had symptoms for approximately 10 years, and is greater in those whose disease starts early in life. It has been confirmed that patients with extensive colitis are most at risk and that those with distal forms of the disease have an almost insignificant chance of developing carcinoma. In a prospective study of patients with extensive colitis, it has been shown that there is no increased cancer risk until the patient has had symptoms for 10 years. Between 10 and 20 years the excess risk was 23 times that expected in the general population and after 20 years, 32 times (11). Patients with symptoms of chronic continuous disease seem to be more prone to cancer than those with the acute relapsing type (7).

Even after the type of patient with ulcerative colitis most susceptible to malignant change has been defined, the treatment of the individual remains a formidable problem. Prophylactic proctocolectomy for all patients with total colitis and a history of symptoms exceeding 10 years would certainly result in colectomies being performed for patients who were not going to develop carcinoma. There is difficulty in persuading a patient who has spent many of the best years of his life adjusting to colitis that a major operation, with permanent ileostomy, is necessary. Moreover, some patients developing carcinoma in colitis have few symptoms and are in remarkably good general health. Panproctocolectomy carries a mortality and morbidity which must be taken into account.

On the other hand, there is sufficient risk to health and life other than cancer in some long-standing colitis on medical treatment alone to make colectomy attractive as a final answer to the whole problem. The prognosis of cancer in colitis is generally regarded as poor (19) but may not be so bad as first reported (7).

MACROSCOPIC FEATURES IN SURGICAL SPECIMENS

Three features distinguish cancer in colitis from ordinary intestinal cancer. First, the tumors are often multiple, which is to be expected in view of the widespread precancerous change described below. The cancers arise predominantly on the left side of the colon and are most common in the rectum (17). Second, they are often flat and infiltrating with an ill-defined edge and sometimes can be felt more easily than they are seen. In many ways, cancer in colitis resembles the macroscopic pathology of carcinoma of the stomach rather than ordinary carcinoma of the colon. Third, there is also a higher incidence of high-grade and colloid carcinomas than in ordinary intestinal cancer. This is one explanation for the poorer prognosis. Many sections from all parts of a colectomy speciman must be examined in the search for small cancers that cannot be seen by the naked eye. Such a policy will also yield examples of misplaced epithelium in the submucosa, which may be important in the pathogenesis of carcinoma in colitis.

It is important to examine the mucosa of surgical specimens with great care in a search for macroscopic evidence of epithelial dysplasia. This can vary from a verrucose appearance (villous change) to a frankly polypoid mucosa, but probably a velvety surface appearance is most common. Such areas should be scanned for evidence of ulceration which may be caused by small microinvasive carcinomas (18).

There have been reports of carcinoma of the terminal ileum in patients with ulcerative colitis in which the ileum showed the same inflammatory changes as in the colon (10). A case of a primary carcinoma occurring in an ileostomy many years after colectomy for ulcerative colitis seems to be unique (19).

EPITHELIAL DYSPLASIA IN ULCERATIVE COLITIS

There are two main histological varieties of epithelial dysplasia in ulcerative colitis: the adenomatous, which is probably more common, and dysplasia in an entirely flat mucosa. Adenomatous dysplasia more often adopts a low villous pattern than a tubular type of proliferation, but in either case manifests itself as a velvety or nodular macroscopic appearance. The resemblance to ordinary villous adenoma and tubular adenoma can be striking except that the lesions are poorly circumscribed, usually cover large areas of mucosa, and are seldom raised up much above the adjacent flat mucous membrane, although large polypoid tumors do occur. Adenomatous dysplasia in colitis rarely produces tumor on a stalk or pedicle. Small, isolated adenomas are discovered occasionally in older patients with colitis and then consideration has to be given whether they are the consequence of the inflammatory disease or a coincidental finding.

The cytological criteria for dysplasia in colitis are similar for the adenomatous histological type and for the changes seen in flat mucous membrane. They are essentially the same as for dysplasia in ordinary adenoma. In most surgical specimens, both the adenomatous type and dysplasia in a flat mucosa are found together and usually merging with one another, so that many sections must be taken from all parts of a surgical specimen in order to categorize the type and extent of dysplasia. Difficulties in the recognition of dysplasia in colitis arise because (a) it is uncommon, and (b) dysplasia is hard to distinguish from reactive hyperplasia, especially when the degree of dysplasia is mild and much active inflammation is also present.

The main criteria for dysplasia (see Table 1) are increase in size and variation in size and shape of nuclei, increase in amount of chromatin and size or number of nucleoli, increase in number of mitotic figures and the presence of abnormal forms, stratification of nuclei and increase in nuclear-cytoplasmic ratio, and presence of goblet cells deep in the epithelial membrane with loss of polarity of the nucleus, giving the appearance of an intraepithelial signet ring cell. The presence of these features along the whole length of the crypt and in the surface epithelium is particularly significant in the distinction from reactive hyperplasia. Some changes special to dysplasia in flat mucosa have been described (17).

TABLE 1. *Individual criteria (percentage incidence) graded as severe or moderate in all 32 biopsies classified as severe dysplasia, all 73 biopsies classified as moderate-mild dysplasia, and representative samples of biopsies with no dysplasia but reactive hyperplasia due to severe inflammation and no dysplasia or hyperplasia with minimal inflammation[a]*

| | Dysplasia | | No dysplasia: reactive (inflammatory) epithelial hyperplasia | |
	Severe (precancer)	Moderate or mild	Present	Absent
Villous change	9	1	0	0
Tubular budding	28	1	0	0
Variation in size of nucleus	81	16	25	0
Increased chromatin	72	32	42	0
Increased number of nucleoli	6	11	17	0
Abnormal mitotic figures	3	0	0	0
Stratification	91	29	46	0
Abnormal position of mucus	69	47	29	0
Abnormal cells in upper third of tubule	94	52	8	0

[a] Full details for all the criteria studied are available from the authors on request.

These include proliferation of enlarged, darkly stained cells arranged in a line along the whole length of the crypt and accompanied by eosinophilic cytoplasm. Goblet cells are absent. This type of dysplasia often gives rise to a very poorly differentiated type of carcinoma in colitis. Another form closely resembles intramucosal carcinoma of the stomach and has been called *in situ* anaplasia. Sometimes the dysplastic cells become vacuolated, stain poorly with mucin stains, and resemble the clear cell type of carcinoma of the stomach and colon; the so-called nephrogenic carcinoma. Finally, a variety known as pancellular dysplasia has large hyperchromatic nuclei with loss of polarity and affects all cell lines including Paneth, argentaffin, and goblet cells.

Dysplasia in colitis can be subjectively graded as mild (Fig. 1), moderate (Fig. 2), and severe (Fig. 3). Severe dysplasia can be regarded as synonymous with carcinoma *in situ*. Grading has been shown to have particular importance in the design of cancer prevention programs for patients at increased risk (see below). The term "precancer" implies only an increased susceptibility to invasive carcinoma, but is used as a clinical counterpart for the grade of severe dysplasia.

The epithelial dysplasia of colitis can be patchy, involve large areas of mucosa

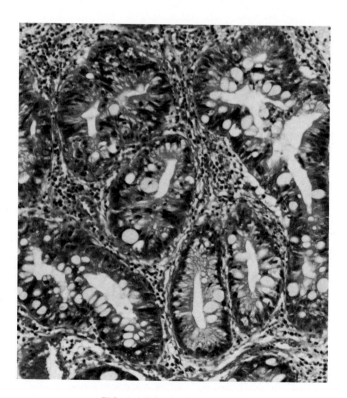

FIG. 1. Mild colonic dysplasia.

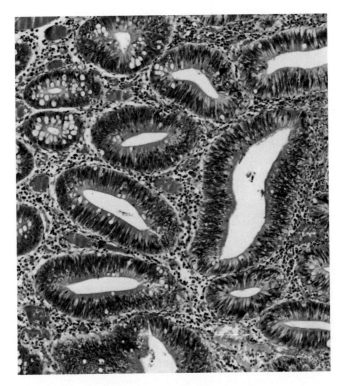

FIG. 2. Moderate colonic dysplasia.

and even the entire bowel. It is often present at a distance from any obvious cancers, but it is generally agreed that severe dysplasia can be present in the absence of invasive carcinoma (3,6,8,14,17,22). The definition and grading of dysplasia so far have been based on conventional histological studies, but cytological techniques (12) and staining for carcinoembryonic antigen (9) may prove useful in the future. Epithelial dysplasia in ulcerative colitis can be recognized by microscopic examination of rectal and colonic biopsies. It has been suggested that all patients with total colitis and a history of symptoms for more than 10 years should have a regular examination, including sigmoidoscopy and rectal biopsy, at least once every 6 months. Such a policy should help to detect those individuals with colitis who have severe dysplasia and should be considered for total proctocolectomy.

Experience has shown that the recognition of severe dysplasia (precancer) in a rectal biopsy is associated with a high incidence of suspected or unsuspected invasive cancer in the more proximal bowel. This may only be because these colitics have not been under previous observation for long enough by this method. It is desirable that all total colitics with a history of symptoms exceeding 10 years should be under indefinite observation using rectal biopsy to see if this

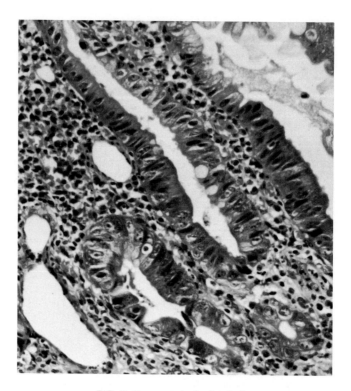

FIG. 3. Severe colonic dysplasia.

will lead to a measurable degree of cancer prevention in this high-risk population.

Because of the patchy distribution of dysplasia in the colon and rectum, it is likely that rectal biopsy will sometimes fail to be helpful. Negative reports should not be regarded as excluding the chance that dysplasia or carcinoma may be present in the proximal bowel beyond the reach of the sigmoidoscope.

Proctosigmoidoscopy is likely to detect about 40% of cancers in colitis, and dysplasia, when it occurs, involves the rectum in 60 to 80% of cases (2,17). This means that although regular rectal biopsy in patients at risk will detect dysplasia in most cases, it will not pick up that minority who may develop dysplasia only beyond the reach of the proctosigmoidoscope. For this reason, it has been suggested that regular follow-up by rectal biopsy of the patient at risk should be supplemented by total colonoscopy and multiple biopsies every 2 years or more frequently if there is any suspicion of dysplasia in the rectum (1). So far it has not been possible to demonstrate that patients pass through increasingly severe grades of dysplasia before carcinoma develops, although this would appear likely. It is clear, however, that if severe dysplasia is absent from rectal and colonic biopsies, the short-term risk of carcinoma is small.

A recent prospective study has shown that the detection of severe dysplasia by sequential rectal and colonic biopsy can detect those patients at special risk of developing cancer and that patients with mild to moderate dysplasia and those without biopsy evidence of dysplasia can safely continue under medical supervision (11). Severe dysplasia is uncommon but is associated with a high risk of carcinoma (14,15,22), but if patients at increased risk—as judged by the length of history of symptoms and the extent of colitis—are identified and carefully followed-up by sequential biopsies, then any carcinomas will be detected at an early and curable stage of development. Ideally, patients should be treated in the precancerous phase, which puts a special responsibility on the pathologist who must screen all biopsies from patients with ulcerative colitis for dysplasia with special care. Knowledge of whether the patient is clinically and statistically at increased risk may not always be available, so that it is essential to acquire experience in recognizing and grading dysplasia and differentiating it, in particular, from the much more common cellular changes which are reactive to the inflammation.

REFERENCES

1. Bargen, J. A. (1928): Chronic ulcerative colitis associated with malignant disease. *Arch. Surg.*, 17:561.
2. Boden, R. W., Rankin, J. G., Goulston, S. J. M., and Morrow, W. (1959): The liver in ulcerative colitis: The significance of raised serum-alkaline-phosphatase levels. *Lancet*, ii:245.
3. Cook, M. G., and Goligher, J. C. (1975): Carcinoma and epithelial dysplasia complicating ulcerative colitis. *Gastroenterology*, 68:1127.
4. Crohn, B. B., and Rosenberg, H. (1925): The sigmoidoscopic picture of chronic ulcerative colitis (non-specific). *Am. J. Med. Sci.*, 170:220.
5. Edwards, F. C., and Truelove, S. C. (1964): The course and prognosis of ulcerative colitis. Part IV. Carcinoma of the colon. *Gut*, 5:15.
6. Evans, D. J., and Pollock, D. J. (1972): In situ and invasive carcinoma of the colon in patients with ulcerative colitis. *Gut*, 13:566.
7. Hinton, J. M. (1966): Risk of malignant change in ulcerative colitis. *Gut*, 7:427.
8. Hulten, L., Kewenter, J., and Ahren, C. (1972): Precancer and carcinoma in chronic ulcerative colitis. *Scand. J. Gastroenterol.*, 7:663.
9. Isaacson, P. (1976): Tissue demonstration of carcinoembryonic antigen (CEA) in ulcerative colitis. *Gut*, 17:561.
10. Jalan, K. A., MacLean, N., Ross, J. M., Surcus, W., and Butterworth, S. T. G. (1969): Carcinoma of the terminal ileum and sarcoidosis in a case of ulcerative colitis. *Gastroenterology*, 56:583.
11. Lennard-Jones, J. E., Morson, B. C., Ritchie, J. K., Shove, D. C., and Williams, C. B. (1977): Cancer in colitis: Assessment of the individual risk by clinical and histological criteria. *Gastroenterology*, 73:1280.
12. Levin, R., Riddell, R. H., and Kirsner, J. B. (1976): Management of precancerous lesions of the gastrointestinal tract. *Clin. Gastroenterol.*, 5:827.
13. MacDougall, I. P. M. (1964): The cancer risk in ulcerative colitis. *Lancet*, ii:655.
14. Morson, B. C., and Pang, L. (1967): Rectal biopsy as an aid to cancer control in ulcerative colitis. *Gut*, 8:423.
15. Myrvold, H. E., Kock, N. G., and Ahren, C. (1974): Rectal biopsy and precancer in ulcerative colitis. *Gut*, 15:301.
16. Perrett, A. D., Higgins, G., Johnston, H. H., Massarella, G. R., Truelove, S. C., and Wright, R. (1971): The liver in ulcerative colitis. *Q. J. Med.*, 40:211.
17. Riddell, R. H. (1976): The precarcinomatous phase of ulcerative colitis. *Curr. Top. Pathol.*, 63:179–219.

18. Riddell, R. H. (1977): The precarcinomatous lesion of ulcerative colitis. In: *The Gastrointestinal Tract,* Monograph of the International Academy of Pathology, edited by J. H. Yardley, B. C. Morson, and M. R. Abell, pp. 109–123. Williams & Wilkins Co., Baltimore.
19. Sigler, L., and Jedd, F. L. (1969): Adenocarcinoma of the ileostomy occurring after colectomy for ulcerative colitis. *Dis. Colon Rectum,* 12:45.
20. Slaney, G., and Brooke, B. N. (1959): Cancer in ulcerative colitis. *Lancet,* ii:694.
21. Welch, C. E., and Hedberg, S. E. (1956): Colonic cancer in ulcerative colitis and idiopathic colonic cancer. *JAMA,* 191:815.
22. Yardley, J. H., and Keren, D. F. (1974): 'Precancer' lesions in ulcerative colitis: A retrospective study of rectal biopsy and colectomy specimens. *Cancer,* 34:835.
23. Yeomans, F. C. (1927): Carcinomatous degeneration of rectal adenomas. *JAMA,* 89:852.

Colorectal Cancer: Prevention, Epidemiology,
and Screening, edited by S. Winawer, D. Schottenfeld,
and P. Sherlock. Raven Press, New York © 1980.

Dysplasia: A Pathologist's View of Its General Applicability

Daniel G. Sheahan

University of Dublin, School of Pathology, Trinity College, Dublin 2, Ireland

A large volume of literature on a subject usually indicates a continuum of confusion or at least controversy about that subject. The concept of dysplastic growth of epithelial mucosae dates back to the latter portion of the last century when interest in precancerous conditions in the uterine cervix was first noted (30). The initial work on early cervical carcinoma from European centers was followed by those from North America in the 1920s and 1930s and received a great impetus from the studies of Papanicolaou (27,28). As a result, there was greater use of cytology and biopsy, and reports on preinvasive carcinoma of the cervix became world-wide and profuse. These observations were extended to the less accessible mucosal surfaces as their availability for study became feasible.

However, in 1980, there is still a lack of uniformity concerning the specific histological diagnosis of dysplasia, carcinoma *in situ* (intraepithelial carcinoma), or of regenerative change in most of these sites, and the biological behavior of the diseases which this spectrum of morphological change identifies is not yet fully established. It is apparent that in some patients, these changes regress and in others, they are associated with progression to invasive malignancy. The separation of these lesions is by histological means and represents an increasingly frequent and on occasion, very difficult problem, especially when the lesions occur in columnar-cell-lined mucosae.

TERMINOLOGY

Numerous terms have been used to describe the changes seen in these lesions, but there is no uniform application of the terms used to specific histological patterns. As an attempt towards simplification, only three terms—dysplasia, regenerative change, and atypia—will be described.

DYSPLASIA

The term dysplasia, from Greek (*dys*—difficult and *plasis*—a forming), means disorganized growth. It was introduced with reference to cervical lesions in 1953

TABLE 1. *Comparison of columnar mucosal dysplasia and regenerative change*

	Mucosal growth pattern	Epithelial cytological atypia
Dysplasia	Usually primary alteration (e.g., adenoma)	Yes
	May be secondary alteration (e.g., ulcerative colitis)	Yes
Regenerative change	Always secondary alteration (e.g., edge of peptic ulcer)	Yes (Active inflammation)

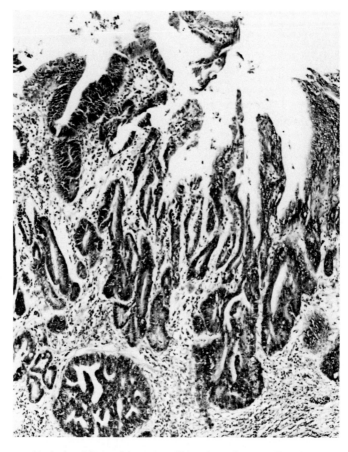

FIG. 1. Severe dysplasia of Barrett's mucosa. There is surface papillary formation with deep glands showing branching and "gland within gland" formation. H and E ×125.

by Reagan (31). It embraces the changes attributable to primary, noninvasive alterations of the mucosal growth pattern, such as an adenoma, as well as to the cytological changes (atypia) of the individual epithelial cells which constitute these lesions (Table 1). These changes are considered secondary when superimposed on a mucosa previously altered by inflammation, e.g., ulcerative colitis. Though the term dysplasia is also applied to mesodermal lesions, e.g., fibrous dysplasia of bone, the term used in the context of this discussion refers only to mucosal changes. The most severe dysplastic changes may be considered similar to carcinoma *in situ* in which the histological pattern is identical to that seen in invasive carcinoma but the lesion remains limited to the mucosa.

The altered growth pattern is readily identified in dysplastic squamous mucosa in which the abnormal basal type cells are seen in a more superficial location than normal, and these dyskaryotic epithelial cells show a disorganized relationship to one another. The pattern in dysplastic columnar cell mucosae is manifest as altered mucosal architecture with branching and budding of glands lined by columnar epithelial cells showing varying degrees of cellular crowding and stratification (Fig. 1). The individual columnar cells show mucin depletion and loss of polarity with nuclear pleomorphism and hyperchromasia. The length of gland lined by these abnormal cells varies, ranging from involvement of the deeper regions of gland crypt only, to situations in which the entire epithelial column to the surface is composed of malignant cells. Similarly, mitotic figures, some of which are abnormal, are found in more superficial locations than usual and can be seen on the surface. The latter features are considered to be a diagnostic criterion of severe dysplasia when the entire epithelial column to the surface is abnormal.

REGENERATIVE CHANGE

Regenerative change is always secondary to injury to mucosal surfaces and consists of a complex of mucosal architectural distortion and epithelial cytological atypical changes seen in inflamed and healing mucosae. It appears during the healing phase of the acute inflammatory response but can persist in certain circumstances of repeated or continuous inflammation e.g., edge of chronic peptic ulcer, chronic ulcerative colitis, or chronic atrophic gastritis.

The histological picture results from the presence of rapidly growing immature epithelial cells which are attempting to cover the surface of the mucosal defect produced by injury. These cells show a wide spectrum of pleomorphism, hyperchromasia, and loss of polarity. The injury also causes destruction of the normal reticular framework of the mucosa which causes the epithelial cell growth to form an irregularly shaped glandular pattern in a background of inflamed and organizing granulation tissue. In columnar-cell-lined mucosae, this results in architectural distortion of the glandular components of the mucosa with fibrosis of the lamina propria. These changes are permanent. As a result, the epithelial cells will be normal in the completely healed stage of columnar cell mucosal inflammation but the architecture of the mucosa will have been altered. This pattern is much more readily recognized in columnar than in squamous epithelial cell mucosae. It must be remembered that dysplastic changes may develop in such mucosae many years later and have been recognized more than 30 years after initial inflammatory insult.

ATYPIA

The term atypia, which describes any change from the typical, is used extensively in cytopathological interpretation and applies to the abnormalities of individual cells as seen in cytological or histological preparations. They range from mild to severe. In mild atypia, the cells show minimal nuclear and cytoplasmic changes in size, shape, and staining character. These changes do not imply immediate sinister significance. They are usually considered reactive and benign in nature, especially when accompanied by an acute and chronic inflammatory reaction. The epithelial cells may be infiltrated by neutrophils. The most severe changes are characterized by greater pleomorphic and hyperchromatic nuclear appearances and alterations in the nuclear:cytoplasmic ratio. The cytoplasm is retained to varying degrees and shows increased basophilia with diminished mucin complement. In this context, the term atypia is nonspecific because the individual epithelial cells in both dysplastic and regenerating lesions may show varying degrees of atypia. It is therefore important to recognize that the cytological appearances of atypia are but one of the components of the histological criteria currently used to establish the diagnosis of carcinoma *in situ,* dysplasia, or regenerative change.

HISTOLOGICAL DIAGNOSIS

The histological recognition of invasive carcinoma is usually simple. Similarly, mucosal acute inflammatory reactions with or without ulceration are also easy to identify. There is some difficulty in the accurate recognition of all stages of the preinvasive spectrum of neoplastic change and of the effects of the inflammatory process on epithelial mucosae. This difficulty increases as the two patterns approach morphological similarity. Features common to dysplasia and regenerative change include irregularly shaped and sized glands with epithelial cytological changes of mucin depletion, nuclear and cytoplasmic hyperchromasia, variations in nuclear size and shape, and prominent numbers of mitoses. Dysplasia is most likely when nuclear stratification, pleomorphism, and apolarity—including signet ring cell apolarity—involve the entire epithelial cell column to the surface with marked architectural disarray, prominent papillary intraglandular budding, and "back to back" gland formation seen in the absence of an inflammatory reaction (Figs. 2, 3, and 4). Features which favor the diagnosis of regenerative change are the presence of active, acute inflammation of the mucosa, especially the presence of neutrophils in the epithelium, and the more orderly, though

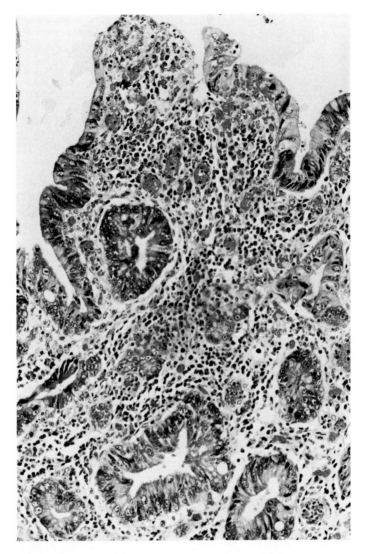

FIG. 2. Moderate to severe dysplasia of columnar cell mucosa. There is irregularity of glandular shape. Glands are lined by irregularly stratified cells showing nuclear pleomorphism and focal loss of polarity. H and E ×550.

focally abnormal, pattern of anatomic arrangement of the mucous glands without prominent papillary budding or back to back glands (Fig. 5).

Some cases of dysplasia and regenerative change are easily recognized. Others are so difficult as to defy distinction on the basis of histological examination of a single biopsy specimen. Though most of the difficult cases can be resolved satisfactorily when subsequent biopsy tissue is examined, there remain a certain

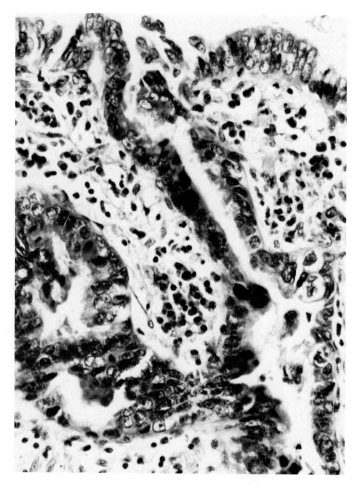

FIG. 3. Severe dysplasia of columnar cell mucosa. There is marked glandular disarray with "gland within gland" formation and minimal lamina propria cell infiltrate. The glands are lined by pleomorphic, hyperchromatic, apolaric columnar epithelial cells. Abnormal cells in stratified arrangement are seen at the surface. H and E ×550.

small number of cases in which the diagnosis remains uncertain or dissenting opinions are rendered when viewed by more than one observer. These uncertainties are more common in lesions of columnar rather than squamous epithelial origin. This reflects to some degree the more recent recognition of lesions arising in columnar cell epithelium.

Such diagnostic variation results from difficulties in establishing uniform histological criteria. These difficulties stem from the intrinsically subjective nature of the art and the differing degrees of observer experience in histopathological

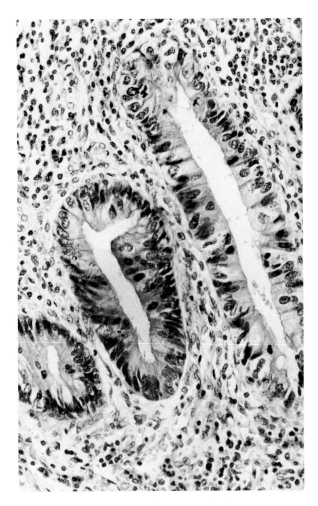

FIG. 4. Moderate to severe dysplasia of columnar cell mucosa. The small gland at left shows mild cellular atypia. The gland at right shows moderate cellular stratification, focal loss of polarity, abnormal mitoses, and loss of goblet cells. H and E ×550.

interpretation. Cases diagnosed as basal cell hyperplasia or "inflammatory atypia" (regenerative change) of squamous mucosae may be interpreted by others as dysplasia. In other circumstances, cases showing a thin zone of surface maturation covering deeper layers of squamous carcinoma may be considered by some to be dysplasia only.

Lack of diagnostic uniformity hinders the optimal patient management. The ideal, whereby histopathological diagnosis dictates therapy, becomes liable to erosion by expedient compliance of histological diagnostic opinion to therapeutic

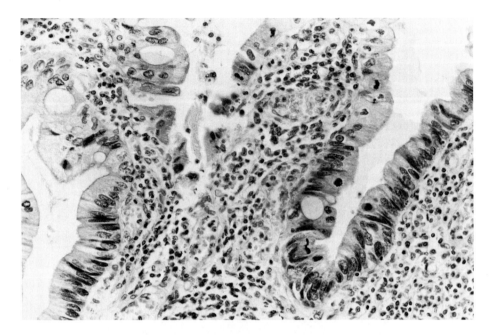

FIG. 5. Regenerative change in columnar cell mucosa showing acute ulcerative inflammation. There is cellular stratification, pleomorphism, and increased mitotic activity in deeper regions of glands. The surface epithelium shows lesser degrees of change. Neutrophils are seen in lamina propria and in epithelium. H and E ×500.

requirement. For example, the currently recommended therapy for severe dysplasia and carcinoma *in situ* of the uterine cervix is similar and as a result, there may be a less stringent requirement for their histological separation. This approach has a number of significant disadvantages. The requirement for accurate application of strict histological criteria remains, but now the pathologist's problem is the separation of carcinoma *in situ*/severe dysplasia from moderate dysplasia which is associated with less urgent therapeutic implication. It will tend to allow pathologists to deemphasize the importance of continued attempts to separate carcinoma *in situ* from severe dysplasia. Such differentiation is important and may become more so if distinct, separate, and selective therapeutic measures become available for each of these lesions. Similar problems are encountered on one hand, when dealing with carcinoma showing superficial "microinvasion" both concerning its histological recognition and its biological significance and on the other, with the requirement to clearly separate the most severe degrees of regenerative change from mild or moderate dysplasia. These problems are compounded in the spectrum of dysplastic and regenerative changes of columnar epithelial-cell-lined mucosae due to the greater lack of experience and the inherent difficulty in dealing with the histopathological appearances of these lesions.

DIFFERENTIATION BETWEEN DYSPLASIA AND REGENERATIVE CHANGE

There are not sufficient objective histological criteria that enable the pathologist in all cases to separate marked regenerative change in an inflammatory background from dysplasia of moderate to severe degree. However, certain general features are helpful in their distinction.

The diagnosis of dysplasia should not be established unequivocally in the presence of active mucosal inflammation. Most cases of diffuse mucosal inflammatory disease with abnormal epithelial cells show a return to normal epithelial cell appearances when the inflammatory response becomes quiescent. If a strong suspicion of dysplasia exists despite the presence of mucosal inflammation, biopsies should be repeated during a quiescent phase of the disease, when there is no morphological evidence of active inflammation, and compared with the original. Remaining cognizant of sampling variation, if the biopsy appearances are improved, the likelihood is that the lesion is reactive and benign. However, if the epithelial cell abnormalities persist in the absence of an inflammatory reaction, the lesion is most probably dysplastic in nature. Identification of dysplasia only in biopsy samples does not preclude the existence of carcinoma *in situ* or invasive carcinoma elsewhere in the lesion. Prior exposure to radiation must always be kept in mind, as atypical cellular appearances that can also resemble dysplasia may be seen even 20 to 30 years after irradiation.

The diagnostic problems posed by these lesions embrace the earlier stages of histologically recognizable neoplastic development. As a result of the growing recognition of their significance, the importance and responsibility of the role of the histopathologist in the initial diagnosis and subsequent follow-up of these patients have increased. A considerable degree of experience is required in the evaluation of these lesions, and it should not be undertaken by those without appropriate morphological training in this area. However, it is stressed that all concerned with the management of these patients should be aware that there are limitations to histopathologic interpretation in this area. Errors in this area of diagnostic pathology can result in extensive but unnecessary extirpitive surgery or failure to recognize and treat effectively a potentially lethal disease in its early form.

DYSPLASIA IN SPECIFIC SITES

Before proceeding to a discussion of dysplasia in the gastrointestinal tract, a brief description of dysplasia in other mucosal surfaces will emphasize the histological similarity between dysplasia occurring in columnar, transitional, and squamous mucosae irrespective of their anatomic location. Many of these mucosal lesions are of relatively recent recognition, a fact probably related to the advent of endoscopic instruments and the capability of biopsying regions which were until then only histologically examined in larger surgical resection specimens or in autopsy material. The resultant advantages include earlier diagnosis for the patient, identification of the earlier stages of disease, and the opportunity to study the morphological changes during the earlier stages of evolution of malignancy in ideally prepared tissue.

BRONCHUS

Squamous metaplasia of the bronchial epithelium was recognized in the 1930s but it was not until 20 years later that the association of carcinoma *in situ* and invasive carcinoma of the bronchus was noted (6). The subsequent detailed studies of Auerbach and colleagues (2) showed that cigarette smoking was associated with a spectrum of histological change in the bronchial mucosa that ranged from goblet cell and squamous cell metaplasia to atypical epithelial proliferation including dysplasia and squamous carcinoma *in situ* identical to that seen in the uterine cervix. Some of the milder hyperplastic and metaplastic changes of bronchial epithelium are known to be reversible if cigarette smoking ceases but if smoking continues, the lesions may progress over a variable course of time to invasive carcinoma.

URINARY BLADDER

Most bladder carcinomas are low grade, papillary transitional cell tumors with a high rate of recurrence. It is now recognized that a certain group of patients present with diffuse transitional cell carcinoma *in situ* and contiguous dysplasia without evidence of papillary formation (7). Total cystectomy apparently provides effective treatment in these patients. However, the presence of carcinoma *in situ* and to a lesser extent, dysplasia contiguous to papillary tumor, significantly increases the likelihood of invasive carcinoma occurring within a few years (1). The biologic behavior and prognostic significance of urothelial dysplasia and carcinoma *in situ* are not clear. It is assumed that dysplasia and carcinoma *in situ* progress to invasive malignancy but how often this occurs and how long it takes to develop invasive capacity is not known. The carcinoma *in situ* lesion may be visible at cystoscopy only as a granular erythematous patch but is frequently not recognizable to naked eye examination (14). Histologically, the lesion shows thickening and disorganization of mucosa which is composed of anaplastic transitional epithelial cells showing loss of normal polarity, nuclear "crowding," pleomorphism, and hyperchromasia with abnormal mitotic figures (Fig. 6). Significantly, the urinary bladder dysplastic lesion was first recognized less than 30 years ago (18) in association with papillary invasive tumors. Thus, the patchy distribution of epithelial dysplasia also has been recognized recently in neoplastic conditions of the bladder but as in other sites, knowledge of extent, frequency of occurrence, and prognostic significance is still being accumulated (14,23).

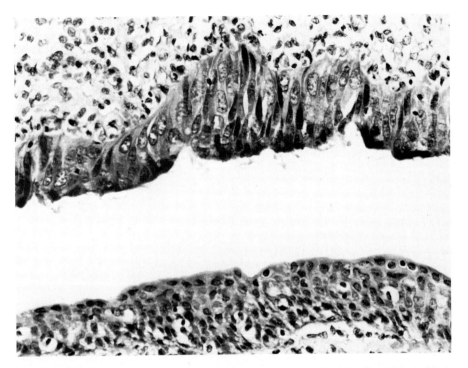

FIG. 6. Severe dysplasia of urothelium contiguous to papillary transitional cell carcinoma. Bladder mucosa *(top)* showing marked cellular pleomorphism and hyperchromatism with some loss of polarity. Note the basement membrane is intact. The mucosa in lower portion shows a lesser degree of dysplasia. H and E ×550.

ENDOMETRIUM

Endometrial hyperplasia may be cystic and benign or adenomatous and considered to be premalignant (9,36). In its mild form, the changes of adenomatous hyperplasia consist of proliferation and crowding of endometrial glands which are of irregular shape and size separated from one another by scant stroma. The lining epithelium shows cellular stratification, frequent mitoses, and minimal pleomorphism. In the more severe cases, termed atypical adenomatous hyperplasia, cellular pleomorphism, stratification, and papillary intraluminal tufting are marked with back to back gland formation, and the epithelial cells become acidophilic rather than basophilic. Histological differentiation between atypical adenomatous hyperplasia and well-differentiated endometrial adenocarcinoma is on occasion very difficult. The evidence that atypical endometrial hyperplasia is premalignant stems from the observations that it often accompanies and frequently antedates endometrial adenocarcinoma. The latter feature has been shown both in retrospective and prospective studies. At the practical level, treatment for atypical adenomatous hyperplasia is very similar to that for well-differentiated adenocarcinoma of the endometrium.

GASTROINTESTINAL TRACT

Mucosal dysplasia and carcinoma *in situ* may be seen in various sites in the alimentary tract. Other than that seen in primary columnar epithelial cell neoplasms (e.g. gastric and colonic adenomas), gastrointestinal dysplasia occurs in association with chronic mucosal inflammation and certain types of metaplastic epithelial response (Table 2). The histological changes of dysplasia are similar in all three areas and are identical to those seen in columnar-cell-lined mucosae elsewhere. The relationship of metaplastic epithelium to the later development of dysplasia is important, as the presence of the former enables identification of patients who as a group have an increased liability to develop dysplasia or carcinoma in that region.

Esophagus

The sequelae of chronic reflux esophagitis include hyperplasia of the squamous epithelium (3,11) and healing of the ulcerated distal squamous esophageal mucosa by a metaplastic columnar epithelial cell lining known as Barrett's mucosa. Behar et al. (4) have shown that such epithelium remains after symptoms have been significantly relieved by surgical means but its total duration is not known. Adenocarcinoma of the distal esophagus is recognized more frequently in patients with a history of chronic reflux esophagitis (10,25). It is now recognized that the carcinoma arises from the Barrett's columnar-cell-lined mucosa which shows areas of columnar cell dysplasia or carcinoma *in situ* (16) and that the premalignant phase can be detected by both biopsy and cytology (5,29). We have noted in our laboratory the occurrence of severe dysplasia on esophageal biopsies of Barrett's mucosa with invasive adenocarcinoma and contiguous carcinoma *in situ* and severe dysplasia in the subsequent resected specimen (Figs. 7 and 8).

Stomach

Atrophic gastritis with intestinal metaplasia is seen in over 90% of cases of cancer of the stomach (20). The gastric remnant of patients who have had

TABLE 2. *Sites of gastrointestinal columnar cell dysplasia*

Esophagus: Barrett's (columnar-cell-lined) mucosa
Stomach: Intestinal metaplasia (atrophic gastritis)
Idiopathic
Pernicious anemia
Mucosa contiguous to epithelial neoplasm
Postsurgical gastric remnant
Intestines: Adenoma
Multiple adenomatosis syndromes
Chronic ulcerative colitis

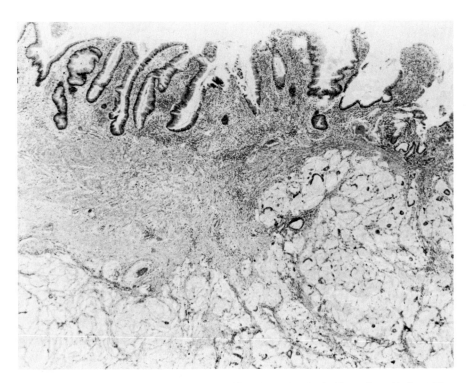

FIG. 7. Mucinous (colloid) adenocarcinoma arising from dysplastic Barrett's epithelium. The mucosa shows papillary formation with architectural disarray. H and E ×55.

gastrectomy or gastroenterostomy for peptic ulcer frequently shows atrophic gastritis and these patients have an increased incidence of gastric cancer 20 to 25 years later (35). Patients with pernicious anemia, who have an increased incidence of gastric carcinoma, have diffuse atrophy of gastric mucosa (22,37). Patients with atrophic gastritis unassociated with pernicious anemia have also been shown to have an increased incidence of gastric carcinoma (34). The underlying lesion which is common to all of the above conditions is atrophic gastritis with intestinal metaplasia. Gastric carcinomas frequently show regions composed of cells with features of intestinal epithelium (26).

The growing Japanese experience (13) shows that early gastric cancer can be diagnosed by endoscopically directed biopsies with resultant curative resection in most patients. At this stage, the carcinoma is not evident as a tumor mass but may be recognized as a slight excavation or minimally raised mucosal plaque. The carcinoma is intramucosal and is frequently associated with varying degrees of dysplasia arranged in patchy distribution throughout the gastric mucosa. The increasing awareness of early gastric cancer has engendered the more frequent and widespread use of gastric biopsy.

Most gastric polyps are hyperplastic (regenerative) in type and have little

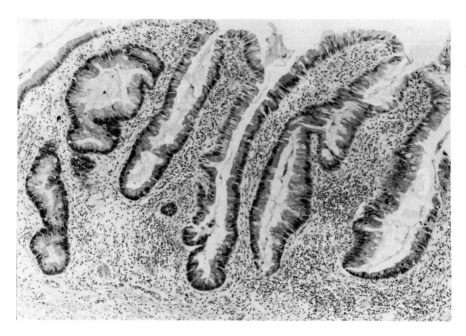

FIG. 8. Higher magnification of portion of mucosa seen in Fig. 7. There is irregularity of glandular shape and size with budding and branching of glands. The muscularis mucosae is intact. The hyperchromatic epithelial nuclei are stratified and apolaric in focal areas as compared to the normal appearing epithelium at top left. H and E ×120.

neoplastic potential (19). The relatively uncommon gastric adenoma which is neoplastic is also frequently associated with intestinal metaplasia and may manifest all grades of dysplasia to intramucosal carcinoma similar to that seen in its colonic counterpart.

Colon

The current concensus of opinion is that colonic adenocarcinomas arise from benign adenomas (33). The increased incidence of colonic carcinoma in patients with multiple adenomatosis syndromes and chronic ulcerative colitis is well recognized. An ominous feature common to these latter conditions is the presence of severe dysplasia. An increased incidence of colonic carcinoma has also been described in radiation colitis following ureterosigmoidostomy and Crohn's colitis but there has not been good documentation of dysplasia in association with these lesions.

The colonic adenoma consists of a primary neoplastic disorder of epithelial cell growth, the epithelium of which may show various degrees of cytological atypia. In ulcerative colitis, the mucosal architecture is altered primarily by the inflammatory disease process with dysplasia becoming manifest years later in a small but significant number of cases. It is not known by what means, under what circumstances, or what length of time it takes for these conditions, one neoplastic and the other inflammatory, to develop severe dysplastic or carcinomatous changes. Therefore, clinical scrutiny of patients with these lesions by repeated endoscopic and mucosal biopsy examinations remain the best means of identifying the extent and severity of dysplastic changes in the colonic mucosa. Because of sampling variation, the patchy nature of the lesions, and the lack of endoscopic gross changes in some colitic conditions, the liability to underdiagnose is continuously present. The therapy of these lesions continues to be controversial. Personally, I believe that there is not much question as to whether or not surgery is indicated when severe dysplasia is identified in colonic mucosa but rather when it should be performed and how extensively.

A number of different properties of colonic adenomas are important in the evaluation of their malignant potential. Quantitative properties such as large size and large number correlate with increased liability of malignant change (8,24). Qualitative properties such as the presence of villous change and severe dysplasia are also associated with increased malignant potential (21). The interrelationship between these quantitative and qualitative properties is not known, but it appears reasonable that the presence of severe dysplasia in colonic adenomas should possess similar significance to that which pertains in panulcerative colitis (15).

Dysplastic lesions are frequently multifocal especially in the stomach and colon. Practical reasons dictate that mucosal biopsy sampling is limited and as a result, the full extent of the degrees of dysplastic change that may be present cannot always be fully ascertained. The correlation of both the quantitative and qualitative degrees of dysplasia with the biological progression of disease appears at present to be a difficult goal to obtain, but when feasible, should represent a valuable contribution of morphology to patient management.

The Pathologist's Contribution and The Endoscopist's Responsibility

Histopathological evaluation of mucosal disease in autopsy material has not been fruitful. The availability of modern endoscopic instruments has, for example, facilitated biopsy evaluation of the mucosa of the esophagus, stomach, and proximal duodenum from above and the entire colon and distal ileum from below. As a result, the amount of well preserved and properly prepared gastrointestinal mucosal tissue available for histological study has greatly increased. The growing expertise of the examining endoscopists at recognizing the more subtle gross changes of neoplastic and inflammatory disease has enabled better selection of the tissues to be biopsied with consequent improvement in the diagnostic yield. Close liaison with clinicians, radiologists, and endoscopists in the management of patients and examination of large amounts of biopsy material contribute to improved diagnostic skills. As the diagnostic expertise grows with experience, it may be expected that the difficulties that are currently being encountered in the interpretation of columnar cell dysplasia in organs such as the alimentary tract will become minimized and less frequent.

The pathologist can only study the tissue submitted for histological evaluation. These tissue samples are usually small and their histological appearances cannot be assumed to be representative of the disease process elsewhere in the lesion or mucosa. This is particularly true for the interpretation of biopsies of colonic polypoid lesions where the invasive malignancy may be missed on biopsy (17). Additional information, including the pertinent clinical history and radiological findings, is also required. Histopathological interpretation of small mucosal biopsies in the absence of appropriate clinical information is fraught with error. It is recommended that biopsies should be from multiple areas of the mucosa irrespective of its endoscopic appearance because it is now recognized that dysplasia and even focal acute inflammation may not show gross endoscopic changes.

The preparation of tissue for examination is important. The endoscopist has the primary responsibility for ensuring the best orientation of the specimen. This is difficult with samples obtained from small endoscopic biopsy forceps. However, endoscopic instruments using forceps with a central spike are helpful as they tend to maintain the mucosal aspect uppermost in the cups with the submucosal aspect beneath applied to the spike. This then allows the specimen to be placed submucosal side down and adherent to a flat, semirigid surface, e.g. cardboard, and then placed gently in fixative with mucosal aspect uppermost. This allows sections to be prepared that show mucosal orientation in a vertical plane. This is important because the true extent of mucosal architectural disarray or invasion of epithelium through muscularis mucosae is best determined in properly oriented sections and the surface epithelium is seen to best advantage in vertical plane sections of the mucosa.

It appears that the major contribution of pathologists to this area of diagnostic controversy lies in the continued attempts to further define generally acceptable histological criteria of the various degrees of dysplasia and of carcinoma *in situ* and their separation from the regenerative changes seen in nonspecific mucosal inflammation. The promotion of the general recognition of the potentially sinister significance of epithelial dysplasia and the pathological environment in which it occurs can also be emphasized by pathologists. All instances of premalignant conditions should be documented. In the gastrointestinal tract lesions such as Barrett's epithelium in the esophagus, intestinal metaplasia in the stomach and panulcerative colitis when recognized morphologically should be recorded, and the presence or absence of dysplasia noted. Awareness of the presence of a premalignant condition in patients even in the absence of dysplasia contributes significantly to their future management, even if it only results in the more frequent assessment of the patient.

CONSISTENCY OF HISTOPATHOLOGICAL DIAGNOSIS

Do all pathologists diagnose squamous and columnar cell dysplasia uniformly, consistently, and accurately and can they easily separate it from carcinoma *in situ* and regenerative change? At the present time, it is probably fair to say that some pathologists do not. Many general pathologists will not see a sufficient number of endoscopically-derived biopsies showing dysplastic lesions in their daily practice to enable them to consistently and accurately diagnose the various grades of columnar epithelial cell dysplasia. Close study of the premalignant mucosa contiguous to an obvious gastric carcinoma, or to a colonic carcinoma arising in ulcerative colitis, or to the neoplastic epithelium of colonic adenomas will provide increased familiarity with the spectrum of dysplastic changes and as a result, should enable a greater degree of accuracy to be applied to the histological separation of carcinoma *in situ,* dysplasia, and regenerative change.

BIOLOGICAL IMPLICATIONS

Opinions concerning prognosis based on morphological grounds alone and without accurate knowledge of the biological progression of the disease have limited value. As has been outlined, there are limitations to the morphological approach to the understanding of these diseases. Our current knowledge of the biological behavior of precancerous lesions of mucosal surfaces is also limited. The possible co-existence of or potential for subsequent evolution to invasive malignancy cannot be excluded in any case in which a mucosal biopsy shows dysplasia. Once a definite histological impression of dysplasia has been established, it constitutes clear indication that the patient's specific organ mucosa has focally undergone significant change with at least potential to develop invasive malignancy, and that close scrutiny with repeated examinations of the mucosa of the entire organ should be maintained thereafter. The optimum frequency of such repeat examinations is not known and there are at present no more than conceptually or arbitrarily derived guidelines on when extirpative surgery should be undertaken in patients shown to have severe dysplasia on mucosal biopsy. For example, in a recent study, the findings of severe dysplasia on colonic biopsy from two separate sites or at sequential examinations in patients with chronic ulcerative pancolitis was considered an indication for total colectomy (15).

CONCLUSIONS

Recent immunohistological studies have indicated that specific blood group isoantigens are deleted from neoplastic and dysplastic colonic epithelium in panulcerative colitis, colonic carcinomas, and adenomas but not from the regenerative epithelium at the edge of ulceration in Crohn's disease (32). As more information is obtained in this area, it is to be anticipated that the histological criteria will become better defined, more knowledge of the biological behavior of the dysplastic lesion will accrue, and better clinical management of these patients will ensue. The earlier recognition of patients with such lesions should result in improved survival rates from neoplastic disease.

There are numerous questions to which we have at best only partial answers.

Does the dysplastic lesion regress and if so can we clearly recognize the type which regresses? Are the dysplastic appearances neoplastic or reactive? How long may dysplastic changes persist? For how long may dysplasia be present before carcinoma changes are recognized? Do all dysplastic lesions necessarily progress to carcinoma? In today's sociomedical circumstances, the answers cannot be satisfactorily derived because of increasingly earlier interference with the biological progression of the lesion as a result of investigation or therapy or both. Stated most simply, the best answer we have at the moment is that some cases diagnosed as carcinoma *in situ* or dysplasia regress, some persist without apparent change, and some progress to invasive carcinoma but we do not know the temporal relationships of the progression of these changes in terms of either duration or frequency of occurrence. The desirable prospective studies will also be difficult to perform.

REFERENCES

1. Althausen, A. F., Prout Jr., G. R., and Daly, J. J. (1976): Non-invasive papillary carcinoma of the bladder associated with carcinoma-in-situ. *J. Urol.,* 116:575–580.
2. Auerbach, O., Gere, J. B., Forman, J. B., Petrick, J. G., Smolin, H. J., Muchsam, G. E., Kassouny, D. Y., and Stout, A. P. (1957): Changes in the bronchial epithelium in relation to smoking and cancer of the lung. *New Engl. J. Med.,* 256:97–104.
3. Behar, J., and Sheahan, D. G. (1975): Histological abnormalities in reflux esophagitis. *Arch. Pathol.,* 99:387–391.
4. Behar, J., Sheahan, D. G., Biancani, P., Spiro, H. M., and Storer, E. H. (1975): Medical and surgical management of reflux esophagitis. *New Engl. J. Med.,* 293:263–268.
5. Belladonna, J. A., Hajdu, S. I., Bains, M. S., and Winawer, S. J. (1974): Adenocarcinoma-in-situ of Barrett's esophagus diagnosed by endoscopic cytology. *New Engl. J. Med.,* 291:895–896.
6. Black, H., and Ackerman, L. V. (1952): The importance of epidermoid carcinoma-in-situ in the histogenesis of carcinoma of the lung. *Ann. Surg.,* 136:44–55.
7. Farrow, G. M., Utz, D. C., and Rife, C. C. (1976): Morphological and clinical observations of patients with early bladder cancer treated with total cystectomy. *Cancer Res.,* 36:2495–2501.
8. Gilbertsen, V. A. (1974): Proctosigmoidoscopy and polypectomy in reducing the incidence of rectal cancer. *Cancer,* 34:936–989.
9. Gore, H. (1973): Hyperplasia of the endometrium. In: *The Uterus. International Academy of Pathology Monograph,* No. 14, edited by H. J. Norris, A. T. Hertig, and M. R. Abell, pp. 255–275. Williams and Wilkins, Baltimore.
10. Hawe, A., Payne, W. S., Weiland, L. H., and Fontana, R. S. (1973): Adenocarcinoma in the columnar epithelial lined lower (Barrett's) esophagus. *Thorax,* 28:511–514.
11. Ismail-Beigi, F., Horton, P. F., and Pope, C. E. II (1970): Histological consequences of gastroesophageal reflux in man. *Gastroenterology,* 58:163–174.
12. Järvi, O., and Lauren, P. (1951): On the role of heterotopias of the intestinal epithelium in the pathogenesis of gastric cancer. *Acta Pathol. Microbiol. Scand.,* 29:26–44.
13. Kawai, K. (1971): Diagnosis of early gastric cancer. *Endoscopy,* 3:23–27.
14. Koss, L. G., Nakanishi, I., and Freed, S. Z. (1977): Non-papillary carcinoma-in-situ and atypical hyperplasia in cancerous bladders. *Urology,* 9:442–454.
15. Lennard-Jones, J. E., Morson, B. C., Ritchie, J. K., Shove, D. C., and Williams, C. B. (1977): Cancer in colitis: Assessment of the individual risk by clinical and histological criteria. *Gastroenterology,* 73:1280–1289.
16. Levin, B., Riddell, R. H., and Kirsner, J. B. (1976): Management of precancerous lesions of the gastrointestinal tract. *Clin. Gastroenterol.,* 5:827–853.

17. Livstone, E. M., Troncale, F. J., and Sheahan, D. G. (1977): The value of a single forceps biopsy of colonic polyps. *Gastroenterology,* 73:1296–1298.
18. Melicow, M. M. (1952): Histological study of vesical urothelium intervening between gross neoplasms in total cystectomy. *J. Urol.,* 68:261–279.
19. Ming, S. -C. (1977): The classification and significance of gastric polyps. In: *The Gastrointestinal Tract,* edited by J. H. Yardley, B. C. Morson, and M. R. Abell, p. 153. Williams and Wilkins, Baltimore.
20. Morson, B. C. (1955): Carcinoma arising from areas of intestinal metaplasia in the gastric mucosa. *Br. J. Cancer,* 9:377–385.
21. Morson, B. C. (1977): Polyps and cancer of the large bowel. In: *The Gastrointestinal Tract,* edited by J. H. Yardley, B. C. Morson, and M. R. Abell, pp. 101–108. Williams and Wilkins, Baltimore.
22. Mosbech, J., and Videbaek, A. (1950): Mortality from and risk of gastric carcinoma among patients with pernicious anaemia. *Br. Med. J.,* 2:390–394.
23. Murphy, W. M., Nagy, G. K., Rao, M. K., Soloway, M. S., Parija, G. C., Cox, C. E., and Friedell, G. H. (1979): "Normal" urothelium in patients with bladder cancer. A preliminary report from the National Bladder Cancer Collaborative Group A. *Cancer,* 44:1050–1058.
24. Muto, T., Ishikawa, K., Kino, I., Nakamura, K., Sugano, H., Bussey, H. J. R., and Morson, B. C. (1977): Comparative histologic study of adenomas of the large intestine in Japan and England with special reference to malignant potential. *Dis. Col. Rectum.,* 20:11–16.
25. Naef, A. P., Savary, M., and Ozzello, L. (1975): Columnar lined lower esophagus: An acquired lesion with malignant predisposition. *J. Thor. Cardiovasc. Surg.,* 70:826–835.
26. Nakamura, K., Sugano, H., Takagi, K., and Kumakura, K. (1971): Conception of histogenesis of gastric carcinoma. *Stomach Intestine,* 6:9–21.
27. Papanicolaou, G. N. (1928): In: *Proceedings of the Race Betterment Conference,* p. 528. Race Betterment Foundation, Battle Creek, Michigan.
28. Papanicolaou, G. N., and Traut, H. (1943): Diagnosis of uterine cancer by the vaginal smear. The Commonwealth Fund, New York.
29. Paull, A., Trier, J. S., Dalton, M. D., Camp, R. C., Loeb, P., and Goyal, R. K. (1976): The histologic spectrum of Barrett's esophagus. *New Engl. J. Med.,* 295:476–480.
30. Petersen, O. (1955): Precancerous changes of the cervical epithelium in relation to manifest cervical carcinoma. *Acta. Radiol. [Stockh. Suppl.],* 127.
31. Reagan, J. W., Seidemann, I. L., and Saracusa, Y. (1953): Cellular morphology of carcinoma-in-situ and dysplasia or atypical hyperplasia of the uterine cervix. *Cancer,* 6:224–235.
32. Sheahan, D. G. (1979): Blood group ABH isoantigens in colonic mucosa of patients with inflammatory bowel disease. *Front. Gastrointest. Res.,* 4:51–64.
33. Sheahan, D. G. (1979): The colonic adenoma-carcinoma sequence. The evidence in favour of the relationship. In: *Screening and Early Detection of Colorectal Cancer,* edited by D. R. Brodie, pp. 80–96. U.S.P.H.S., National Institutes of Health Publication No. 80-2075.
34. Siurala, M., and Seppälä, K. (1960): Atrophic gastritis as a possible precursor of gastric carcinoma and pernicious anemia. Results of follow-up examinations. *Acta Med. Scand.,* 166:455–474.
35. Stalsberg, H., and Taksdal, S. (1971): Stomach cancer following gastric surgery for benign conditions. *Lancet,* ii:1175–1177.
36. Welch, W. R., and Scully, R. E. (1977): Precancerous lesions of the endometrium. *Human Pathol.,* 8:503–512.
37. Zamcheck, N., Grable, E., Ley, A., and Norman, L. (1955): Occurrence of gastric cancer among patients with pernicious anemia at the Boston City Hospital. *New Engl. J. Med.,* 252:1103–1106.

Colorectal Cancer: Prevention, Epidemiology, and Screening, edited by S. Winawer, D. Schottenfeld, and P. Sherlock. Raven Press, New York © 1980.

Surveillance of Patients with Ulcerative Colitis: Lahey Clinic Results

F. Warren Nugent

Department of Gastroenterology, Lahey Clinic Foundation, Boston, Massachusetts 02215

Patients with ulcerative colitis have long been known to be at a greater risk for the development of carcinoma of the colon than the general population of the same age (1–3, 5, 7–9). Only patients with long-standing disease involving most of the colon are thought to be at risk (5). These patients represent a relatively small group in the large pool of those suffering from ulcerative colitis. Perhaps as many as 50% of all patients with ulcerative colitis have their disease confined to the rectum or sigmoid or both (ulcerative proctitis, distal colitis, or proctosigmoiditis); studies have shown that these patients are not at increased risk (4,12). Although occasionally a patient has been reported in whom cancer developed in the course of ulcerative proctosigmoiditis, these have invariably been elderly patients in the peak age incidence for cancer of the colon, and their disease is considered coincidental. Figure 1 shows the entire range of neoplastic and hyperplastic changes that may occur in the colon in ulcerative colitis.

DURATION AND EXTENT

Only those patients who have suffered from ulcerative colitis for a long duration have been found to be at risk. Whereas the incidence in the first 10 years is approximately 2 to 3%, it increases sharply after the first decade and reaches 2% per year—10-fold the incidence in the first 10 years (3). All series of patients with ulcerative colitis in whom cancer developed include a minority who have had colitis fewer than 10 years. In a recent study of 23 patients in whom cancer developed during the course of ulcerative colitis, we found that 5 (22%) had suffered from their disease 10 years or less (11). No patient with ulcerative colitis has been reported in whom cancer developed after seven or fewer years of disease. Approximately half of all patients with disease involving most of the colon (universal colitis) will require total colectomy at some time because of the severity or complications of their disease. Thus only those patients who have universal disease and who have escaped colectomy for at least 7 years are in the group that is prone to the development of colonic cancer.

All authors agree that duration and extent of disease are firm criteria for

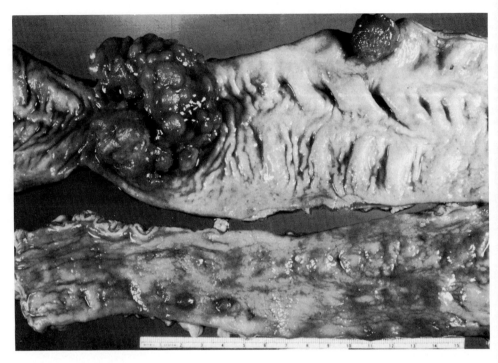

FIG 1. "Burned-out" ulcerative colitis. *Upper left,* carcinoma; *upper right,* adenomatous polyp with focus of carcinoma; *lower left,* adenomatous polyp; *lower right,* hyperplastic polyp. From Nugent and Haggitt (10).

selection of patients who are at high risk. Other criteria, such as onset at an early age, or the characteristics of the clinical course of the disease have been suggested by some but are questioned by others.

Some patients with ulcerative colitis suffer from acute attacks during their early years and then enjoy prolonged remission of their disease. With the remarkable mobility of present-day society, these patients, whose active disease may have occurred when they were very young, may find themselves in an entirely different part of the country with different medical contacts. They may reject the fact that they had a serious intestinal disease at an earlier age or may forget it in the sense that they have no reason to believe that it is still a problem. This group is important if long-term surveillance for cancer in patients with ulcerative colitis is to be effective, and the physician must be aware and take a careful history to identify these patients.

MANAGEMENT

The management of patients with long-standing ulcerative colitis who are considered at risk for cancer has varied a great deal over the years and from

TABLE 1. *Possible components of a surveillance program*

Clinical evaluation
Proctoscopy
Barium enema
Air contrast barium enema
Colonic cytology
Carcinoembryonic antigen level
Reversal of sialomucin/sulfomucin ratio in colonic mucosa
Reversal of LSH isoenzyme ratios
Decrease in secretory component production
Colonoscopy
Dysplasia

center to center. The problem was simply ignored by many as it is not frequently seen. Others have proposed, and some still do, that proctocolectomy is the treatment of choice for all patients after the first decade of disease. Still others have chosen to carry out surveillance programs of one type or another (Table 1). Clinical evaluation, proctoscopy, and routine barium enema study at regular intervals have simply not proven adequate to the task. Cytologic, serologic, and histochemical studies are being investigated. Air contrast barium enema study performed after a thorough cleansing of the colon is proposed by some, but, here again, the differentiation of inflammatory, pseudopolypoid, and neoplastic changes is difficult. Clinically, the signs and symptoms of carcinoma of the colon and of the underlying ulcerative colitis may overlap greatly. Approximately 25% of these cancers are difficult if not impossible to identify macroscopically when the colon has been removed, and it is therefore not surprising that they are not recognized on barium enema examinations. Although strictures in ulcerative colitis are always suspect, in fact, only one in three radiologically evident strictures proves to be malignant.

DYSPLASIA

Retrospective pathological study of colons that have been removed for cancer complicating ulcerative colitis has demonstrated that practically all, if not all, of these colons have had atypical changes in the mucosa in areas distant from the cancer. These changes have been called dysplasia or precancer. Although the changes of dysplasia may be scattered in a spotty fashion throughout the colon, and may even be confined to localized areas in a minority, it seems likely that the large majority of patients with dysplasia could be identified by periodic colonoscopy and multiple biopsies of the colonic mucosa. Prospective studies, although of limited duration, have suggested that this is a satisfactory method of surveillance.

Only a limited number of patients have had their colons removed because of the finding of dysplasia without any other evidence, either radiologic or endoscopic, of cancer. In this small group, more than one-third already have a cancer in the colon that was not discovered before operation (6).

The evidence leaves little question that dysplasia occurs in the colons of some patients with ulcerative colitis whereas it is not known to occur in patients with other inflammatory diseases. It is also clear that cancer of the colon develops in patients with ulcerative colitis in a setting of dysplasia. It is therefore highly suggestive that dysplasia is, in fact, a precancerous lesion and should be sought for in patients with long-standing, universal disease.

Dysplasia can be present in one of three patterns: flat mucosa with crypts lined by dysplastic epithelium, mucosa with a villous surface configuration and dysplastic epithelium, and polypoid excrescences containing dysplastic epithelium and resembling adenomas.

Dysplasia may include cytologic or histologic changes or both. Epithelial cells lose their mucin, nuclei are stratified, mitoses may be present in the upper half of the crypt, and nuclei become larger and hyperchromatic and may lose their polarity. The crypt architecture may be distorted with branching and lateral buds, villous configuration, and "back-to-back" glands without interposed stroma. These dysplastic changes may be graded as mild, moderate, or marked.

BIOPSY SURVEILLANCE

Every effort should be made to orient biopsy specimens carefully. With rectal biopsies a large specimen may be obtained, which may easily be oriented and result in optimal conditions for histologic interpretation. This is more difficult to do with the small biopsy specimens obtained via the colonoscope. The ideal time to perform biopsies for dysplasia is when the mucosa is healed or nearly healed. The presence of acute inflammation in the crypt epithelium is confusing and makes it extremely difficult to make a diagnosis of dysplasia with certainty. Patients should therefore undergo biopsy when disease is clinically quiescent, and biopsy specimens should be taken from those areas that look most normal as well as from abnormal areas that arouse suspicion.

In the past 5 years, we have studied 80 patients with chronic ulcerative colitis who have undergone at least one colonoscopy with multiple biopsies as well as large bite rectal biopsy. Duration of disease was longer than 5 years in all patients and averaged 16 years.

Dysplasia was found in 17 patients (Table 2), and 10 of these patients underwent colectomy. Four of the 10 had carcinoma at the time of colectomy. None of the four malignancies was suspected by radiologic or endoscopic examination.

TABLE 2. *Five-year surveillance study*

No dysplasia	55
Dysplasia	17
Borderline dysplasia	8
Total	80

Two of the lesions had already metastasized. The other six patients all had severe dysplasia in the resected specimen but no carcinoma. Of the four who were found to have carcinoma, preoperative biopsy revealed mild dysplasia in one and severe dysplasia in the other three. Thus 4 of 10 patients (40%) with dysplasia who underwent colectomy already had cancer. It is obvious that patients with long-standing universal ulcerative colitis should be watched carefully. We hope that large numbers of patients will be entered into surveillance studies so that greater experience can be gained and so that the gradation and significance of dysplasia can be defined better.

During the past few years increasing experience and improved technology have resulted in a preference by most investigators for routine rectal and colonoscopic biopsies performed at regular intervals to detect the presence or absence of dysplasia. Periodic rectal biopsy should be performed in patients with ulcerative colitis beginning at the fifth year of disease. Total colonoscopy with multiple biopsies (preferably 10 to 20) should also be carried out at the seventh year and all histologic sections carefully studied for the presence of dysplasia. Colonoscopy should be performed when the inflammatory disease is relatively inactive, and biopsy samples should be taken approximately every 10 cm throughout the colon. For the most part, the biopsies should be taken from areas of least active inflammation endoscopically. Specimens should also be taken from areas showing suspicious changes of color, texture, or morphology. If histologic studies show no evidence of dysplasia, rectal biopsy should be repeated yearly. If no dysplasia is found in these subsequent rectal biopsies, colonoscopy with biopsies should be carried out again the third year of surveillance, and this cycle should be repeated every 3 years. If at any time moderate or marked dysplasia is found on biopsy, proctocolectomy should be carried out. If questionable or mild dysplasia is found, colonoscopy should be repeated yearly and biopsies taken.

If a colonoscopist who can consistently examine the entire colon is not available, an alternate surveillance program would include yearly rectal biopsy and a careful air contrast barium enema examination. The high correlation between the histologic findings in the rectum and in the remaining colon suggests that this might be a reasonable program of surveillance. Rectal biopsy specimens showed dysplasia in 16 of 17 of our patients in whom dysplasia was found on colonic biopsies. This is similar to the findings of Riddell (13), whose retrospective study identified dysplasia in the rectum in 92% of patients in whom cancer of the colon or rectum developed as a complication of ulcerative colitis. Thus rectal biopsy alone may yield a high degree of accuracy in detecting dysplasia in ulcerative colitis, suggesting that colonoscopic biopsies add additional information in only a limited number of patients.

If the finding of dysplasia is a key part of the surveillance program, it is essential to have the histologic sections reviewed by a pathologist interested in and knowledgeable about dysplasia in colonic mucosa. Some confusion still exists among interested pathologists regarding the definition and gradation of dysplasia, but increasing experience is resulting in a resolution of most of these problems of interpretation.

The program of surveillance outlined here is to some extent arbitrary, but if effectiveness, patient compliance, and cost effectiveness are considered, it seems reasonable in light of today's understanding of the problem of long-standing ulcerative colitis and development of cancer.

REFERENCES

1. Dawson, I. M., and Pryse-Davies, J. (1959): The development of carcinoma of the large intestine in ulcerative colitis. *Br. J. Surg.,* 47:113–128.
2. Devroede, G., and Taylor, W. F. (1976): On calculating cancer risk and survival of ulcerative colitis patients with the life table method. *Gastroenterology,* 71:505–509.
3. Devroede, G. J., Taylor, W. F., Sauer, W. G., Jackman, R. J., and Stickler, G. B. (1971): Cancer risk and life expectancy in children with ulcerative colitis. *N. Engl. J. Med.,* 285:17–21.
4. Farmer, R. G., and Brown, C. H. (1966): Ulcerative proctitis: course and prognosis. *Gastroenterology,* 51:219–223.
5. Goligher, J. C., de Dombal, F. T., Watts, J. M., Watkinson, G., and Morson, B. C. (1968): *Ulcerative Colitis,* pp. 150–174. Williams & Wilkins Co., Baltimore.
6. Lennard-Jones, J. E., Morson, B. C., Richie, J. K., Shove, D. C., and Williams, C. B. (1977): Cancer in colitis: Assessment of the individual risk by clinical and histological criteria. *Gastroenterology,* 73:1280–1289.
7. MacDougall, I. P. M. (1964): The cancer risk in ulcerative colitis. *Lancet,* 2:655–658.
8. Michener, W. M., Gage, R. P., Sauer, W. G., and Stickler, G. B. (1971): The prognosis of chronic ulcerative colitis in children. *N. Engl. J. Med.,* 265:1075–1079.
9. Morowitz, D. A., and Kirsner, J. B. (1969): Mortality in ulcerative colitis: 1930 to 1966. *Gastroenterology,* 57:481–490.
10. Nugent, F. W., and Haggitt, R. C. (1980): Long-term follow-up, including cancer surveillance, for patients with ulcerative colitis. *Clin. Gastroenterol. (in press).*
11. Nugent, F. W., Haggitt, R. C., Colcher, H., and Kutteruf, G. C. (1979): Malignant potential of chronic ulcerative colitis: preliminary report. *Gastroenterology,* 76:1–5.
12. Nugent, F. W., Veidenheimer, M. C., Zuberi, S., Garabedian, M. M., and Parikh, N. K. (1970): Clinical course of ulcerative proctosigmoiditis. *Am. J. Dig. Dis.,* 15:321–326.
13. Riddell, R. H. (1976): The precarcinomatous phase of ulcerative colitis. In: *Topics in Pathology,* edited by B. C. Morson, pp. 179–219. Springer-Verlag, Berlin.

Colorectal Cancer: Prevention, Epidemiology, and Screening, edited by S. Winawer, D. Schottenfeld, and P. Sherlock. Raven Press, New York © 1980.

Evaluation of Cancer Risk in Chronic Ulcerative Colitis: University of Chicago Experience

*Bernard Levin, **Robert H. Riddell, †Paul Frank, and *Jane E. Gilpin

Departments of *Medicine, ** *Pathology, and* † *Radiology, University of Chicago Hospitals and Clinics, Chicago, Illinois 60637*

The dreaded complication of carcinoma in ulcerative colitis accounts for only a small proportion of large bowel carcinomas; the true figure is probably about 1%. Although few in number, these patients pose difficult problems in management. There are multiple reasons for this, but the most disturbing ones are that carcinomas may develop insidiously even when the patients are under active medical care, that the tumors are frequently multiple, and that they may not become clinically apparent until they are advanced. These tumors may escape detection in the hands of even the most experienced radiological or endoscopic observers because they may be flat or plaque-like.

The average age at which these tumors are discovered is 40 to 45 years, which is much younger than that of patients with noncolitic cancer (1). These patients are in their most productive period of life.

A subgroup of patients with ulcerative colitis in whom most of these carcinomas occur has been identified. This highly predisposed group consists of those patients with total or extensive colitis especially with an early age of onset and a long history (2). However, patients with left-sided disease predominantly and long duration of illness also may be at increased risk (3).

The identification of this high-risk group has placed the clinician in a dilemma. A safe approach would be to recommend prophylactic proctocolectomy after 10 to 12 years of the disease. Certain disadvantages arise if such a course were to be followed, and these include a small mortality from the operation, and the slight but definite disability of a permanent ileostomy. However, it should be recognized that only a small proportion of the high-risk group will develop carcinoma, approximately 12 to 15% after 20 years of disease (4). A recent study by Lennard-Jones and co-workers (5) from St. Mark's Hospital, London, failed to detect a single carcinoma in 578 patient years of follow-up within 10 years of onset of the colitis, but the risk in the second decade was approximately 1 to 200 years, and in the third 1 in 60 patient years. Some clinicians view any risk of carcinoma as unacceptable and will therefore follow an aggressive course of management. Others tend to follow a middle course, i.e., although not routinely recommending proctocolectomy, they become eager to advise surgical removal when exacerbations occur, which they might otherwise have treated medically.

Additional approaches are required to identify those ulcerative colitis patients within this high-risk group who are at greatest risk from developing carcinoma. One such approach involves the use of multiple biopsies in an attempt to identify dysplastic or precarcinomatous changes (5–10). Fine detail, double contrast radiological studies may offer another way of demonstrating dysplastic lesions in the colon (11).

UNIVERSITY OF CHICAGO EXPERIENCE—PROSPECTIVE STUDY

Entry Criteria

1. Ulcerative colitis.
2. Inactive or minimally active disease.
3. Total colonic involvement demonstrated radiologically or endoscopically at some stage of illness.
4. Duration of symptoms of longer than 7 years.

Because of the long-standing interest of Dr. Joseph B. Kirsner and his associates, patients with inflammatory bowel disease are referred to the University of Chicago largely from the greater Chicago area, but also from all parts of the United States. A geographical analysis of our study patients is as follows: Chicago—10 patients, Chicago-suburban—27 patients, Illinois (excluding 1, 2 above)—4 patients, Indiana—6 patients, Michigan—1 patient, Wisconsin—3 patients, Missouri—1 patient, California—2 patients.

RESULTS

Since the beginning of this project, 196 studies have been performed in 91 patients. The mean duration of symptoms in those 54 patients still actively involved in the study is 19.7 years with a range of 7 to 38 years. The mean age of onset on the same group of patients is 20.8 years with a range of 3 to 43 years. Most patients undergo total colonoscopy with biopsies every 10 cm above the anal verge. Large forceps are used to obtain multiple rectal biopsies in patients who are new to the program and those who have shown evidence of dysplastic changes in past biopsies. Rectal biopsies are obtained at proctoscopy on the day following the colonoscopy (Tables 1 and 2).

Our preliminary data confirm that the dysplastic lesions may be patchy, reinforcing the need for multiple biopsies. In addition, reversibility may occur, reinforcing a need for repetition of biopsies on several occasions in the same area.

Patients 1 through 10 were advised to undergo colectomy because of the presence of moderate dysplasia on colonic and/or rectal biopsy. In only one,

TABLE 1. *Biopsy findings in patients with ulcerative colitis*

	No. studies	
Histology	Colon	Rectum
No abnormality (apart from ulcerative colitis)	102	106
Epithelial hyperplasia	31	39
Borderline dysplasia	30	23
Mild dysplasia	22	17
Moderate dysplasia	11	4
Total	196	189

TABLE 2. *Characterization of dysplasia in patients with ulcerative colitis*

Patient no.	Site of dysplasia	Age at onset	Duration (years)	Postcolectomy findings
1	Transverse colon	27	10	Cancer—sigmoid colon
2	Hepatic flexure	23	23	Cancer—hepatic flexure
3	Colon and rectum	23	20	No cancer found
4	Colon	25	10	No cancer found
5	Colon and rectum	12	37	No cancer found
6	Colon and rectum	27	10	—(Colectomy advised)
7	Colon	26	37	—(Colectomy advised)
8	Colon	12	19	—(Colectomy advised)
9	Colon	29	26	—(Colectomy advised)
10	Right colon	23	12	Cancer—ascending colon

patient 10, was there a high clinical suspicion of cancer preoperatively. Patients 6 through 9 have not yet undergone colectomy because of patient unwillingness or other medical consideration. Of patients 1 through 5, a carcinoma was discovered in two (1 and 2) after removal of the specimen and examination by the surgical pathologist. In one of these (1), the site of the cancer was different from that of the dysplasia.

The staging (modified Dukes' classification) of these lesions was B_2 in patients 1 and 2 and C_2 in patient 10.

COMMENT

Based on these data we have been using the following *interim* operational guidelines:

1. No abnormality (other than changes of ulcerative colitis), epithelial hyperplasia, or borderline dysplasia: continued surveillance at 12- to 18-month intervals by endoscopic biopsy; double contrast barium enema every 24 to 36 months.
2. Mild dysplasia: repeat studies in 6 to 12 months.

3. Moderate dysplasia which is persistent on several studies or mild dysplasia overlying a mass lesion seen endoscopically or radiologically, with endoscopic correlation: proctocolectomy advised (12).

Safety

Five patients have reported an exacerbation of their colitis associated with the radiological and endoscopic studies. These patients responded to conventional medical therapy.

Cytology

To date, lavage cytology and brush cytology have been disappointing. In only two instances were atypical cells found in individuals with moderate dysplasia.

In an attempt to characterize further possible metabolic or biochemical abnormalities which may indicate individuals predisposed to the development of cancer, stools from some of these patients are being submitted for mutagen analysis (Drs. W. G. Bruce and P. Dion, Ontario Cancer Institute, Toronto).

SUMMARY

These surveillance techniques have been safe in our hands. In the absence of dysplasia, it appears to be satisfactory to monitor such patients at regular intervals. The low incidence of cancer detected in this group of individuals so far may reflect the low level of inflammatory activity in this particular population. Newer biochemical and radiological methods should be evaluated as supplemental techniques to currently employed biopsies.

This study confirms the lack of need for prophylactic proctocolectomy in the majority of these patients and suggests that patients with long-standing colitis can safely be monitored at regular intervals using these methods.

ACKNOWLEDGMENTS

This study was supported by the University of Chicago Cancer Research Center Grant USPHS CA-19266. We acknowledge the expert endoscopic contributions of Drs. B. H. G. Rogers and M. O. Blackstone, the interest and support of Dr. Joseph B. Kirsner, and cytologic analyses by Mr. Leroy Cockerham.

REFERENCES

1. Mottet, N. K. (1971): Histopathologic spectrum of regional enteritis and ulcerative colitis. In: *Major Problems in Pathology, Vol. II,* pp. 217–235. W. B. Saunders, Toronto.
2. Devroede, G. J., Taylor, W. F., Sauer, W. J., Jackman, R. J., and Stickler, G. B. (1971): Cancer risk and life expectancy of children with ulcerative colitis. *N. Engl. J. Med.,* 285:17–21.

3. Greenstein, A. J., Sachar, D. B., Pucillo, A., Vassilades, G., Smith, H., Kreel, I., Geller, S. A., Janowitz, H. D., and Aufses, A. H. (1979): Cancer in universal and left-sided ulcerative colitis: Clinical and pathologic features. *Mt. Sinai J. Med. (N.Y.)*, 46:25–32.

4. Edwards, F. C., and Truelove, S. C. (1964): The course and prognosis of ulcerative colitis. IV. Carcinoma of the colon. *Gut*, 5:15–22.

5. Lennard-Jones, J. E., Morson, B. C., Ritchie, J. K., Shove, D. C., and Williams, C. B. (1977): Cancer in colitis: Assessment of the individual risk of clinical and histological criteria. *Gastroenterology*. 73:1280–1289.

6. Morson, B. C., and Pang, L. S. C. (1967): Rectal biopsy as an aid to cancer control in ulcerative colitis. *Gut*, 8:423–427.

7. Riddell, R. H. (1976): The precarcinomatous phase of ulcerative colitis. *Curr. Top. Pathol.*, 63:179–219.

8. Nugent, F. W., Haggitt, R. C., and Colcher, H. (1979): Malignant potential of chronic ulcerative colitis: Preliminary report. *Gastroenterology*, 76:1–5.

9. Levin, B., and Riddell, R. H. (1977): Evaluation of cancer risk in chronic ulcerative colitis: Progress report of a prospective study. *Gastroenterology*, 72[5]:1088 (abst.).

10. Ransohoff, D. F., Riddell, R. H., and Levin, B. (1979): Mucosal dysplasia in patients with ulcerative colitis and colon cancer: How universal? *Gastroenterology*, 76:1223 (abst.).

11. Frank, P., Riddell, R. H., Feczko, P., and Levin, B. (1978): Radiological detection of colonic dysplasia (precarcinoma) in chronic ulcerative colitis. *Gastrointest. Radiol.*, 3:209–219.

12. Blackstone, M. O., Riddell, R. H., Rogers, B. H. G., and Levin, B. (1980): Dysplasia associated masses detected by colonoscopy in long standing ulcerative colitis—an indication for colectomy. *Gastroenterology, (in press)*.

Colorectal Cancer: Prevention, Epidemiology, and Screening, edited by S. Winawer, D. Schottenfeld, and P. Sherlock. Raven Press, New York © 1980.

Role of Colonoscopy in Surveillance for Cancer in Patients with Ulcerative Colitis

Jerome D. Waye

Mt. Sinai School of Medicine of the City University of New York, Gastrointestinal Endoscopy Unit, Mt. Sinai Hospital, New York, New York 10028

Cancer in ulcerative colitis may develop insidiously causing little change in the patient's symptoms until the tumor has grown to a large size. Patients at risk are those with extensive colitis for 7 years duration. In this high risk group, stool testing for occult blood loses its specificity since the underlying inflammatory disease may cause spontaneous mucosal surface bleeding; pseudopolyps may also bleed without provocation. In the high risk patient with chronic ulcerative colitis, the goal is discovery of the malignant tumor before it becomes symptomatic—indeed, even before it can be demonstrated roentgenographically. As in any high risk population, extrapolation of attempts at early cancer detection inevitably lead to the desire for discovery of "premalignant" changes so that curative steps can be taken before metastases occur. Pursuit of these goals in ulcerative colitis has focused on the use of dysplasia as an indicator of maligancy risk in patients with ulcerative colitis (1). The chapter by Dr. Morson in this book details the current approach to dysplastic findings on mucosal biopsies in ulcerative colitis. The original studies (2) were based on sigmoidoscopic biopsies in the intact colon or on colectomy specimens received at operation. The colonoscope rapidly became an accepted method (3) of obtaining tissue specimens since advances in optics permitted magnified direct visual inspection of the entire colonic mucosal surface. Based on histopathologic findings (1,4–6), colonoscopy with multiple biopsies may allow the selection of a subpopulation within the high risk group that should have total colectomy for cancer prevention prior to its actual development. This chapter deals with the technique of surveillance colonoscopy and biopies of patients with chronic long-standing ulcerative colitis, the preparation of the bowel, the locations where biopsies should be taken, and the frequency of colonoscopy.

Colonoscopy as a tool for cancer surveillance in patients with ulcerative colitis represents a considerably different use than when colonoscopy is employed for diagnostic purposes. Patients for surveillance colonoscopy are preselected by the criteria of duration of colitis, not by the clinical parameters of illness nor the degree of inflammatory activity. All patients have the previously established diagnosis of ulcerative colitis, and most have universal involvement. Data are currently being collected from multiple centers (6–9) concerning colonoscopic biopsy in the detection of cancer and pre-cancer in patients with ulcerative colitis. In order to be able to properly interpret the results of such studies, it is important for gastroenterologists, clinicians, and pathologists to separate data obtained from surveillance studies from those obtained by diagnostic colonoscopy.

Diagnostic colonoscopies in ulcerative colitis are usually performed for the investigation of an abnormality seen on a previous barium enema X-ray examination (10). The two most common problems requiring endoscopic resolution are the investigation of a stricture or a mass lesion. Although most strictures are benign, some may be malignant, and carcinoma may spread submucosally narrowing the lumen circumferentially. Multiple biopsies may fail to reveal the presence of carcinoma within such a stricture (11). Endoscopies and biopsies performed for resolution of such a radiographic abnormality must be categorized as "diagnostic" rather than surveillance, even if the patient has had ulcerative colitis for many years. In a similar manner, colonoscopies performed for the investigation of a mass lesion whether it be a pseudopolyp, a neoplastic polyp, or carcinoma should be considered in the "diagnostic" category. Colonoscopic examinations and biopsies for the sole purpose of surveillance should be performed only on those patients who are endoscoped by nature of their having had extensive colitis for more than 8 years duration, but who do not have a specific problem requiring resolution.

Dobbins (12) reviewed the literature up to 1977 concerning dysplasia and cancer in ulcerative colitis. He reported dysplasia in 88% of all colectomies in which carcinoma of the colon was found. The distribution of dysplasia was not uniform, with only 66% of patients having this histological finding in the rectum. Reviewing all colectomy specimens in which no cancer was found revealed that 13% had dysplasia. Up to 1977, dysplasia was reported in 5.7% of rectal biopsies in ulcerative colitis, and one-third of these patients had associated carcinoma of the colon. Since the review article by Dobbins, two articles (5,7) have reported retrospective data (Table 1) and both of these and one additional study (4) have discussed prospective data concerning dysplasia (Table 2). The recent retrospective literature has confirmed that colectomy specimens

TABLE 1. *Retrospective data in ulcerative colitis patients with known cancer who have dysplasia*

Reference	Patients with cancer	Colectomy specimens with dysplasia	% Cancer having dysplasia
Dobbins (12) (review)	108	95	88
Riddell (5)	80	65 ⎱	80.6
Nugent et al. (7)	23	18 ⎰	

TABLE 2. *Prospective data in ulcerative colitis patients with dysplasia found to have cancer*

Reference	Patients with dysplasia	Patients with cancer at operation	% Dysplasia having cancer
Dobbins (12) (review)	53	17	32
Riddell (5)	26	15 ⎫	
Lonnard-Jones et al. (4)	33	5 ⎬	31
Nugent et al. (7)	7	1 ⎭	

for cancer demonstrate a high incidence of dysplasia; however, approximately 20% of patients will show no dysplastic foci throughout the colon mucosa. Recent prospective data also correlate well with previous published reports that one-third of patients with moderate to severe dysplasia on biopsy will have a colon cancer discovered when colectomy is performed. These data may be interpreted to show that some cancers in ulcerative colitis may develop as a unifocal pathologic aberration without diffuse colonic histologic abnormalities, but the majority (80%) will be associated with dysplasia elsewhere in the colon. Therefore, biopsies that do not reveal dysplastic changes are no assurance that cancer does not exist in that colon (such as in an unexamined portion of the right colon or beyond a tight stricture).

Surveillance studies are usually started after ulcerative colitis has affected the colon for over 10 years (4,6). Some investigators have found cancer of the colon in patients whose disease has been present for only 8 years (7), suggesting that long-term surveillance should begin at that time. There is evidence (13) that patients with less than total colitis—that is, with only left-sided disease—also have an increased risk for the development of carcinoma with a longer precancerous phase of their disease. Therefore, patients with only left-sided colitis should be entered into long-term surveillance on the 15th anniversary of their illness onset. The degree of colitic activity throughout the patient's clinical course does not bear any relationship to the propensity for the development of carcinoma. It must be recognized that relatively few patients with continuous symptoms or intermittently severe colitis retain their colons for 10 years. However, patients with quiescent disease must be observed as closely as those with active colitis, as there are no clear-cut predictors between the group which will and those which will not develop carcinoma.

The use of colonoscopy extends the ability of the clinician to visualize the colon mucosa further than the traditional 25 cm reached by the rigid proctosigmoidoscope. The entire colon to the tip of the cecum can usually be evaluated with the colonoscope in almost every patient in whom the examination is performed for surveillance purposes. Although reports (7,8) indicate that dysplasia found throughout the colon on endoscopy is concomitantly associated with a positive rectal biopsy for dysplasia, there are several reasons to perform colonoscopy rather than rely on repeated proctosigmoidoscopy. A major advantage is that total endoscopy permits evaluation of the right colon, where one-quarter of all carcinomas are located (13) in chronic ulcerative colitis. Since dysplastic changes may be patchy in distribution, the ability to visually identify mucosal abnormalities and biopsy them at any location throughout the colon represents a distinct advantage (6). The magnified image allows the endoscopist to precisely identify and biopsy tiny lesions and bumpy mucosal irregularities. Because ulcerative colitis is characteristically a disease with the most severe inflammation located distally, the ability to biopsy proximal areas may permit more precise differentiation of dysplasia unhindered by artifacts induced by the distal mucosal inflammatory changes. The use of the shorter "flexible sigmoidoscope" provides only a limited extension of the range of vision of the rigid proctosigmoidoscope, and has no application in the endoscopic surveillance of patients with chronic ulcerative colitis.

During the colonoscopic examination, the endoscopist need not biopsy pseudopolyps since they have no malignant or premalignant potential (14–16). However, when multiple polypoid masses are present throughout the colon, it may not be possible for the endoscopist to visually differentiate between a pseudopolyp, a neoplastic polyp, or a carcinoma. Polypoid lesions seen on colonoscopy during the surveillance of patients with chronic ulcerative colitis should be biopsied when they meet the following criteria (10): (a) larger than 1 cm in diameter, (b) surface friability, (c) different color than adjacent pseudopolyps, and (d) irregular surface configuration. Pseudopolyps have a characteristic histologic configuration, and biopsies of any portion of their surface will permit a definitive pathologic diagnosis. Since pseudopolyps have their genesis in inflammation, biopsies may contain various degrees of inflammatory changes, some bearing a striking similarity to dysplastic changes noted in noninflamed mucosa. The closest of histologic features may prevent accurate pathological interpretation, and biopsies taken from pseudopolyps should be so noted by the endoscopist. This will ensure that the finding of mild to moderate dysplasia on the surface of a pseudopolyp can be correctly interpreted as an inflammatory response, as opposed to the diagnosis of dysplasia on a biopsy taken from a flat, uninvolved area of mucosa. The endoscopist should strive to take an average of eight biopsies in patients during surveillance studies. Biopsies should be taken from the following areas:

1. Cecum
2. Ascending colon
3. Hepatic flexure/proximal transverse colon
4. Mid-transverse colon
5. Distal transverse colon/splenic flexure area
6. Descending colon
7. Sigmoid colon
8. Rectum

Each site and the presence or absence of inflammation should be recorded for reference by the clinician and pathologist. More biopsies may be necessary if any abnormalities are seen in the course of colonoscopy. Although dysplastic changes may be reported in biopsies taken from completely flattened and normal appearing areas of mucosa, the endoscopist should attempt to "target-biopsy" segments of mucosa that are slightly irregular or bumpy in configuration. These areas will produce the greatest yield of dysplastic changes (17). In some instances, biopsies of such "minimally elevated" and normal-colored mucosa may detect actual intraepithelial carcinoma rather than just dysplasia.

The quest for precancer mucosal changes in patients with chronic ulcerative colitis is directly linked with the endoscopist's ability to visualize minor aberrations of mucosal contour. This therefore implies that the colon be absolutely clean at the time of surveillance endoscopy. The preparation of the bowel must be individualized for each patient, but the "standard" 2 oz of castor oil may be too vigorous for all but the completely asymptomatic patient. In the presence of diarrhea with more than three bowel movements daily, a 48-hr liquid diet (full fluids) and 5 oz of citrate of magnesia are sufficient. In the relatively asymptomatic patient with less than three bowel movements per day, a 24-hr clear liquid diet and 10 oz of citrate of magnesia produce adequate bowel cleansing. All patients should have enemas on the day of the examination (none the night previously) until the returns are clear. Usually two tap water enemas will suffice. Since total colonoscopic examination is desired, the smaller volume phospho-soda enemas are usually not sufficient.

The technique of examination is exactly similar to other diagnostic examinations of the colon. Since the surveillance population group is destined to have multiple colonoscopic examinations over the remainder of their lifetime, special attempts should be made to counsel the patient in the necessity of repeated examinations. An unpleasant endoscopic experience may deter the patient from undergoing repeated endoscopic surveillance. Although the colon may be straight and tubular in chronic colitis, the majority of patients have a colon of normal configuration and may require sedation with meperidine and diazepam prior to the performance of endoscopy. The interval for the performance of colonoscopic examinations is unknown at the present time. Reports have ranged from 1 to 3 years in the high risk patient category with or without interval sigmoidoscopic biopsies. Suggestions have been made for sigmoidoscopy every 6 months with colonoscopy every year, or sigmoidoscopy yearly with colonoscopy every 3 years. In articles written within the past 2 years, Nugent and Lennard-Jones suggest colonoscopy every 2 years, and Dobbins, Williams, and Waye suggest yearly colonoscopies. When dysplasia is found on biopsies, it is suggested that repeat endoscopic examinations be performed to corroborate these findings. The repeat examinations may be performed within 3 to 6 months. At our present level of knowledge, when moderate to severe grades of dysplasia are a consistent finding on biopsies, colectomy should be recommended, since one-third of patients in this category have an undetected cancer of the colon.

SUMMARY

The role of colonoscopy in the surveillance for carcinoma in patients with ulcerative colitis is to aid in the detection of carcinoma at a curable stage. It is too early to predict the exact time interval for the performance of repeated surveillance colonoscopy, but there is general agreement among physicians and pathologists that colonoscopy and multiple biopsies have a role in providing visual and histological material in patients at high risk for the development of colon cancer.

REFERENCES

1. Morson, B. C. (1974): The technique and interpretation of rectal biopsies in inflammatory bowel disease. *Pathol. Annu.,* 179–219.
2. Morson, B. C., and Pang, L. S. C. (1967): Rectal biopsy as an aid to cancer control in ulcerative colitis. *Gut,* 8:423–434.
3. Williams, C. B., and Waye, J. D. (1978): Colonoscopy in inflammatory bowel disease. *Clin. Gastroenterol.,* 7:701–717.
4. Lennard-Jones, J. E., Morson, B. C., Ritchie, J. K., Shove, D. C., and Williams, C. B. (1977): Cancer in colitis—assessment of the individual risk by clinical and histological criteria. *Gastroenterology,* 73:1280–1289.
5. Riddell, R. H. (1976): The precarcinomatous phase of ulcerative colitis. *Curr. Top. Pathol.,* 63:179–219.
6. Yardley, J. H., Bayless, T. M., and Diamond, M. P. (1979): Cancer in ulcerative colitis. *Gastroenterology,* 76:221–225.
7. Nugent, F. W., Haggit, K. C., Colcher, H., and Kutteruf, G. C. (1979): Malignant potential of chronic ulcerative colitis. Preliminary report. *Gastroenterology,* 76:1–5.
8. Riddell, R. H. (1977): Endoscopic recognition of early carcinoma in ulcerative colitis. *JAMA,* 237:2811.
9. Waye, J. D. (1978): Colitis, cancer and colonoscopy. *Med. Clin. North Am.,* 62:211–224.
10. Waye, J. D. (1980): Endoscopy in inflammatory bowel disease. *Clin. Gastroenterol.,* 9(2).
11. Crowson, T. D., Ferrante, W. F., and Gathright, J. B., Jr. (1976): Colonoscopy: Inefficacy for early carcinoma detection in patients with ulcerative colitis. *JAMA,* 236:2651–2652.
12. Dobbins, W. O. (1977): Current status of the precancer lesion in ulcerative colitis. *Gastroenterology,* 73:1431–1433.
13. Greenstein, A. M., Sachar, D. B., Pucillo, A., Vassiliades, G., Smith, H., Kreel, I., Geller, S. A., Janowitz, H. D., and Aufses, A. H. (1979): Cancer in universal and left-sided ulcerative colitis: Clinical and pathologic features. *Mt. Sinai J. Med. (N.Y.),* 46:25–32.
14. Dawson, I. M. P., and Pryse-Davies, J. (1959): The development of cancer of the large intestine in ulcerative colitis. *Br. J. Surg.,* 47:113–128.
15. Schneider, R., Dickersin, R. G., and Patterson, J. F. (1973): Localized giant pseudopolyposis: A complication of granulomatous colitis. *Am. J. Dig. Dis.,* 18:265–270.
16. Teague, R. H., and Read, A. E. (1975): Polyposis in ulcerative colitis. *Gut,* 16:792–795.
17. Yardley, J. H., and Keren, D. F. (1974): "Precancer" lesions in ulcerative colitis: A retrospective study of rectal biopsy and colectomy specimens. *Cancer,* 34:835–844.

Colorectal Cancer: Prevention, Epidemiology, and Screening, edited by S. Winawer, D. Schottenfeld, and P. Sherlock. Raven Press, New York © 1980.

Commentary: Difficulties in Interpretation of Dysplasia

*,**William O. Dobbins III and **Henry D. Appelman

*ACOS for Research, VA Medical Center, Ann Arbor; and **University of Michigan Medical School, Ann Arbor, Michigan 48105*

Data in regard to surveillance for early detection of carcinoma of the colon in patients with chronic ulcerative colitis (CUC) were reported in abstract form to the International Symposium on Colorectal Cancer from six centers (Johns Hopkins University, George Washington University, The University of Chicago, The Cleveland and Lahey Clinics, and St. Mark's Hospital in London). The cumulative data from these abstracts covered 567 patients, most with 10 or more years of disease, all of whom had surveillance colonoscopy with multiple colonic and rectal biopsies. These biopsies were evaluated morphologically for changes which have been considered to be markers of epithelial neoplasia in ulcerative colitis, changes which have been designated as dysplasia. Depending on the extent of the cytologic and architectural deviations from normal epithelium, this dysplastic epithelium may be separated into various grades of intensity, usually termed mild, moderate, and severe. In general, but not uniformly, such grading of dysplasia was done by the six centers reporting, and, as a result, there were 41 cases of mild dysplasia, 34 patients with the moderate variety, and 33 with the severe form. About half of each grade was found in the rectum, the remainder being distributed elsewhere in the colon. Colectomies were performed in 18 patients with severe dysplasia, none of whom had clinical evidence of carcinoma, and in 11 cases an unsuspected carcinoma was found. In 16 patients defined as having moderate dysplasia, colectomy was performed, and 5 cancers were discovered. These cumulative data tabulate in the following fashion:

Degree of dysplasia	No. of colectomies	No. of carcinomas	% Carcinomas
Severe	18	11	61
Moderate	16	5	31

It is clear that there is a distinct trend toward greater cancer risk with higher grades of dysplasia found on biopsy. These figures are supported by previously published data from St. Mark's (1) in which four cancers were found in 7 patients with severe dysplasia on biopsy (57%), as compared to one cancer among 5 patients with moderate dysplasia (20%).

In general, in the surveillance studies, in which there are frequent, regularly scheduled follow-up visits by the patients once the dysplasia is detected and the colectomies performed, the carcinomas which are discovered tend to be small or early and quite limited in extent. This is the optimal time, then, to detect and remove carcinomas, when they have just developed and have not metastasized.

From the cumulative data, it would appear that once severe dysplasia is discovered, colectomy is indicated. However, unfortunately, this issue is too complex for such simplistic solutions (2,3). Optimally, colectomy should be performed when one or more markers are present which indicate that the patient is more at risk of dying if the colon is left *in situ* than if it is removed. One such marker might be the presence of severe dysplasia if the cumulative numbers (as quoted above) continue to be confirmed. Dysplasia becomes an important marker when its presence incidates a cancer risk above and beyond the clinical risk defined in several studies by clinical markers such as duration and extent of colitis and age of onset.

However, there are several problems in placing total dependence on such data at present. First, data from the literature indicate that the average duration of CUC in patients with severe dysplasia is about 5 to 6 years less than the average duration of disease in those with carcinoma. This suggests that there is a 5- to 6-year lag time from the onset of severe dysplasia to carcinoma, if, indeed, dysplasia is a precursor of invasive cancer. It is not at all clear just when during this 5- to 6-year period colectomy should be performed. Unfortunately, there is no way of knowing how long the dysplasia has been present already.

Second, the dysplastic changes encountered in CUC form a morphologic continuum, with arbitrary points separating the various grades. In fact, it has become clear that even among these pathologists who have studied these colitic dysplasias and published their results, there are broad areas of disagreement on the grading of severity of dysplasia. As a result, a group of 10 such pathologists have begun an intense cooperative study of the spectrum of epithelial alterations in CUC in an attempt to define and standardize a nomenclature for dysplasias, inflammatory-induced hyperplasias, and carcinomas. The first phase of their study, a review of 73 coded specimens from CUC colons, resulted in the discovery that even this group of pathologists differed markedly in their interpretations. Therefore, at present, the validity of using pooled data from different centers, data such as are summarized from the six reporting institutions above, must be considered highly questionable. Until there are uniformly accepted morphologic standards for the different grades of dysplasia and uniformly acceptable ways of separating them from inflammatory hyperplasias or regenerating epithelium, we must be cautious in our clinical use of the finding of dysplasia. Certainly, if experienced gastrointestinal pathologists are having trouble agreeing in this area, the busy general surgical pathologist is not likely to lessen the confusion.

Epithelial dysplasia is considered to be a neoplastic alteration, comparable to anaplastic epithelium found in colonic adenomas. The milder degrees of dysplasia are considered to be on the benign side of the neoplastic spectrum, whereas the more severe forms are thought to be closer to carcinoma. We suspect that the milder forms give rise to the more severe forms which in turn ultimately lead to carcinoma. Therefore, if the factors allowing dysplastic epithelium to develop in one site are active, then, theoretically, they also are likely to act at other sites which also may become dysplastic and eventually carcinomatous. Thus the finding of dysplasia in one site raises suspicions of the status of the epithelium elsewhere in the colon. In order to give rise to carcinoma, dysplasia must not be a transient event, but must persist. Therefore, for dysplasia to serve as an indicator for colectomy, it must remain once it develops; it must be found in repeat biopsies. Similarly, we suspect that the greater the amount of dysplasia, the greater the cancer risk, since more epithelium has become neoplastic. As a result, another requirement might be that dysplasia be found in multiple biopsy sites. Both these prerequisites were cautiously used as indicators for colectomy in the St. Mark's prospective study reported in December 1977 (1).

We recommend that before every pathologist begins making diagnosis of dysplasia in CUC and before every clinician starts recommending colectomy on the finding of dysplasia, additional hard data be obtained. We need a uniformly accepted set of histologic criteria of dysplasia which can be easily used by all surgical pathologists. We need to know the risk for colon cancer in the presence of varying grades of dysplasia, and we need to determine if these risks are greater or less than the risks previously identified on the basis of clinical factors alone. Only then will we know what dysplasia in CUC truly means (2,3).

REFERENCES

1. Lennard-Jones, J. E., Morson, B. C., Ritchie, J. K., Shove, D. C., and Williams, C. B. (1977): Cancer in colitis: Assessment of the individual risk by clinical and histological criteria. *Gastroenterology,* 73:1280–1289.
2. Dobbins, W. O., III (1977): Current status of the precancer lesion in ulcerative colitis. *Gastroenterology,* 73:1431–1433.
3. Yardley, J. H., Bayless, T. M., and Diamond, M. P. (1979): Cancer in ulcerative colitis. *Gastroenterology,* 76:221–225.

Colorectal Cancer: Prevention, Epidemiology, and Screening, edited by S. Winawer, D. Schottenfeld, and P. Sherlock. Raven Press, New York © 1980.

Commentary: Colon Cancer and Precancer in Ulcerative Colitis

Theodore M. Bayless, John H. Yardley, Mark P. Diamond, and Moses Paulson

Departments of Medicine and Pathology, The Johns Hopkins University School of Medicine, The Johns Hopkins Hospital, Baltimore, Maryland 21205

The increased risk of colon carcinoma development is now a well-accepted fact of life for patients with ulcerative colitis (UC). There is some evidence that the lag before the appearance of carcinoma may be shorter in patients with adolescent and preadolescent onset of ulcerative colitis (1), but this has not been found by other groups (2). Although some surgeons recommend "prophylactic" colectomy for patients with severe pancolitis, it is our observation that most physicians do not advise total colectomy in patients simply because they have had pancolitis for over 10 years. This group of noncolectomized high-risk patients definitely needs a surveillance program to identify those individuals at greatest risk of cancer development, including some who may already have developed an early potentially curable malignancy.

TERMINOLOGY

Various definitions and terms for histologic changes that precede or correlate with the onset of carcinoma have been used by different investigators. Mucosal lesions that are considered precarcinomatous occur in many histologic patterns (3). Dobbins (4) has pointed out that there is much variation in the terminology currently employed by various pathologists. Obviously, this variation creates difficulties for clinicians who must make decisions about their individual patients, and it also complicates efforts to try to generalize from results described in the literature.

Generally, most investigators now describe degrees of epithelial dysplasia in ulcerative colitis. There is agreement that dysplasia in UC consists primarily of cytologic changes comparable with those seen in malignant transformation in other organs such as the lung or cervix; these changes can be readily appreciated by an experienced pathologist. However, a lesion described as "moderate dysplasia" by one investigator may be described by another as "severe dysplasia." This inconsistency comes about in part because grading is a subjective and inherently imprecise process. More importantly, however, inconsistent grading results from differences in the scales used by various workers. Some investigators use a mild–moderate–severe scale which is specifically applied to dysplasia in ulcerative colitis with only severe dysplasia being viewed as the point at which colectomy may be advised (5,6). Others also seem to define moderate dysplasia as ominous (2,3). Riddell (7) bases his grading scale on one used for adenomas in noncolitis patients. He would argue for this view since the villiform change in glandular proliferation in dysplastic mucosa does indeed appear adenomatous and, secondly, an advantage is obtained because only one scale is used for all forms of adenomatous epithelium. Another cause of uncertainty and confusion was the variation in the way the term "carcinoma *in-situ*" was applied. Yardley and Keren (6) had considered this a separate lesion lying above severe dysplasia, but now they and most authors incorporate such lesions into the severe dysplasia group.

Morson and Pang (8) introduced the term "precancer" in their landmark article to cover, in a broad way, mucosal lesions that they found to correlate with the presence of cancer. These included villiform thickening, polyp formation, and other adenomatous features as well as epithelial dysplasia. It is true that the word "precancer" should not be construed as implying more knowledge about a patient's colon than we can actually claim. It is clear that lesions judged to be precancerous will not always lead to cancer, whereas many patients with precancer are found to already have invasive cancer in their colectomy specimens.

Some workers have avoided using the word "precancer" because of the threatening connotations. Nevertheless, we strongly support its use or a related term such as "precarcinomatous." Utilization of such a term overcomes many of the problems created by varied grading scales and terminology. It provides a common "go-no-go" reference point for discussion and decision making in a presumed continuum of increasing dysplasia in UC.

It is obvious that a continued exchange of materials and additional dialogue between pathologists are needed to develop terms and definitions for describing the high risk histologic changes in a standardized form. The conference held by the National Foundation for Ileitis and Colitis at Tarrytown, New York was helpful as a first step in this type of surveillance program for "precancer" and carcinoma.

SURVEILLANCE PROGRAMS

Patients with Pancolitis

It is generally agreed that the occurrence of precancer and carcinoma increases markedly beginning about 8 to 10 years from the onset of pancolitis, but that a few cases are seen in an even shorter period. Surveillance requires not only ongoing awareness by the physicians but also patient education and increasingly vigorous and regular efforts as time progresses. Clearly, awareness of the potential for precancer and carcinoma should intensify greatly by the 8th year of colitis and beyond the 10th year; strict compliance with a surveillance program is needed if it is to be successful. The reader should realize that there is no firm basis currently available for determining the optimal frequency of cancer surveillance in pancolitis. Currently different groups employ ranges varying from 6 months to 3 years. The latter may be too long a waiting period because one study may not provide a complete examination, and carcinoma arising or progressing between studies could easily reach an untreatable stage in that span of time. If there is no evidence of dysplasia, a follow-up once a year seems reasonable for a patient with pancolitis. On the other hand, once definite dysplasia is seen, even if it is not severe enough to be judged precancerous, more frequent surveillance is needed.

Patients with Left-Sided UC or Long-Standing Inactive Disease

Inactivity of a patient's UC definitely does not eliminate the risk of cancer. Many physicians and patients are not aware of this, but the data strongly support this concept. At present, we are uncertain whether or not long-term inactive pancolitis can be safely dealt with by modified surveillance and currently apply the same program to all patients with demonstrated pancolitis at any time in their history. Even though patients with left-sided colitis are statistically at lower risk of cancer development, this group also has to be considered for regular follow-up. The lag time before cancer appearance is apparently longer for these patients, perhaps because there is less mucosal injury. The onset of the risk apparently appears 10 years later, and after that point the risk gradually becomes equal to that of the patient with pancolitis. At present there are no data on which to decide on a cost-effective surveillance program for patients whose radiologic changes of UC are limited to the left half of the colon. As a working approach, one might consider a program for patients with left-sided UC to consist of an air contrast barium enema as a baseline and then colonoscopy with multiple biopsies to obtain histologic information on the extent of involvement, which is usually beyond that seen on the X-ray. Whether the onset of this program could be delayed until the person has had colitis for 15 years or so is not yet known. Subsequently, somewhat less intensive surveillance with yearly proctosigmoidoscopy and rectal biopsies and with colonoscopy and multiple biopsies at 2- or even 3-year intervals could be considered if no evidence of dysplasia is found on the preceding studies. Serial stool guaiac examinations and serial serum CEA levels might be obtained, although recurrence of UC activity would interfere with the interpretation of both. Patients with easily controlled proctitis are reportedly not at increased risk of cancer, and presumably, occasional proctoscopy and rectal biopsy are adequate.

Role of Colonoscopy

Proctosigmoidoscopic study with biopsy may prove to be an adequate surveillance technique for precancer in some patients. The use of the flexible sigmoidoscope makes this even more feasible. Nugent and his co-workers (2) found dysplasia in the rectum of all 8 patients who underwent colectomy. Furthermore, Riddell (7) noted dysplastic changes in the rectum of 91% of the colectomy specimens in patients with UC and carcinoma at St. Mark's Hospital. Nonetheless, there are several advantages to colonoscopy, and these lead us to believe that it should remain an integral part of the surveillance. Precancerous changes often occur as scattered patches, and this may be especially true at early stages of precancerous transformation when the rectum is less likely to be involved. Thus colonoscopy provides the opportunity for early diagnosis of precancer. In addition, the presence of dysplasia in a mass clearly seems much more significant in terms of an underlying carcinoma than finding the dysplasia in a flattened area. Also, the sigmoidoscope does not reach the more proximal carcinomas that develop in UC, and these can also be undetected by conventional barium enema. Additionally, precancerous dysplasia may be more readily recognized histologically from active colitis by colonoscopy because in the proximal colon inflammatory changes are usually less marked.

It is hoped that endoscopists will be able to learn to recognize dysplastic lesions and to perform biopsies in areas that are most likely to result in precancer detection. Although confirmatory histologic changes are usually essential, gross endoscopic findings alone can on occasion be the chief means for detecting precancer. Indeed, we have seen instances where endoscopic judgment was more accurate than histologic assessment of small, distorted biopsy specimens. Thickened, heaped-up areas of mucosa that are plaque-like or nodular may prove to be precancer and should be biopsied. Large polypoid lesions often turn out to be inflammatory pseudopolyps, which are unrelated to precancer, but precancerous lesions clearly also can be polypoid. These probably are the most ominous lesions. Unfortunately, perfectly flat mucosa will on occasion be found to contain precancer. Thus, in the final analysis, a combination of selected biopsies and multiple, more or less random biopsies at regular intervals of 10 to 20 cm is necessary.

RECOMMENDATIONS FOR COLECTOMY

A number of prospective surveillance studies are currently under way in high-risk patients, and several groups are gaining experience with patients in whom rectal or colonic biopsies reveal definite precancer. At present, it appears that approximately half of the patients in these initial surveillance studies with precancer detected by rectal or colonic biopsy have subsequently been found to have colon cancer in the colectomy specimen; it is possible that this figure may drop as precancer is detected at an earlier and earlier stage. The workers at St. Mark's Hospital in London report that they advocate colectomy only if severe dysplasia equivalent to precancer is found at multiple sites in the colon or on repeated examinations (2). We agree, and would add to this the additional indication of the finding of dysplasia in a grossly polypoid lesion or in a strictured area. On the other hand, the Lahey Clinic group is apparently recommending colectomy for all patients with precancer (3). Thus guidelines for advising colectomy are still flexible and will probably continue to change as more experience is gained with colonoscopy, multiple biopsies, and pathologic detection of precancer.

ACKNOWLEDGMENTS

This work was supported by a grant from the National Foundation for Ileitis and Colitis, Inc., as well as funds from the Aaron and Lillie Strauss Foundation, the Harvey M. Meyerhoff Family, the Himmelrich Fund, and the Marvin Schapiro Family.

REFERENCES

1. Diamond, M. P., Yardley, J. H., Bayless, T. M., et al. (1978): Colon carcinoma and severe epithelial dysplasia in patients with ulcerative colitis. *Gastroenterology,* 74:1120.
2. Nugent, F. W., Haggitt, R. C., Colcher, H., et al. (1979): Malignant potential of chronic ulcerative colitis. Preliminary report. *Gastroenterology,* 76:1–5.
3. Riddell, R. H. (1977): The precarcinomatous lesion of ulcerative colitis. In: *The Gastrointestinal Tract,* edited by J. H. Yardley, B. C. Morson, and M. R. Abell, pp. 109–123. Williams & Wilkins Co., Baltimore.
4. Dobbins, W. O., III (1977): Current status of the precancer lesion in ulcerative colitis. *Gastroenterology,* 73:1431–1433.
5. Lennard-Jones, J. E., Morson, B. C., Ritchie, J. K., et al. (1977): Cancer in colitis: Assessment of the individual risk by clinical and histological criteria. *Gastroenterology,* 73:1280–1289.
6. Yardley, J. H., and Keren, D. F. (1974): "Precancer" lesions in ulcerative colitis: A retrospective study of rectal biopsy and colectomy specimens. *Cancer,* 34:835–844.
7. Riddell, R. H. (1976): The precarcinomatous phase of ulcerative colitis. *Curr. Top. Pathol.,* 179–219.
8. Morson, B. C., Pang, L. S. C. (1967): Rectal biopsy as an aid to cancer control in ulcerative colitis. *Gut,* 8:423–434.

Subject Index